Surgical patient care for veterinary technicians and nurses

D1063474

Surgical patient care for veterinary technicians and nurses

Gerianne Holzman, CVT, VTS (Dentistry)

Orthopaedic and Renal Transplant Coordinators
UW Veterinary Care
School of Veterinary Medicine University of Wisconsin
Madison, WI
USA

Teri Raffel, CVT, VTS (Surgery)

Laboratory Coordinator
Veterinary Technician Program
Madison Area Technical College
Madison, WI
USA

WILEY Blackwell

Library of Congress Cataloging-in-Publication Data applied for

A catalogue record for this book is available from the British Library.

Wiley also publishes its books in a variety of electronic formats. Some content that appears in print may not be available in electronic books.

Typeset in 8.5/12pt MeridienLTStd by Laserwords Private Limited, Chennai, India

Printed and bound in Singapore by Markono Print Media Pte Ltd

1   2015

Contents

Foreword

It is a privilege to write the Foreword to *Surgical Patient Care for Veterinary Technicians and Nurses* by Gerianne Holzman and Teresa (Teri) Raffel. The objective of the authors was to create a comprehensive text targeted to the Veterinary Technician interested or involved with all aspects of veterinary surgical practice. This text follows a logical progression beginning with deciphering clinical information by history taking and physical examination, then onto preoperative planning, asepsis, infection control, a description of common surgical procedures, a description of common surgical instruments and finishing with postoperative patient care. The authors support each chapter with eloquent details and illustrations derived from their clinical experience, highlighting the crucial role played by the Veterinary Technician at each step. This text offers a unique perspective for Veterinary Technicians by two very capable Veterinary Technicians and educators.

The authors, Gerianne Holzman and Teresa Raffel bring a wealth of clinical experience to this book.

Both graduates of Madison Area Technical College, they quickly brought their combined talents to the academic environment of the newly created School of Veterinary Medicine in Madison, Wisconsin in the mid 1980s. When I was recruited at University of Wisconsin in 1984, I was a young and relatively naïve veterinary surgeon specializing in orthopaedic surgery. Geri and Teri were instrumental in the refinement and development of my skills, both inside and outside of the operating room. Over the ensuing years, the authors have continued to educate and groom thousands of veterinary surgeons, veterinary students, and Veterinary Technicians. This book will stand as a legacy to their perseverance and endurance and will serve as a primer for all those interested in the practice of veterinary surgery.

Paul Manley, DVM, MSc, DACVS
Professor Emeritus
School of Veterinary Medicine
University of Wisconsin, Madison

Preface

Welcome to our book *Surgical Patient Care for Veterinary Technicians and Nurses*. This book came together to address the needs of veterinary professionals in their daily patient care. Books are available for surgical assisting, surgical techniques, emergency care, anesthesia, and for other similar subjects; however, there are few books for veterinary technicians interested in expanding their knowledge of taking care of patients during the entire perioperative period. Patient care begins before the animal even enters the hospital. Triaging a condition over the phone provides information to the client and allows for a more efficient use of time and resources upon the patient's arrival. The art of history taking helps to focus the client on the specific presenting complaint as well as to determine if underlying issues may also be present. While veterinary technicians do not provide a diagnosis of a patient's condition, their ability to perform a physical exam is an invaluable resource for the veterinary surgeon. Preoperative testing varies with an individual patient's needs. Technicians possess the ability and knowledge to carry out most of these tests. Perioperative medications may include non-steroidal anti-inflammatories, antibiotics, narcotics, and other pain medications. Determination of a patient's needs by the veterinarian, prior to the procedure, helps the technician in providing ultimate care.

Surgical assisting begins the moment a patient is anesthetized. While some practices may have the veterinary technician monitor anesthesia while performing other surgical duties, ideally, enough staff are present to decrease this need for multitasking. (Anesthesia monitoring and care is not covered in this text.) Aseptic preparation of the patient, surgical suite, equipment and personnel are important responsibilities for technicians. Whether serving as a circulating technician or scrubbing-in to assist in surgery, veterinary technicians play an integral role in the surgical team. A general knowledge of common surgical procedures, the condition being addressed, special equipment needed, and postoperative care gives the technician an edge in preparing the patient and client for surgery.

Postoperative care starts when the patient leaves the operating room. The animal must be monitored and provided with special care to stay warm, decrease swelling, and experience minimal pain. Clients give extended care following any surgical procedure. Delivering explicit, well-understood discharge instructions is imperative for a good surgical outcome. Following up to assure compliance with rehabilitation, medications, and recheck appointments while allaying client fears is a valuable service to the surgeon and the client. This book aims to help veterinary technicians and other veterinary professionals to achieve all of the above facets of patient care as members of the surgical team. As the authors, we saw a need for this book for novice veterinary technicians as well as for people who are more experienced.

After graduation from Madison Area Technical College, we both started our careers in private practice but soon had the desire to get into the heart of veterinary medicine. Teri traveled to Purdue University where she worked as a surgical technician. A new veterinary medical school opened in Wisconsin and Gerianne became part of the original group of technicians to staff the brand new Veterinary Medical Teaching Hospital. Teri and Gerianne's paths crossed when Teri traveled back to Wisconsin to join the original surgical staff at the University of Wisconsin Veterinary Medical School. Gerianne began her university career performing preoperative and postoperative patient care. She eventually broadened her expertise to include dentistry – becoming a charter member of the Academy of Veterinary Dental Technicians. Currently, Gerianne coordinates the orthopedic section and renal transplant team at the UW Veterinary Care. Both Teri and Gerianne enjoyed teaching hands-on skills to fourth year veterinary students while instructing these future veterinarians of the need for great technical assistance. Teri eventually moved on to teaching these same skills to veterinary technician students in the veterinary technician program at Madison College. She is a charter member of the Academy of Veterinary Surgical Technicians. Our career paths took similar routes into organized veterinary medicine with each of us serving as Presidents of the Wisconsin Veterinary Technician Association. (Teri, also, went national as the President of NAVTA.) Over both of our long careers, we have received recognition and honors from our peers and students. We both have lectured around the country and written journal articles and book chapters before tackling this, our final contribution to our profession.

This book has been a dream for both of us. While writing it, we each experienced extreme personal challenges causing several delays in publication. However, the strong desire to provide a great resource for technicians, and a very understanding literary staff, helped us to persevere and finish the long journey to completion. Our combined experience, of over 60 years, shows in the personal knowledge conveyed in these pages. However, we could not have completed this book without the help of many individuals. We thank and acknowledge, in particular, the following people for their inspiration, assistance, guidance, time, patience, and knowledge: Paul Manley, Susan Schaefer, Peter Muir, Jason Bleedorn, Robert Hardie, Dale Bjorling, Jonathan McAnulty, Eb Rosin, CC Sheldon, Krystal Telfer, the staff of Wiley-Blackwell especially Nancy Turner and Erica Judisch and the many surgeons, residents, and technicians we have had the pleasure of working with through our careers. The thousands of students, who taught us many lessons as we shared our knowledge with them, were instrumental in our growth as veterinary technicians. Finally, we thank our families for their support and encouragement: Rob Zimmerman, Sherry Freiberg, Carole Vick, Penny Lamb, Bob Holzman, Tony Raffel, Patrick Raffel, Peter Raffel, Gerry Stoeberl, Carol Sliwka, Peggy Marvin, Tom Stoeberl and our late parents.

We encourage all veterinary technicians and veterinary professionals to pursue their dreams, advance their careers, explore new challenges but most of all have fun while they enjoy one of the best jobs in the world!

Gerianne and Teri
July 2014

From Gerianne: "Life is a daring adventure or nothing at all." Helen Keller

From Teri: "Don't be afraid your life will end: be afraid that it will never begin" Grace Hansen

About the companion website

This book is accompanied by a companion website:

wiley.com/go/holzman/surgical

The website includes:

- Review questions and answers
- PowerPoints of all figures from the book for down-
loading

CHAPTER 1

History and Physical Examination

The history and physical exam provide the basis for all patient care. Without this information, a diagnosis and treatment plan cannot be formulated by the veterinarian. Veterinary technicians provide an invaluable service in deciphering a client's perception of a problem while determining their true concerns. These may not be the same as the patient's actual medical condition. For example, a client brings a pet in for behavioral problems of urinating in the house. The client thinks the cat is "mad" because it is left alone for many hours. The client's concern is for the cat to stop urinating in the house. Questions are asked about litter pan behavior, urine color, and the cat's attitude. The patient shows pain on abdominal palpation and a distended bladder. After consultation with the surgeon, it is decided to perform abdominal radiographs on this patient. Radiographs show the cat has cystic calculi (Figure 1.1). After discussing medical versus surgical options with the client, it is decided to surgically remove the stones.

History

Surgical patients may present with many or no other medical conditions other than the original complaint. A careful medical history contributes to the patient's diagnosis, prognosis, and care. A complete history includes:

- Vaccinations
- Heartworm testing/preventative
- Diet
- Allergies
- Current medication
- Patient's lifestyle
- Medical and surgical history

Vaccinations

Hospitalized patients may be exposed to many communicable diseases. Suggested canine vaccinations include Distemper, Adenovirus, Parainfluenza, Parvovirus, Leptospirosis, Rabies, and possibly Bordatella. Feline vaccinations include viral Rhinotracheitis, Calicivirus, Rabies, and Panleukopenia. Care is taken to protect unvaccinated emergency patients with minimal inter-patient contact. Hospital policy and local regulations dictate vaccination requirements.

Parasites

Every state reports cases of heartworm disease. Preventative treatment promotes patient good health. Patients with active or prior heartworm disease pose an anesthetic risk. The client is quizzed to determine the status of heartworm testing and preventative. Flea infestation is avoided in the veterinary hospital with appropriate prevention; therefore, determining a client's use of flea and tick preventative is imperative.

Diet

Diet affects all aspects of a patient's health. Knowledge of a patient's dietary habits aids treatment plans. For example, young puppies fed with a high calcium diet can succumb to developmental orthopedic conditions. Obesity causes stress to most body systems including heart, lungs, and joints. Determining if a patient's feeding schedule is free choice or meal feeding aids in formulating weight management plans. Between-meal snacks contribute to obesity. Maintaining a patient's current diet while hospitalized avoids gastrointestinal upset from food change. However, client-provided, raw food diets might create an in-hospital storage problem

Surgical Patient Care for Veterinary Technicians and Nurses, First Edition. Gerianne Holzman and Teri Raffel.
© 2015 John Wiley & Sons, Ltd. Published 2015 by John Wiley & Sons, Ltd.
Companion Website: wiley.com/go/holzman/surgical.

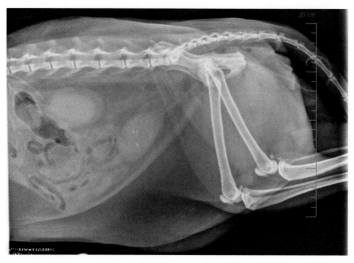

Figure 1.1 Lateral radiograph of a cat with cystic calculi. (Amy Lang, University of Wisconsin Veterinary Care, Madison, WI. Reproduced with permission from Amy Lang).

and hazard for hospital personnel. Patients undergoing oral surgery may need a softened diet, postoperatively. Crushing a normal diet of dry kibble and soaking for a short time in water maintains the animal's normal diet.

Allergies

Food allergies are prevalent in the veterinary patient population. Determining a patient's food allergies avoid gastrointestinal problems while hospitalized. Unidentified medication allergies can cause very serious complications during hospitalization, surgery, and recovery. Obtaining information on past sedation and anesthetic episodes provides guidelines for future needs. Patients with a history of a poor response to anesthesia must be more closely monitored during any surgical procedure. Anesthetic drug complications include vomiting, diarrhea, cardiac arrhythmias, breathing difficulties, blood pressure changes, and slow recovery. Other allergic reactions to medications or environmental conditions must also be noted.

Current medication

A patient's current and prior medications, and other supplements and history influences future treatment plans. For example, patients receiving anti-inflammatory medications need a "wash-out" period prior to starting a different anti-inflammatory drug to avoid gastrointestinal problems including stomach ulceration. Medications for many medical conditions influence the choice of

perioperative drugs. Dietary supplements, such as glucosamine chondroitin, calcium, and vitamins, affect patients' health and food needs.

Patient's lifestyle

Clients have different expectations for patients leading a sedentary life versus working or service animals. If a dog's main job is to sit on the couch most of the day, recovery from a ruptured cranial cruciate ligament (CCL) and its attending arthritis is much different from a search and rescue animal. If a patient lives in a city dwelling apartment, it will have different experiences during recovery than a dog, living in the country, with acres of freedom. The same holds true for an indoor cat versus an outdoor cat. Will the client be able to medicate a mostly outdoor cat postoperatively?

Medical history

A complete medical history begins with the signalment: age, breed, sex (intact or neutered), and presenting complaint. A preconceived diagnosis may affect physical exam findings. (E.g., a patient presented for hip dysplasia may actually have a cranial cruciate rupture causing more lameness than poor hip conformation.) Carefully interviewing the client provides much information to aid in the veterinarian's diagnosis. In addition to the presenting complaint, for example, lameness, the entire patient is taken into consideration with inquiries into coughing (C), sneezing (S), vomiting (V), diarrhea (D), increase in thirst or urination –polyuria/polydipsia(PU/PD), and appetite(A). These parameters are easily recorded in the medical record as C, S, V, D, PU/PD, and A with notations made accordingly. Note all current and previous medical problems as they may influence the surgical experience. Form questions to prevent leading a client into a specific "yes or no" answer. For instance, asking a client "Is Lily more lame today?" provides a yes or no answer as opposed to asking, "When do you see Lily's lameness increase?" With the second question, the client needs to give a more detailed answer providing the clinician with better historical information. Record all prior surgical procedures. A patient may present for a second opinion of a recurrent problem. Historical knowledge influences a treatment plan.

Current exercise regimen determines the client and patient's ability or lack of ability to provide appropriate postoperative rehabilitation. While delicate to obtain, a client's personal situation – time, finances, other obligations – also influences the surgical plan. A client with many commitments may not have the time required for extensive postop rehab. For this person, a more conservative plan betters fit the client's lifestyle. A mnemonic for obtaining a history is using the OLD CHARTS method (Figure 1.2).

Physical exam

A complete physical exam covers the patient from the tip of the nose to the tip of the tail. Failure to recognize

patients' underlying medical problems can lead to devastating consequences. (The extent of the exam performed by a veterinary technician varies with individual veterinary practices.) A complete physical exam includes the following parameters:

- Temperature, pulse, respiration (TPR), and weight
- Body condition score (BCS)
- General appearance
- Attitude
- Locomotion
- Head and Face
- Oral pharynx
- Lymph nodes
- Integument
- Musculoskeletal
- Perineum
- Abdominal cavity
- Respiratory
- Cardiovascular
- Nervous system

Use of a paper or electronic physical exam form serves as a reminder to examine all body systems. See an example of a useful physical exam form in Figure 1.3.

Temperature, pulse, respiration, and weight

Obtain a TPR and weight at every visit. Clients appreciate knowing if their pet's TPR is in the normal range (Table 1.1). Knowledge of a patient's pre-surgical TPR influences the anesthetic protocol. Changes in TPR affect intraoperative and postoperative care. Accurate weight provides proper medication dosing. Monitoring obese patients aids in weight management.

Body condition score

Many charts help determine a patient's body condition score (BCS). Determining a patient's level of obesity or thinness influences treatment plans. BCS varies with the source – one style of chart uses a scale of one to nine with one being emaciated and nine being extremely obese. Describing a pet's BCS score to a client helps in understanding the nutritional needs of the animal. Dogs and cats within a breed can vary greatly. (Figures 1.4a, b–1.5a, b) Printing copies of the BCS images and providing them to clients allows for a visual reminder of a healthy state. See Chapter 8 for examples of BCS charts.

```
O = Onset

L = Location

D = Duration

Ch = Character (better/worse/static)

A = Alleviating/Aggravating factors

R = Rx (medications, other therapies)

T = Temporal pattern

S = Symptoms associated
```

Figure 1.2 OLD CHARTS: a mnemonic device to remember important aspects of a patient's history.

UNIVERSITY OF WISCONSIN - MADISON
SCHOOL OF VETERINARY MEDICINE
VETERINARY MEDICAL TEACHING HOSPITAL

Date: _____

Prev. Weight _____ Kg.
_____ Lb.

T _____ P _____ R _____ Weight _____ Kg.
_____ Lb.

Body Condition Score: _____/9 (1=emaciated, 5=normal, 9=obese)

DETAILED EXAMINATION
(Auscultation, Percussion, Rectal, etc.)

	Normal	Abnormal	No Exam
1. General Appearance	☐	☐	☐
2. Attitude	☐	☐	☐
3. Locomotion	☐	☐	☐
4. Head & Face	☐	☐	☐
Eyes	☐	☐	☐
Ears	☐	☐	☐
Nose	☐	☐	☐
5. Oral Pharynx	☐	☐	☐
Mucous Membrane	☐	☐	☐
Gingiva	☐	☐	☐
Teeth	☐	☐	☐
Tonsils	☐	☐	☐
6. Lymph Nodes	☐	☐	☐
7. Integument	☐	☐	☐
8. Musculoskeletal	☐	☐	☐
Joints	☐	☐	☐
Muscles	☐	☐	☐
9. Perineum	☐	☐	☐
Anus	☐	☐	☐
Vulva/Testicles	☐	☐	☐
Mamm. Gland/Penis	☐	☐	☐
Prostate	☐	☐	☐
10. Abdominal Cavity	☐	☐	☐
11. Respiratory	☐	☐	☐
12. Cardiovascular	☐	☐	☐
13. Nervous System	☐	☐	☐

Signed: _____

VMTH-45 MEDICAL RECORD

PHYSICAL EXAMINATION

Figure 1.3 An example of a physical exam form used at the UW Veterinary Care, Madison, WI. (Ruthanne Chun, University of Wisconsin Veterinary Care. Reproduced with permission of Ruthanne Chun.).

Table **1.1** Normal feline and canine TPR.

Parameter	Feline	Canine
Temperature	101–102.5 °F	101–102.5 °F
Pulse	160–240 beats/min	70–160 beats/min
Respiration	20–30 breaths/min	10–39 breaths/min

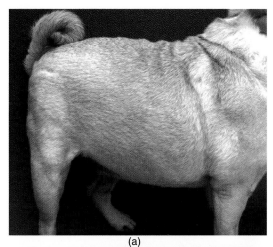

(a)

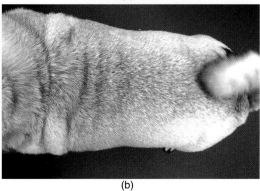

(b)

Figure 1.4 (a) An obese pug (BCS 7) shown in lateral view. (b) An obese pug (BCS 7) shown in dorsal view.

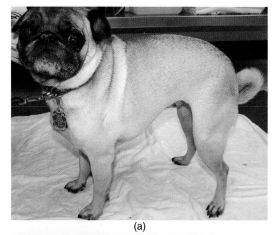

(a)

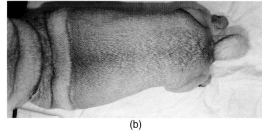

(b)

Figure 1.5 (a) A thin pug (BCS 4) shown in lateral view. (b) A thin pug (BCS 4) shown in dorsal view.

General appearance

A patient's general appearance may be a sign of its overall health. Ill patients often have an unkempt appearance, poor hair coat, and so on. They generally are not grooming themselves as normal or may be over grooming (chewing or licking) a painful or irritated area. Obese or hypothyroid patients may be sluggish. Emergent patients may be obtunded, comatose, painful,

and so on. However, a patient may be in perfect condition except for its presenting complaint.

Attitude

Patients come with all personalities. They may be bright, alert, and responsive (BAR) or quiet, alert, and responsive (QAR). Unusual environments and pain produces fear and concern or may cause aggression. Careful reading of a patient's attitude prevents misunderstandings and provides a safe working environment. Dogs, by nature, hide their pain. Cats are often over aroused in an unfamiliar environment.

Maintaining a calm, quiet environment alleviates patients' fears and client concerns. Keeping cats in crates helps them to feel safe. Often time, much of the initial exam can be carried out with the cat within the crate. Providing a mat or blanket on the floor for a dog may help it to relax. Dogs, unlike cats, prefer to be at ground level. Performing a physical exam on the floor alleviates dogs' fears of being off the ground. Patients can "get away" if too stressed instead of leaping

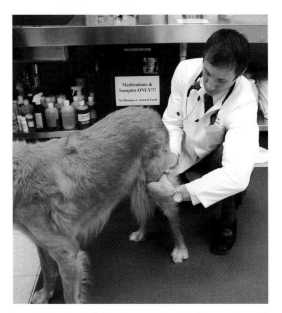

Figure 1.6 A physical exam on a comfortable floor mat provides patient and staff stability and comfort.

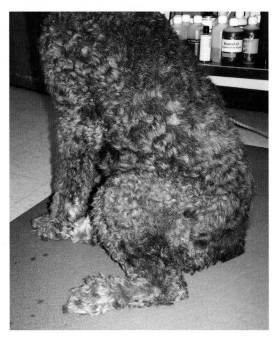

Figure 1.7 The "sit test" often indicates a ruptured cranial cruciate ligament as the patient is uncomfortable flexing its stifle.

from an exam table and possibly sustaining an injury. Performing physical exams on the floor also helps to maintain a healthy working environment by avoiding back injuries from lifting heavy dogs and providing an easy way to back away from aggressive patients. Small dogs, however, are more used to lifting and carrying by their owners. Physical exams on tables are useful for these patients provided they are safe and the client or an assistant can aid in restraint. Providing a mat on the floor or table provides sturdy footing for the patient. A mat or blank also adds comfort and cushioning for the patient and staff (Figure 1.6).

Locomotion

Allowing a patient to roam the exam room during history taking provides an assessment of a patient's uncontrolled movement. (Ensure that all doors are closed.) Note any lameness or gait abnormalities. If a hallway or outside area is available, ask the client to walk a dog on a leash. Request a variety of speeds, as lameness maybe more prevalent at faster or slower speeds. For example, a patient with hip dysplasia may walk relatively normally but "bunny hops," with both rear feet moving as one, when at a rapid gait. Observe the patient sitting in the exam room. Patients with cranial cruciate rupture may sit with one leg slightly extended due to pain induced when flexing the stifle (Zeltzman 2009) (Figure 1.7).

Most cats do not walk on a leash and provide a challenge in locomotion assessment. Placing a crate or box at one end of a closed exam room and the cat at the other end provides the cat with a destination. It may run or slink to the crate or box allowing for gait evaluation. Keep all people away from the crate to aid in letting the cat think it is "getting away."

Always ask the client if and when they note any lameness at home. Patients in an unfamiliar setting or on slippery hospital tiled floors may walk differently than at home. Ask clients which leg they believe is causing the problem but do not assume they are correct. Patients with front-leg lameness, drop their head when putting weight on the unaffected limb (Piermattei *et al.* 2006a). The degree of lameness is graded on a scale of 0–5 as follows (Kerwin, 2012):

- Grade 0/5: no lameness, stands normally
- Grade 1/5: stands with abnormal posture, no lameness
- Grade 2/5: mild lameness
- Grade 3/5: moderate lameness
- Grade 4/5: severe lameness
- Grade 5/5: consistent non-weight bearing lame

Head and face

Assess all parts of the head. Palpate the bone and musculature of the head for asymmetry. Neuromuscular diseases may cause muscle atrophy of one or both sides of the face. Trauma of the head may cause fractures. Young patients may have an open fontanel at the top of the skull. Monitor the patient for any pain or discomfort when moving the head and neck from side to side and up and down.

Observe the eyes for nystagmus, symmetry, pupil dilation and constriction, light response, eyelid masses, tear production, ectropion, and entropion. Examine the ears for debris, odor, masses, aural hematoma, intact tympanic membrane, discharge, and color change. Palpate and observe the nose for changes including masses, deviated septum, stenoic nares, and drainage. Check for a cough while palpating the trachea. Palpate the thyroid gland for size abnormalities.

Oral pharynx

Begin the oral exam by lifting the lip; if the patient does not protest, continue the exam with caution to avoid injury. Assess the teeth for correct number (42 teeth in the adult dog, 30 in the adult cat), retained deciduous teeth, calculus and plaque, mobility, and color. Observe the gingiva and oral mucosa for color (red, pink, or various shades of black), gingivitis, periodontal disease, masses, and bleeding. Check capillary refill time by pushing on the mucosa to blanch the color. Normal color should return in 1–2 seconds. Assure the tongue is normal color and does not contain any masses. The tongue may be dark pigmented in addition to the normal pink color. If possible, examine the tongue for abnormalities and check the gag reflex. Check the tonsils for inflammation and location within their crypts. Check the palate for elongation, redness, and ulceration.

Lymph nodes

Palpate lymph nodes for enlargement. The most accessible nodes are the submandibular (not to be confused with the submandibular salivary glands), prescapular, axillary, inguinal, and popliteal. Lymph node enlargement may be an indication of infection, inflammation, or neoplasia.

Integument

The skin can indicate underlying conditions. Allergic patients may bite or lick any part of the body; however, feet and legs are especially vulnerable. Check for alopecia, redness, or irritation from self-trauma. Check the skin for erythema, rashes, excess moisture, dryness, or flakiness. These may indicate conditions ranging from allergies to fleas to Lyme disease. Observe any parasites such as fleas and ticks. If present, provide the client with prevention and control information.

Discern any indication of pyoderma. It may be indicated by the presence of pustules, rash, or skin odor. Skin infections present at the time of surgery can lead to surgical site sepsis. Pyoderma must be treated appropriately. If possible, delaying the procedure until after the skin has healed may be indicated. Alternatively providing antibiotic therapy at the time of surgery may prevent bacterial infection of the surgery site.

Musculoskeletal

Patients presenting for lameness receive a complete orthopedic exam. This includes all legs not just the injured area. If an exam begins with the painful leg, the patient anticipates discomfort and may react to minimal stimulus of other legs creating false exam findings. Beginning the exam with the unaffected side provides for a more comfortable patient. Ideally, a musculoskeletal exam is performed with the patient in lateral recumbency to provide a non-weight bearing exam. However, uncooperative patients may be examined while standing or may need sedation to complete manipulation of all limbs.

The orthopedic exam begins with the toes, feeling for any swelling, tenderness, or pain. Look between the toes for foreign materials, redness, or injures. Each toe is moved, checking for normal range of motion (ROM). Examine the toenails for abnormal or asymmetric wear indicating unusual gait or dragging the foot. Observe the bottom and between the pads for injuries or foreign objects such as glass shards, sticks, or thorns.

Examine the carpus for swelling and pain. Discern the range of motion. Normally a dog or cat is able to flex its carpus until the toes touch the caudal side of the ulna. The normal degree of extension is 10–12 degrees (Piermattei *et al.* 2006b). Extending beyond this range indicates damage to the palmar fibrocartilage (Figure 1.8).

Deviation from standard is a cause for concern and may indicate an acute or chronic condition. Carpal

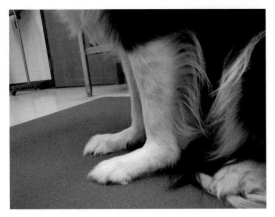

Figure 1.8 A Border Collie with carpal hyperextension.

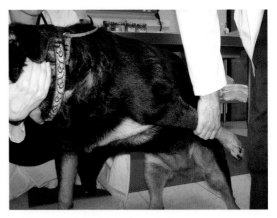

Figure 1.9 Patients with biceps tendon conditions become more lame after performing the biceps flexion test as shown. The shoulder is flexed for 2 minutes, leg is released, and patient is allowed to walk.

valgus is present when the carpus deviates laterally. Carpal varus indicates medial deviation of the carpus. Both of these conditions may result from trauma or genetics. They often occur with the bowing of the radius due to premature closure of the distal ulna growth plate (Piermattei *et al.* 2006c). Some breeds of dogs have naturally occurring carpal valgus such as the Shih Tzu, Lhasa Apso, and English Bulldog. Other conditions to monitor in the carpus are fractures and luxations. (Note: if the forelimb is the area of concern, begin the exam on the rear limb.)

Inspect the elbow for pain and swelling. Edema of the elbows is more easily palpated while the patient is standing to allow for comparison of left and right sides. Observe the elbow range of motion. Normal elbow flexion permits the carpus to touch, almost, the cranial area of the shoulder. Pain on hyperextension of the elbow may indicate an ununited anconeal process while pain on rotation can be indicative of osteochondritis dissicans.

Evaluation of the shoulder is more difficult due to its extensive muscle mass. Begin by checking the range of motion and observing for any pain response. Examine for pain in the biceps tendon by fully flexing the shoulder and extending the elbow (Figure 1.9). Lameness caused by biceps injury exacerbates with this maneuver.

Moving to the rear legs, examine the toes and foot as with the front legs. The tarsus is palpated for pain and swelling. Observe range of motion. Hyperflexion of the tarsus can accompany an avulsion or laceration of the common calcaneal tendon (Achilles mechanism)

(Figure 1.10). Palpate the full length of the tendon for swelling, pain, and laxity.

Palpate the stifle for pain and effusion. Swelling of the medial side of the stifle is often indicative of cranial cruciate ligament (CCL) rupture. Move the stifle through a full range of motion observing for discomfort. To assess joint stability, perform a cranial drawer test. Grasp the distal femur with one hand and the proximal tibia with the other; attempt to move the tibia cranially. If movement is present, the cranial cruciate may be torn. Another test for CCL problems is the tibial thrust. Place a hand over the stifle with the forefinger resting

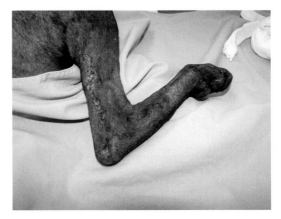

Figure 1.10 Labrador Retriever showing the breakdown of surgical repair of a lacerated Achilles tendon – note hyperflexion of the tarsus.

on the tibial crest, with the other hand flex the tarsus. If the CCL is torn, the tibia moves cranially.

Assess the location of the patella. Determine if it is lays within the patellar groove or if it lays medially or laterally to normal. If outside the normal location, ascertain the patella's ability or inability to return to normal position and stay there. Patella luxation has four levels:

- Grade 1: Patella intermittently luxates but spends most of the time in the normal position
- Grade 2: Patella easily luxates but is readily put back into place, spends most of the time in normal position
- Grade 3: Patella often luxates but is able to be put back into place with effort, most often out of place
- Grade 4: Patella is always luxated and is unable to be moved back into normal position

As with the shoulder, the deep musculature of the hips prevents palpation of swelling. Evaluate the range of motion of the hips and determine if pain is present on flexion or extension. Place a hand over the hip while taking it through a ROM to help evaluate if a hip luxation is present. A sedated exam is indicated to evaluate a patient, completely, for hip dysplasia by performing an Ortolani exam.

Perineum

Evaluate the external urogenital system. Examine the prepuce for swelling and discharge. The scrotum in neutered animals should be flat. Intact dogs and cats' testes are symmetrical. Note any abnormalities. Altered animals normally display minimal to no drainage; however, record any vaginal swelling or secretions. Examine the rectum for irritation, masses, ulcerations, and swelling. Palpate the anal glands to determine fullness.

Abdominal cavity

Systematically palpate the abdominal cavity using the flats of both hands to examine each organ. (It may be better to palpate small dogs and cats with one hand, cupping the abdomen between the thumb and fingers.) Begin just behind the ribs feeling for masses, distension, and abnormal positioning of the liver, stomach, spleen, kidneys, bladder, small intestine, and bowel. An irritated and enlarged gall bladder or pancreas may also be palpable. Observe the patient for a pain response. This may display as flinching, restlessness, biting, and/or vocalizing. Pain may also be associated with pupil dilation. Palpate the mammary chain for any masses. Pregnant

and nursing animals may discharge milk upon examination. Normal milk is white or cream colored.

Respiratory system

Listen to all lung quadrants and the trachea for breath sounds. Cats normally have quieter lung sounds than dogs. Cat lung sounds are heard only during inspiration (McCurnin and Bassert 2002a). Abnormal breathing may express as wheezing, gasping, crackles, coughing, or lack of breath sounds. Observe whether a breathing difficulty is on inspiration or expiration. If panting, close the animal's mouth to assess true lung noises.

Cardiovascular system

Auscultate the heart for murmurs, arrhythmias, and muffled heart sounds. Sinus arrhythmia is a common finding where the heart rate changes during breathing. While this is noted in the medical record, it is not a sign of cardiac pathology. Palpate the femoral pulse while listening to the heart. A pulse should be present for every heartbeat. Areas of the heart to listen for murmurs are the aorta, mitral, and pulmonic valves on the left side and the tricuspid valve on the right side. Record murmurs in quality, grade, location of intensity, timing, and radiation.

Nervous system

Along with examining locomotion for lameness, neurologic disorders are also noted. Observe the patient for scuffing or dragging the feet, inability to bear full weight (knuckling) and inability to lift itself fully when rising. It is often difficult to determine if weakness or lameness is the result of an orthopedic or neurologic condition. Assess the patient's brain and mental status by observing the following

- Strong smells (alcohol) reactivity
- Menace, pupillary light response, and ability to follow the movement of a finger
- Corneal and palpebral reflexes
- Noise reaction
- Moving the head normally and the ability to "right" itself
- Gag and laryngeal reflexes
- Tongue retraction

Assessment of the spinal cord involves testing the spinal reflexes, postural reactions, and pain response. Use a reflex hammer to tap the appropriate tendon to check for response. The triceps tendon behind the

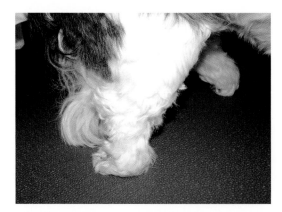
Figure 1.11 Shih Tzu with intervertebral disc disease demonstrating absent conscious proprioception or CP deficits.

elbow, the patellar tendon of the stifle, and the gastrocnemius tendon of the hock are most commonly tested reflexes. Note if the reflex is normal, hyper-reflexive, or not present. Check for conscious proprioception of the limbs by turning each of the feet under, forcing the patient to stand on the dorsal area of the foot. A patient with a normal postural reaction will immediately move the foot into a typical plantar/palmar position. This test is often repeated to confirm the response. Delayed response indicates a neurologic condition (Figure 1.11).

Other postural reactions include hopping – holding three legs in the air and walking the animal sideways toward the one down leg to allow the animal to move the leg laterally. Wheel-barrowing is holding the rear legs in the air and allowing the patient to walk forward and maintain weight and hemi-standing or hemi-walking is holding both legs of one side in the air while allowing the patient to walk with the other two legs. Any abnormality of the above may indicate a neurologic condition.

Evaluate pain response by pinching the toes. Gauge the response as a reflex (pulling the leg away) or a true pain response noted when the patient turns to look at the source of pain, vocalizes, or the pupils dilate. The panniculus aids in localizing the area of a spinal lesion. Pinch the skin of the back just off midline beginning at the tail and slowly moving forward to the head. Watch for a contraction of the skin. The spinal lesion is located one vertebra cranial to the location of the first skin contraction (McCurnin and Bassert 2002b).

Complete the neurologic exam by observing the anus for tone; it is normally closed and gap free. Evaluate the perineal reflex by stimulating the skin around the anus and watching for a contraction of the sphincter.

References

Kerwin, S.C. (2012) Tips and Tricks for the Orthopedic Exam at www.dcavm.org/12febnotes.pdf [accessed on 6 November 2014].

McCurnin, D. & Bassert, J. (2002a) *Clinical Textbook for Veterinary Technicians*, 5th edn. WB Saunders, St. Louis, MO.

McCurnin, D. & Bassert, J. (2002b) *Clinical Textbook for Veterinary Technicians*, 5th edn. WB Saunders, St. Louis, MO.

Piermattei, D., Flo, G. & DeCamp, C. (2006a) *Handbook of Small Animal Orthopedics and Fracture Repair*, 4th edn. Saunders-Elsevier, St. Louis, MO.

Piermattei, D., Flo, G. & DeCamp, C. (2006b) *Handbook of Small Animal Orthopedics and Fracture Repair*, 4th edn. Saunders-Elsevier, St. Louis, MO.

Piermattei, D., Flo, G. & DeCamp, C. (2006c) *Handbook of Small Animal Orthopedics and Fracture Repair*, 4th edn. Saunders-Elsevier, St. Louis, MO.

Zeltzman, P. (2009) How to Confirm Partial ACL Tear Veterinary Practice News, September 2009.

CHAPTER 2

Preoperative Planning

Preparation for surgery includes evaluation of the entire patient not just the specific area of concern. Assuring the patient is otherwise healthy for anesthesia and surgery, performing laboratory, and imaging tests all provide a comprehensive assessment of the patient's health status. Assessing the need for perioperative antibiotic therapy depends on the type of procedure, its duration and the patient's general condition. Planning for the patient's pre, intra and postoperative pain control is an essential aspect of patient care. Veterinary technicians play an important role in preoperative planning by performing tests and providing the veterinary surgeon and anesthesia staff with the results. They also follow the veterinarian's orders by calculating medication dosage, filling prescriptions, and administering medications.

Laboratory tests

A preoperative assessment is performed on each individual patient to determine its anesthetic risks and general physiologic status. Knowledge of a patient's condition aids in creating an anesthetic protocol. **Common** preoperative tests include complete blood count (CBC), serum chemistry panel, and urinalysis. A database of a packed cell volume (PCV), total protein and blood urea nitrogen (BUN—performed with a chemistry strip), and blood glucose via a glucometer provides the minimal information required prior to surgery. A patient's age, physical condition, and surgical procedure determines the need for more extensive testing. Patients suffering a traumatic event, undergoing a complicated operation or in a debilitated condition also lend themselves to additional laboratory tests.

Certain breeds may signify a need for other tests. For example, Doberman Pinschers may carry the trait for von Willebrand disease, indicating the need for a buccal mucosal bleeding time or other clotting tests.

Complete blood count

A CBC measures the actual number and percent of specific blood cellular components: red blood cells (including cell morphology), white blood cells (including all cell types), hemoglobin, hematocrit, PCV, and platelet count/estimate. This test is performed on whole blood collected with an anticoagulant. Normal values are determined for each individual analyzer machine (Table 2.1).

Serum chemistry panel[1]

A serum chemistry panel or metabolic panel determines the current level of chemicals within the body. These establish the health of the liver, kidneys, and pancreas as well as the body's electrolyte status. The test is preferably run on serum but may be performed on plasma. Normal values are determined for each individual analyzer machine (Table 2.2).
- Alkaline phosphatase (Alk Phos): an enzyme that may be elevated in certain cancers, muscle, and liver diseases
- Alanine aminotransferase (ALT) or Serum glutamic pyruvic transaminase (SGPT): an enzyme involved in liver function, elevations indicate liver damage or disease
- Aspartate aminotransferase (AST) or Serum glutamic oxaloacetic transaminase (SGOT): an enzyme associated with liver parenchymal cells as well as red blood cells and cardiac and skeletal muscle. The ratio of AST

[1] Foster, Race, peteducation .com (Doctors Foster and Smith)

Surgical Patient Care for Veterinary Technicians and Nurses, First Edition. Gerianne Holzman and Teri Raffel.
© 2015 John Wiley & Sons, Ltd. Published 2015 by John Wiley & Sons, Ltd.
Companion Website: wiley.com/go/holzman/surgical.

Table 2.1 Complete blood count reference values.

Test	Units	Canine	Feline
RBC	×10⁶/μL	4.95–7.87	5.0–10.0
Hemoglobin	g/dL	11.9–18.9	9.8–15.4
Hematocrit	%	35–57	30–45
MCV	fL	66–77	39–55
MCH	pg	21.0–26.2	13–17
MCHC	g/dL	32.0–36.3	30–36
Reticulocyte	%	0.0–1.0	0.0–0.6
Platelets	×10³/μL	211–621	300–800
MPV	fL	6.1–10.1	12–18
WBC	×10³/μL	5.0–14.1	5.5–19.5
Segs	×10³/μL	2.9–12.0	2.5–12.5
Bands	×10³/μL	0.0–0.45	0.0–0.3
Lymphocytes	×10³/μL	0.4–2.9	1.5–7.0
Monocytes	×10³/μL	0.1–1.4	0.0–0.9
Eosinophils	×10³/μL	0.0–1.3	0.0–0.8
Basophils	×10³/μL	0.0–0.14	0.0–0.2

Adapted from Latimer, K.S. (2011) Duncan and Prasse's Veterinary Laboratory Medicine: Clinical Pathology, Fifth Edition pg 372 Wiley-Blackwell, 2011.
Reference values are derived from University of Georgia College of Veterinary Medicine only as examples, reference values are not appropriate for interpretation for other laboratories.

Table 2.2 Serum chemistry reference values.

Test	Units	Canine	Feline
Albumin	g/dL	2.3–3.1	2.8–3.9
ALKP	U/L	1–114	0–45
ALT	U/L	10–109	25–97
Ammonia	μg/dL	19–120	0–90
Amylase	U/L	226–1063	550–1458
AST	U/L	13–15	7–38
Bile Acids (fasting)	μmol/L	0–8	0–5
Bilirubin, total	mg/dL	0.0–0.3	0.0–0.1
Calcium	mg/dL	9.1–11.7	8.7–11.7
Chloride	mEq/L	110–124	115–130
Cholesterol	mg/dL	135–278	71–156
CK	U/L	52–368	69–214
Creatinine	mg/dL	0.5–1.7	0.9–2.2
Globulin, total	g/dL	2.7–4.4	2.6–5.1
Glucose	mg/dL	76–119	60–120
Iron	mg/dL	94–122	68–215
Lipase	U/L	60–330	0–76
Magnesium	mg/dL	1.6–2.4	1.7–2.6
Phosphorus	mg/dL	2.9–5.3	3.0–6.1
Potassium	mEq/L	3.9–5.1	3.7–6.1
Sodium	mEq/L	142–152	146–156
Total CO₂	mEq/L	14–26	13–21
Total protein (serum)	g/dL	5.4–7.5	6.0–7.9
Triglycerides	mg/dL	40–169	27–94
Urea nitrogen (BUN)	mg/dL	8–28	19–34

Adapted from Latimer, K.S. (2011) Duncan and Prasse's Veterinary Laboratory Medicine: Clinical Pathology, Fifth Edition pg 374 – 375 Wiley-Blackwell, 2011.
Reference values are derived from University of Georgia College of Veterinary Medicine only as examples, reference values are not appropriate for interpretation for other laboratories.

to ALT may differentiate causes of liver damage but is also a cardiac marker.

- Blood Urea Nitrogen (BUN): a by-product of protein breaking down in the body consists of urea compounds containing nitrogen. The kidneys excrete these by-products. Kidney malfunction due to disease or urine blockage causes the compounds to remain in the blood resulting in an elevated BUN. Dehydration can reduce kidney function and cause a rise in this test. Liver disease may demonstrate as a lower than normal blood urea nitrogen.
- Calcium: an abundant mineral aids in bone growth, muscle contraction, blood vessel expansion and contraction, and secretion of hormones and enzymes.
- Cholesterol: a lipid or fat produced by the liver, cholesterol is vital for normal body function. Although elevated cholesterol contributes to arteriosclerosis in people, this is not a concern in the small animal patient. Poorly functioning thyroid glands may show an elevated cholesterol level.
- Creatinine Kinase (CK): an enzyme expressed in many tissues and cells, it helps to evaluate tissue damage particularly in muscles.

- Creatinine: a by-product of muscle metabolism, it is excreted by the kidneys, elevations of this chemical indicates kidney malfunction.
- Glucose: a monosaccharide or sugar, carbohydrates convert to glycogen in the body when an animal's energy level dictates – glycogen converts to glucose. Glucose monitors metabolism and physiology. Low blood sugar (glucose) or hypoglycemia may manifest as weakness, incoordination, or even seizures. High blood sugar or hyperglycemia can come about from stress but in certain disease conditions, particularly diabetes mellitus, excess glucose is excreted in the urine. Blood glucose levels above 180 mg/dl must be investigated further.

- Magnesium: an electrolyte involved in muscle, nerve and enzyme function, helps to move other electrolytes into and out of cells.
- Phosphorus: a nonmetallic chemical element, phosphorous helps to build and repair bones, aids in nerve function and muscle contraction. Phosphorus works in combination with calcium: if calcium levels rise, phosphorous levels decline. Phosphorus levels increase in patients with renal dysfunction.
- Total Bilirubin: a by-product of the breakdown of hemoglobin Elevations occur when excess red blood cells break down, when the liver is diseased and unable to clear the bilirubin or if the bile duct is occluded keeping it from sending bilirubin into the intestine.
- Total Protein: a combined measurement of albumin (produced in the liver) and globulin (produced in the immune system), these proteins can be elevated or decreased in infectious diseases. They may elevate when a patient is dehydrated.
- Triglycerides: a type of fat that stores energy and provides energy to the muscles.
- Electrolytes
  - Sodium: a chemical element, sodium controls the amount of water in the body. The transmission of sodium into and out of cells generates electrical signals. These signals control body processes within the brain, nervous system, and muscles. Increased sodium levels can indicate dehydration and kidney disease. Decreased sodium can be found in patients with liver, kidney, and heart disease.
  - Potassium: a chemical element inside of cells, potassium regulates heartbeat and muscle functions. Increased potassium (hyperkalemia) and decreased potassium (hypokalemia) can be found in patients with kidney disease along with those taking certain medications.
  - Chloride: an ion formed from the element chlorine, it is found in fluid outside of cells, chloride helps to maintain normal fluid balance in the body. Increased chloride levels can be found with diarrhea, kidney disease, and hyperparathyoid conditions. Decrease in chloride can occur with vomiting, adrenal, and kidney disease.
  - Carbon Dioxide (CO_2): a chemical compound, it is a by-product of cellular metabolism, it travels through the body with the hemoglobin and leaves the body through the lungs. Poor respiratory function, kidney disease, and metabolic conditions affect its level.

Urinalysis

Urine for testing is obtained by free catch, manual expression, catheterization, or via cystocentesis. For samples requiring a culture and sensitivity test to check for bladder infection, cystocentesis is preferred to avoid urethral or catheter contamination. To perform a cystocentesis, the patient may lay in lateral or dorsal recumbency. The sample may also be obtained with the patient standing but this position is difficult for the technician working underneath the dog while cats are not likely to stand still. Samples are easily obtained from female dogs laying in dorsal recumbency. The patient is held comfortably on her back by one or two assistants. Alcohol is poured onto the caudal abdomen to form a "pool" along the midline (Figure 2.1).

Using a 22-gauge x 1 – 1 ½" needle on a 10 ml syringe, the needle is inserted straight perpendicular to the body, directly through the pool of alcohol. Usually, one can feel the needle puncturing the bladder. The syringe is aspirated slightly to check for successfully obtaining urine. If present, the syringe is filled, suction released, and the syringe is removed. If blood is noted in the syringe, aspiration ceases and the needle is withdrawn. (Blood contaminates the sample and may cause a false positive on a urinalysis.) Moving cranially or caudally to the original site depending on the expected size of the bladder may yield success. Full bladders tend to be

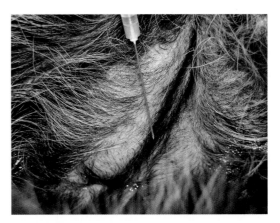

Figure 2.1 "Puddle" of alcohol on a female dog prior to performing a cystocentesis. The needle is directed perpendicular to the body through the puddle and into the bladder.

more cranially located while smaller diameter bladders tend to reside nearer to the pelvis. Palpating the bladder may help in locating it but sometime this is difficult in patients with distended abdomens. Ultrasound is a useful tool for imaging the bladder and obtaining urine samples for all patients.

A similar technique is useful in male dogs; however, the prepuce keeps the alcohol from pooling. The needle is inserted at more of an angle to the body aiming for the midline below the prepuce. Another technique is to move the prepuce to the side and inserting the needle directly perpendicular to midline.

Small dogs and cats have more easily palpable bladders. The patient lays in lateral recumbency with an assistant holding the front and back legs, while the patient is stretched in a comfortable position. Using one hand to palpate the bladder, the hair is smoothed down with alcohol. Keeping the bladder isolated in one hand, the needle is inserted directly perpendicular to the body and into the bladder. Urine is aspirated into the syringe. If blood is seen, the procedure is stopped and tried in another location.

Free catch and expressed samples are acceptable for routine urinalysis without a bacterial culture. Nonabsorbent litter in a plastic litter pan aids in collecting free catch urine from cats.

Urine catheterization is obtained through a variety of catheters. Red rubber and Foley catheters create less urethral trauma and have a decreased risk of bladder perforation than polypropylene catheters. Catheters are inserted using an aseptic technique. The penis or vulva is cleaned with dilute antiseptic of choice. After applying sterile lubricant to the tip of the urinary catheter, the technician (wearing sterile gloves) inserts the catheter. Success is evident when urine flows out of the catheter. If planning for an indwelling (Foley) catheter, the catheter's balloon is filled with the appropriate amount of media (saline or air) depending upon the manufacturer's recommendation. For short-term catheterizations, either to obtain a urine sample or to empty the bladder one time, the catheter is removed immediately following the procedure. Urine from a catheter may be used for bacterial testing but may contain urethral contaminants.

Urinalysis tests include the following (Kahn 2011):

- Specific Gravity (SG) – using a refractometer determines the urine's concentration. Dilute urine may indicate renal disease, adrenal problems, high calcium, diabetes or hyperthyroidism. High SG may be a sign of dehydration. Normal feline SG range: 1.020–1.040; canine SG range: 1.016–1.060)
- pH – measures the acidity level of the urine, bacterial infections create alkaluria, struvite crystals form in alkaline urine and cystine crystals in acidic urine. Normal pH values: feline (6.0–7.0) canine (6.0–7.0).
- Protein – may indicate inflammation, hematuria or glomerular disease. Normal protein values in dogs and cats are "negative to trace."
- Glucose – indicates the presence of sugar in the urine, may be indicative of diabetes (perform blood glucose to confirm). Normal urine glucose test for felines and canines is "negative."
- Ketones (acetone) – checks for the presence of acetate and acetoacetate, may be present in diabetes or starvation. Normal value for cats and dogs is "negative."
- Bilirubin – positive test may indicate liver dysfunction, bilirubin (old blood cells) normally metabolizes through the liver into the colon, when the liver does not function properly, bilirubin is discharged through the kidneys. Normal urine bilirubin value for canines and felines is "trace – 1+" (more often seen in concentrated urine).
- Blood – indicates hematuria, may be an artifact of cystocentesis or catheterization. Urine sediment confirms or disputes this finding. Normal value for dogs and cats is "negative – trace."

Urine sediment exam looks for microscopic components in the urine. This may be crystals, casts, red blood cells, white blood cells, epithelial cells, or bacteria. If present, these entities may be indicative of a medical condition and are investigated along with clinical signs and other tests such as bloodwork and urine cultures.

Other diagnostic tests

In addition to the common blood and urine tests, a variety of conditions benefit from preoperative sampling. These include fine needle aspirates (FNA) of joints, abdomen, pulmonary spaces, masses, cysts, and abscesses for cytologic exam. Prior knowledge of the make-up of a surgical site (joint, mass, etc.) aid the surgeon's preoperative planning. Blood clotting (coagulation) tests may be indicated if excessive bleeding is expected during surgery.

Abdominocentesis

This test may be performed with the patient standing or in lateral recumbency. Sampling from a standing position allows gravity to move any fluid to the most ventral aspect of the abdomen for ease of sampling. After clipping and prepping the area to tap, a needle (attached to a syringe) is inserted through the abdominal wall to obtain the sample. Some patients may need evacuation of large quantities of fluid. For these animals, insertion of an intravenous catheter, with the stylet removed, attached to extension tubing and a 3-way stopcock decreases potential for organ trauma. One person holds the catheter in place while an assistant uses the stopcock and a syringe to remove the abdominal fluid. Fluid is analyzed for blood or urine as well as a microscopic exam.

Arthrocentesis

Tapping a joint or arthrocentesis provides the surgeon with valuable information for diagnosis, presurgical planning, and for postoperative complications. Combined with radiographs, the joint fluid may indicate the need or lack of need for surgery. Bacterial presence indicates a septic joint, while a high cell count may indicate immune mediated polyarthritis (IMPA). These two conditions are treated very differently – one with antibiotics and the other with steroids. Joint taps are readily performed on the carpi, elbows, tarsi, and stifles. It is difficult to accomplish an arthrocentesis of the shoulder or hip due to the depth of the joint and the overlying musculature.

Arthrocentesis is most often carried out on a sedated or anesthetized patient with added pain control medications. Usually, the patient is in lateral recumbency to facilitate access to the joints. The affected side is up except when tapping the elbow, which is accessed from the medial side. The joint(s) of choice is clipped and surgically scrubbed (Figures 2.2 and 2.3). A towel or drape beneath the leg provides a clean surface to avoid contamination from the patient's hair and surroundings. An assistant holds the leg in the desired position (Figure 2.4). The technician or doctor dons sterile gloves to avoid contaminating the arthrocentesis site. A needle is inserted into the joint and may or may not be attached to a syringe (Figure 2.5). It is personal preference on

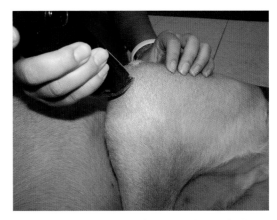

Figure 2.2 Arthrocentesis of a stifle step 1: clipping the hair.

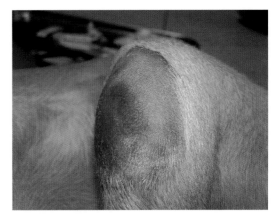

Figure 2.3 Arthrocentesis of a stifle step 2: prepping the skin.

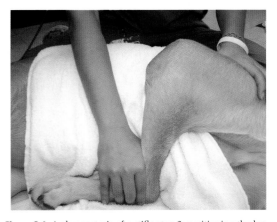

Figure 2.4 Arthrocentesis of a stifle step 3: positioning the leg.

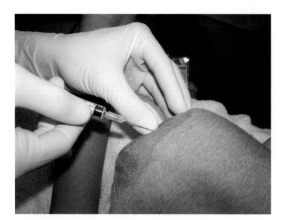

Figure 2.5 Arthrocentesis of a stifle step 4: inserting the needle 2/3 distally between the patella and the tibial crest.

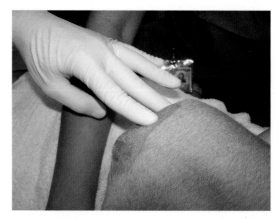

Figure 2.7 Arthrocentesis of a stifle step 6: applying pressure to the tap site.

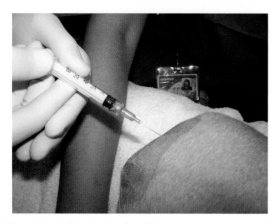

Figure 2.6 Arthrocentesis of a stifle step 5: aspirating synovial fluid.

which technique to employ. The gauge and length of the needle is determined by the joint being sampled and by the size of the patient. After inserting the needle into the joint and fluid is seen in the needle hub, the fluid is slowly aspirated (Figure 2.6). If blood is noted, the procedure is immediately stopped to avoid sample contamination and thus false positive readings of blood in the synovial fluid. (However, depending on the patient's condition, blood MAY be present in the course of the disease.) After obtaining the desired sample, aspiration is stopped prior to removing the needle and digital pressure is applied to the arthrocentesis site if drainage is present (Figure 2.7). The syringe and needle are disconnected and air drawn into the syringe. After reconnecting the needle and syringe, the sample is

squirted onto a microscope slide (Figure 2.8). Small amounts of fluid are smeared on a slide and examined for its cytologic properties. Larger quantities of fluid are put into an EDTA (purple top) microtainer for cytology and fluid analysis. The EDTA prevents clotting of the synovial fluid. If a culture is desired, a quantity of fluid is kept separate from the EDTA preservative.

Arthrocentesis of the most common joints are performed through the following techniques. (Piermattei *et al.* 2006) Effusive joints provide easier access.

1 Carpus – palpate the joint at the base of the accessory carpal bone, flexion and extension of the joint aids in localizing this access space; the needle is inserted from the dorsal cranial aspect, occluding the cephalic vein avoids inadvertent venipuncture.

2 Elbow – a variety of techniques is described for accessing the elbow – medially, laterally, caudally and with the elbow flexed and extended – personal preference comes with experience; however, the goal is to gain access to the joint between the humeral condyles.

3 Tarsus – the joint is hyperextended and the needle is inserted lateral or medial to the fibular tarsal bone aiming for the middle of the joint.

4 Stifle – the stifle is flexed to open up the joint space, the needle is inserted medially or laterally to the patella ligament about two-thirds of the way distally between the patella and the tibial crest, the needle is at a slight angle to the stifle with the goal to insert it caudal to the patella.

Whenever performing an arthrocentesis, if a bone is encountered, the needle is "walked" off the bone to

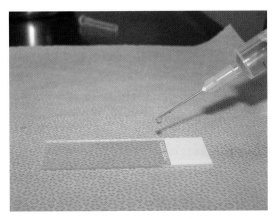

Figure 2.8 Applying needle aspirate to a slide for cytology.

enter the joint space. Repeated attempts increase the likelihood of blood contamination of the sample.

Fine needle aspirate

FNA obtain samples for cytologic examination to aid in diagnosis and treatment plans. Sites to be tested include masses, cysts, surgery sites, abscesses, and so on. If infection or fluid is expected, the FNA site is clipped and cleaned with an antiseptic solution. When aspirating a solid mass, minimal prep, by wetting the hair with alcohol, better visualizes the mass. While steadying the mass with one hand, a needle alone or attached to a syringe is inserted into the desired site. If fluid is seen, it is immediately aspirated and treated in the same manner as synovial fluid described under arthrocentesis. When performing an FNA on a solid mass, after inserting the needle into the mass, the needle is moved in several directions to increase the likelihood of obtaining a diagnostic sample. There may be enough cells within the bore and hub of the needle without aspiration. The rest of the technique for cytologic exam is as previously described.

Imaging

Preoperative, intraoperative and postoperative imaging – radiographs, computed tomography (CT), magnetic resonance imaging (MRI), contrast studies, and ultrasound – aid in diagnosis, surgical planning, and evaluation. Individual and combined modalities provide the surgeon and veterinary technician with specific information.

Personal protection

X-rays produce radicals in exposed cells that may break or change chemical bonds within molecules. Cells may be damaged, die, or mutate. Parameters that contribute to biological effects include radiation dose rate, total dose received, energy of the radiation, part of body exposed, individual sensitivity, and cell sensitivity. The blood-forming, reproductive, and digestive organs are most sensitive to radiation effects. The nervous system, muscles, and connective tissue are less sensitive.[2]

Veterinary technicians performing radiographs must take precautions to assure their own safety. The level of exposure is minimized with proper safety measures. The X-ray tube is the primary source of radiation exposure. Elimination of direct contact with the primary beam is essential. The most common source of X-ray exposure is scatter radiation bouncing off the patient. The amount of scatter increases when a patient receives a high dose of radiation. Therefore, keep patient dosing to the minimum level needed to achieve desired results. Maintaining a distance from the patient while taking a radiograph is ideal but this usually requires sedation or full anesthesia to retain proper positioning. Standing behind shielding provided by a specially reinforced wall or window and lead curtains and screens provides the best protection. If patient contact is required, personal safety is essential. Lead aprons come in a variety of shapes and thicknesses. Depending on its lead equivalence, an apron can block 90% or more of scattered radiation (Le Heron *et al.* 2010). Thyroid shields must always be in place. The lens of the eye is also sensitive to radiation. Protective eyewear with side protection can reduce scatter to the eyes by 90%. Gloves provide excellent protection but care is still taken to keep the hands out of the primary beam. Proper positioning of the patient and the use of devices such as V-troughs, foam rubber, and sand bags help to keep hands away from the primary beam.

Gloves, aprons, and lead shields must be periodically examined for cracks, bite marks, and tears that limit their effectiveness. Replace any damaged protection device as it is ineffective.

[2]http://xrayweb.chem.ou.edu/notes/safety.html, 2011.

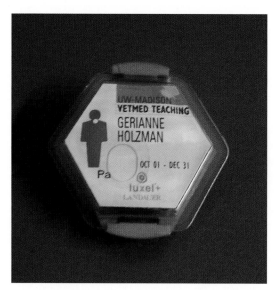

Figure 2.9 Dosimeter for measuring radiation exposure.

All personnel responsible for taking radiographs or monitoring patients during an imaging procedure must wear a dosimeter to track occupational exposure. Individual dose limits must not be exceeded. Calibrated dosimeters, provided by a monitoring service, record exposure and an evaluation is provided on a routine basis (Figure 2.9).

Individuals routinely exposed to scatter radiation wear one dosimeter under the apron to assess the effectiveness of the protective clothing. Another dosimeter worn at shoulder or collar level provides information on exposure of unprotected body parts. A combination of the two readings provides an accurate measurement of the effective dose. When hands are routinely near the primary beam, ring or bracelet dosimeters may also be employed. The current occupational dose limits according to the United States Nuclear Regulatory Commission (USNRC) are an annual limit of: *"the total effective dose equivalent being equal to 5 rems (0.05 Sv); or the sum of the deep-dose equivalent and the committed dose equivalent to any individual organ or tissue other than the lens of the eye being equal to 50 rems (0.5 Sv). The annual limits to the lens of the eye, to the skin of the whole body, and to the skin of the extremities, which are:(i) A lens dose equivalent of 15 rems (0.15 Sv), and (ii) A shallow-dose equivalent of 50 rem (0.5 Sv) to the skin of the whole body or to the skin of any extremity (United States Nuclear Regulatory Commission 2014)."*

Radiographs

Radiographs are created from intensifying screens containing phosphor crystals that emit light when struck by X-ray photons. The light from the screens creates over 95% of the radiograph image. Slower speed screens provide better detail due to their smaller phosphor crystals. However, using too slow screens cause blurring due to patient motion. Use 100–150 speed screens for most tabletop extremities and 400–600 speed film for large body parts such as the pelvis, spine, and shoulder. These areas also require the use of a grid. Excellent detail of very small extremities can be obtained with mammography cassettes – available through X-ray supply companies (Lang 2012).

Exceptional detail is required for orthopedic imaging to allow for evaluation of osteoarthritis, degenerative changes, multiple fracture lines, osteochondritis dissicans (OCD) lesions, and so on. The films need to be of high contrast – bones white, background black, and soft tissue gray. KVP's (kilovoltage peak) are set lower than for a thorax or abdomen. Enough milliamperes is used to provide a diagnostic amount of blackness on the image. A technique chart is created for each individual radiography unit (Table 2.3). Radiography texts are best referenced for specific patient positioning information and will not be covered here.

Computed tomography scan and magnetic resonance imaging (Thrall 2007)

All radiographic imaging aids in the determination of a structure's normalcy or pathology. The advantage of CT and MRI is the tomographic nature of the images. This allows for cross-sectional, three-dimensional, and anatomic localizations of lesions. Comparisons can be made between radiographs and CT scans for preoperative planning. CT scans also allow for three-dimensional reconstruction of fractures to view all angles (Figures 2.10 and 2.11).

Cross sections eliminate the superimposition of structures inherent in a two-dimensional "flat" film/routine radiograph. CT and MRI provide images of greater contrast than traditional films due to the computer technology providing deeper blacks, brighter whites, and more intense grays. The biochemical environment creating the MR image also provides greater contrast and better diagnostics.

CT and MRI images are created with electronic technology. Flowing electrons (or current) carry information

Table 2.3 Sample radiograph technique chart.

All American Animal Hospital

With grid   Regular screens

Thorax

10	11	12	13	14	15	16	17	18	19	20	21	22	23	24	25	26	27	28	29	30	cm
68	70	72	74	76	78	80	82	85	88	91	94	97	100	103	106	109	112	115	118	121	kVp

2.5 mAs*
300 mA × 8.33 msec*

*For obesity or fluid increase to 5 mAs. For Very thin pts decrease to 240 mA and 2.0 mAs

Abdomen

10	11	12	13	14	15	16	17	18	19	20	21	22	23	24	25	26	27	28	29	30	cm
66	68	70	72	74	76	78	81	83	86	89	83	85	87	89	81	83	85	87	89	91	kVp

7.5 mAs	15 mAs	30 mAs
300 mA × 25 msec	300 mA × 50 msec	300 mA × 100 msec

For VD abds on deep-chested or thin pts, you may need a decrease in kVp by 10% or decrease time by half

Spine/skull pelvis large extremities

10	11	12	13	14	15	16	17	18	19	20	21	22	23	24	25	26	27	28	29	30	cm
61	63	65	67	69	71	73	75	77	79	81	77	79	81	83	85	87	90	92	94	96	kVp

25 mAs	45 mAs
300 mA × 83.3 msec	300 mA × 150 msec

For VD pelvis decrease lateral pelvis technique by 4 kVp

Non-grid   Fine screens

Thorax

4	5	6	7	8	9	10	11	12	13	cm
47	49	51	53	55	57	59	61	63	65	kVp

8 mAs
240 mA × 33.3 msec

Abdomen

4	5	6	7	8	9	10	11	12	13	cm
50	52	54	56	58	54	56	58	60	62	kVp

8 mAs	16 mAs
240 mA × 33.3 msec	240 mA × 66.7 msec

Spine/skull pelvis

4	5	6	7	8	9	10	11	12	13	cm
50	52	54	56	58	54	56	58	60	62	kVp

15 mAs	30 mAs
300 mA × 50 msec	300 mA × 100 msec

Extremities* (and turtle bodies)

0.5	1	2	3	4	5	6	7	8	9	10	11	12	cm
42	44	46	48	50	52	54	56	58	54	56	58	60	kVp

15 mAs	30 mAs
300 mA × 50 msec	300 mA × 100 msec

*For avian and reptile extremities subtract 3 kVp

Avian & reptile whole bodies

2	3	4	5	6	7	8	9	10	11	12	cm
46	48	50	52	54	56	58	54	56	58	60	kVp

15 mAs	30 mAs
300 mA × 50 msec	300 mA × 100 msec

Use the extremity chart above minus 3 kVp for extremities

This chart was designed for Kodak lanex regular and fine screens with green film.

Amy Lang, University of Wisconsin Veterinary Care, Madison, WI. Reproduced with permission from Amy Lang.

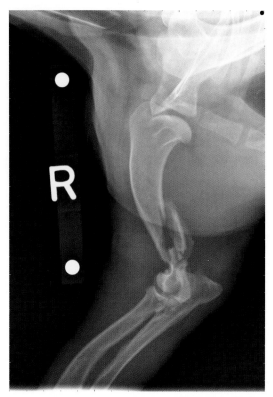

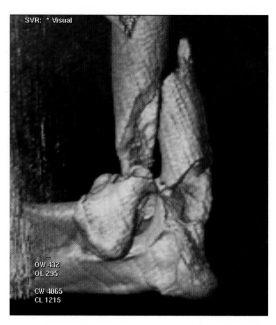

Figure 2.11 Computerized Tomography (CT) three dimensional reconstruction of the same fracture seen in Figure 2.10. When viewed in motion, the reconstruction aids in planning the surgical repair.

Figure 2.10 Radiograph showing the lateral view of a severely comminuted distal humeral fracture.

about the subject to a computer screen creating an image. During an MRI, the patient's hydrogen protons – which possess magnetic fields – directly induce voltage in a conductor by electromagnetic induction. In CT, X-ray photons pass through the patient and convert to electric signals. A computer then processes these signals to create a digital image.

Ultrasound

Ultrasound imaging supports many diagnostic needs. Most common areas of ultrasound are abdomen (including all organs), heart, tendons, and joints. Ultrasounds guide the diagnostician in obtaining biopsies and FNA of organs and masses. Prior to undergoing an ultrasound procedure, the patient's hair is shaved. Insufficient shaving allows hair to interfere with the contact between the ultrasound transducer and the skin. For abdominal ultrasounds, shave the patient cranially to the sternum and caudally to the pubis. The lateral sides are shaved dorsally to midway between the ventral midline and the spine (Figure 2.12). This provides full imaging of the entire abdominal contents.

Ultrasound is defined as sound waves greater than 20,000 Hertz (Hz) per second. Human hearing range is 20–20,000 Hz. Diagnostic ultrasound employs frequencies of two to fifteen megahertz (1 MHz = 1,000,000 Hz). To create the ultrasound wave, electricity is sent to piezoelectric crystals within an ultrasound transducer where it is converted into sound creating a pulse (Lopchinsky *et al.* 2000). The pulse travels to the body part being viewed creating an echo. The echo returns to the transducer where it is converted back to electricity, creating an image on the ultrasound machine. Ultrasound works best in soft tissue, as they do not penetrate air (lungs) or bones well. Unlike other diagnostic imaging, no radiation is used in ultrasounds and only sound waves are used. Thus, no personal or patient protection is required.

Transducers come in a variety of frequencies – higher frequencies create better image resolution. However, the higher frequency allows less penetration of deep tissues. Transducers are mechanical or electronic. Mechanical transducers contain single or multiple

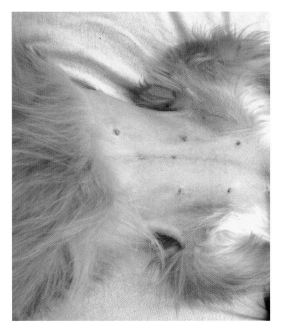

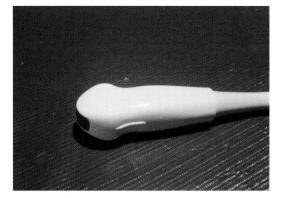

Figure 2.13 Sector ultrasound transducer.

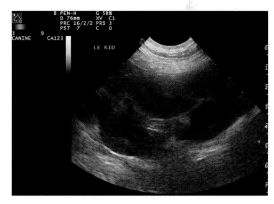

Figure 2.12 Shaving a patient for an abdominal ultrasound covers the distance from the sternum to the pubis and half way up the sides.

Figure 2.14 Left kidney ultrasound image using a sector transducer. (Image courtesy of Fern Delaney, RDMS.).

crystals within an acoustic coupling medium. The crystals oscillate or rotate within the transducer head creating the ultrasound wave and receiving the echo. Mechanical transducers are subject to wear. Electronic transducers contain piezoelectric material arranged in arrays: linear or sector (curved or phased).

a. Sector array
  i. Parallel or concentric rings of crystals
  ii. Curved transducer face (Figure 2.13).
  iii. "Sector" or pie-shaped image (Figure 2.14).
  iv. Deep application or narrow area, e.g. intercostal spaces for thoracic images
b. Linear array
  i. Parallel crystals
  ii. Flat transducer face (Figure 2.15).
  iii. Rectangular image (Figure 2.16).
  iv. Superficial application or to cover larger areas
  Ultrasound is performed in two modes: brightness mode (B-mode) or motion mode (M-mode). B-Mode is a single point in time. M-mode is monitoring an ultrasound over time such as an echocardiogram.

  In traditional radiographs, artifacts are undesired. However, in ultrasound, artifacts can be used to enhance imaging of certain tissues. For example, ultrasounds

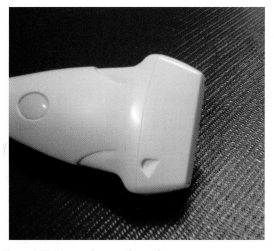

Figure 2.15 Linear ultrasound transducer.

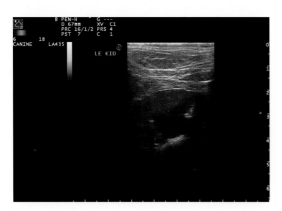

Figure 2.16 Left kidney (same as in Figure 2.14) ultrasound image using a linear transducer. (Image courtesy of Fern Delaney, RDMS.).

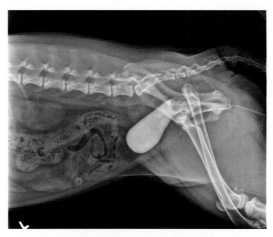

Figure 2.17 Contrast Cystogram of patient hit by a car resulting in pelvic and femur fractures. Radiograph is to determine if bladder trauma is present.

travel well through fluid filled structures (bladder) and can create better visualization of structures located distally (uterus).

Contrast studies

Varieties of radiographic contrast studies are performed to diagnose potential surgical conditions. The insertion of contrast media or air into organs can aid in diagnostics. Prior to performing any contrast radiographs, survey films are taken to view any gross abnormalities.

Cystogram

1 Indicated for dysuria, polyuria, and hematuria
2 May diagnose cystic calculi, neoplasia, rupture, ectopic ureters, urethral, or ureteral damage
3 Procedure: fast patient, perform enema to empty colon, use sterile catheterization technique, empty bladder, inject contrast material to moderate bladder distension, radiograph patient
4 Contrast media: carbon dioxide or nitrous oxide (negative contrast) or water-soluble, organic iodide in 20% iodine solution (positive contrast – preferred), quantity based on patient's weight (Figure 2.17).

Esophogram

1 Indicated for dysphagia
2 May diagnose neoplasia, functional swallowing abnormalities (with fluoroscopy), foreign body, strictures, megaesophagus

3 Procedure: avoid sedation to maintain swallowing, administer contrast media to patient by it eating/licking or via oral syringe, perform a series of radiographs to assess transport of media through the esophagus
4 Contrast media: barium paste, barium liquid, oral aqueous iodine, nonionic organic iodine agents; depending upon the study – contrast may be given in food boluses

Arthrogram

1 Indicated for enhanced visualization of articular cartilage and synovium
2 May diagnose OCD, lesions associated with trauma, joint mice, biceps tenosynovitis, FMCP
3 Procedure: sterilely prep joint, perform arthrocentesis using sterile technique to assure positioning within joint, inject contrast, perform imaging
4 Contrast media: dilute isotonic iodine (positive contrast), air or carbon dioxide through a filter (negative contrast)

Enterogram

1 Indicated for vomiting, palpable mass, pain, weight loss, melena **do not** perform if bowel obstruction or leakage is suspected

2 May diagnose foreign bodies, decreased or increased intestinal lumen size, intestinal content, mucosal abnormalities, peristaltic speed

3 Procedure: fast patient for 24 hours, administer enema 2–4 hours prior to imaging if patient's condition is stable; acute crisis may not permit intestinal emptying, feed or stomach tube appropriate dose of contrast media to patient assuring esophageal and not tracheal placement of media

4 Sedation: avoid medications that affect gastrointestinal motility such as fentanyl, dexmedetomidine, and xylazine. If sedation is required, ketamine (2.7 mg/kg) mixed with diazepam (0.09 mg/kg) given intramuscularly 20 minutes prior to the procedure for cats and acepromazine (0.05 mg/kg) intravenously for dogs are appropriate tranquilizers (Thrall 2007).

5 Contrast media: barium sulfate (preferred for routine studies), ionic organic iodine, and nonionic organic iodine (use if perforation is suspected)

With the increased use of endoscopy, clinicians perform less gastrointestinal contrast studies. Endoscopic and colonoscopic exams assess all structures of the stomach and small and large intestine while potentially removing foreign material causing a blockage. Serial contrast radiographs, however, still aid in evaluating stomach and intestinal motility. The contrast media is monitored and timed as it passes through the gastrointestinal system.

Medications

Antibiotics

The use of perioperative antibiotics is a controversial subject. Overuse or misuse of antibiotics can lead to resistant bacterial infections. Patients on continuous courses of antibiotics may cause a mutation of a specific organism leading to its resistance to that particular antibiotic.

The currently accepted guidelines for perioperative antibiotics are to provide injectable broad-spectrum antibiotics (e.g. Cefazolin 22 mg/kg) at the beginning of a procedure and every 2 hours until the surgery is completed. The use of antibiotics is not usually required in surgeries expecting to last less than 2 hours (Johnson 2007). Common examples of short procedures are a routine ovariohysterectomy or castration.

In the face of obvious infection – contaminated wounds, abscesses, and septic joints – the wound is sterilely swabbed for a bacterial culture and sensitivity prior to administering antibiotics. This procedure allows for maximum culture results, thus providing specific information on drug susceptibility. Highly infected patients may be maintained on a very short course of a broad-spectrum antibiotic while awaiting culture findings prior to surgery.

Analgesics

Pain control is an important aspect of every surgical patient's care. All patients undergoing any procedure will have some discomfort ranging from mild and tolerable to unbearable pain. Veterinary patients cannot describe their pain level but subtle signs can determine a patient's pain score (Figure 2.18).

Nociception or pain is defined as "an unpleasant sensation which may be associated with actual or potential tissue damage and which may have physical and emotional components." In nature, as a survival technique, animals do not readily display pain. However, they will learn to avoid a stimulus that causes a painful response (Holzman 2009).

Pathophysiology of pain

In order to manage pain, it is important to have a basic understanding of the complex interactions coming together to create the pain response. This will allow for formulating a plan to control pain prior to a procedure, during surgery and postoperatively. Nociception is the processing of a noxious stimulus resulting in the perception of pain by the brain. Nociception divides into three parts – transduction, transmission, and modulation. *Transduction* is the conversion of the unpleasant sensation into electrical impulses by a free afferent nerve ending. *Transmission* transports these impulses along nerve fibers to the nucleus caudalis of the brain. These trigeminal afferent nerves subdivide into two categories:

- A-delta or fast fibers, responsible for sharp stabbing pain as in a fracture
- C or slow fibers, responsible for dull throbbing pain as in a chronic condition

Modulation is the synapse of the neurons in the nucleus caudalis in the medulla of the brain. This leads to the perception of pain. The goal of patient analgesia is to block this perception.

University of Wisconsin pain scale

0–1 No pain to probably no pain Dog or cat demonstrates normal behavior for a score of 0
A score of 1 demonstrates normal behaviors but with anxiety being more of an issue
- Sitting and walking normally, sleeping comfortably, normal affectionate responses, normal gromming, normal posture

2- Mild discomfort
- Patient will eat
- Dogs will sleep but may not dream
- Cats may sleep for short periods of time

- Patient may resist palpation of suspected area of discomfort (surgical wound, abdomen...)
- Animal is not depressed

3- Mild pain or discomfort
- Patient gaurds suspected area of discomfort
- Dogs look slight depressed and are unable to get comfortable
- Dogs may tremble or shake

- Cats may sit in a sphinx-like position for extended periods
- Charactr of respiration may change for both species
- Dogs may be intersted in food but only eat small amounts (may be picky)

4- Mild to moderate pain
- Patient resist palpation of suspected painful area
- Patient may lick or chew at wound
- Patient my site or lie in an abnormal position (not curled up or relaxed)
- Patient may be slow to rise and appear somewhat depressed

- Dogs may not appear interested in food they may take a few bites and then stop
- Cats are not usually interested in food
- Dogs may whimper or cry occasionally (animal may respond to quite voice and petting)

5- Moderate pain
- Patient may be reluctant to move and may be recumbent for hours without moving
- Patient may be depressed
- Patient may be inappetant
- Patient may bite or attempt to bite when painful area is approached

- Dog may vocalize when attempts are made to move it or when it is approached
- Cats may growl, hiss and attempt to hide or escape
- Abdominal splinting is present (in abdominal cases)
- No interest in food, minimal sleep, decreased active
- Dogs may tremble or shake with head held low

6- Moderate pain+
- Same criteria as above but dog vocalizes more frequently and without provocation
- Cats may not move from one position for extended periods of time
- Cats may face the back of cage

- Patient may have glazed eyes
- Cats may squint their eyes
- Respiratory character may be increased with an abdominal lift
- Pupils may be dilated

7- Moderate to severe pain
- Same criteria as 5 or 6 but patient is also depressed and uninterested in it's surroundings.
- Dogs will cry out when moved, will spontaneously or continuously whimper (although some dogs may not vocalize)

- Cats appear frozen, frightened and attempt to hide, growl, hiss or bite when approached
- Dogs may urinate/defecate without attempting to move

8- Severe pain
- Same criteria as for a score of 7 but vocalizing may be more of a feature
- Grunting on expiration may be appreciated

- Patient may thrash around the cage intermittently
- Patient may be so consumed With pain that they do not notice caretaker's presence

9- Severe to excruciating pain
- Same criteria as for a score of 8~ but dog is also hyperesthetic, hyperalgesic or allodynic
- Cats may growl, freeze, bite or attempt to escape

- Patient may attempt to escape or bite 1f picked up
- Patient may tremble involuntarily when any part of the body near the painful area is touched

10- Excruciating pain
- Same criteria as a score of 9 but dog or cat is emitting semi-conscious or continuous sounds unless the dog is almost comatose

- The patient is hyperesthetic or hyperalgesic or allodynic
- The patient's entire body is trembling and sign of pain are elicited whenever the dog is touched or approached

Observe patient, interact with them, palpate the suspected painful area and communicate with others who have been working with the patient (technicians, students, interns ...). Take into account the patients physiologic parameters like heart rate, respiratory rate and blood pressure but do not base the presence or absence of pain on those factors alone (opioids and vagal tone can decrease heart rate while hypovolemia and anxiety can increase it). Consider the species and breed; cats and certain dog breeds are more stoic (Newfoundlands, Pitbulls) than others (Northern breeds).

Dogs will often wag their tails in response to commands or touch and many cats will continue to purr even when they are experiencing moderate to severe pain. Tail wagging and purring should not be used as an indication that an animal is not in pain.

Scores of 0-3 may not require additional analgesics but may benefit from low dose anxiolytics. Scores of 4-7 will likely benefit from a multi-modal approach to analgesia. Scores of 8-10 should consider additional analgesics and an alteration in the pain management plan. If the patient exhibits most of the behaviors in a certain category but also exhibits a behavior in a higher category, the patient gets bumped up to the higher score (dog is moderately painful and scores a 5 but is also hyperesthetic, that dog gets a pain score of 9). Use multi-modal or balanced analgesia for the best results. Please consult with the Anesthesia and Pain Management Department if you have questions or concerns.

Figure 2.18 University of Wisconsin (UW) Veterinary School Pain Scale. (Lesley Smith and the staff of the UW Veterinary Care Anesthesia and Analgesia Section.).

Where to control pain

Different modalities of treatment can be combined, or used alone, to produce the desired analgesic effect in a specific area. Local and regional anesthetics and Alpha-2 agonists block the transmission of pain. Anti-inflammatory drugs work at the site of transduction and also modulate the pain response. Opioids modulate pain perception centrally and locally.

When to control pain

It is documented that preventing pain will decrease the total volume of required analgesics (Shaffran, 2011). If pain control is not started until after a patient is showing discomfort, a higher level of drugs is needed to stop this increased sensitivity to noxious stimuli in the central nervous system. This is also known as "wind-up." A multi-modal approach to pain management before, during, and after a procedure will reduce "wind-up" and provide a more comfortable patient. Combining pain medications and sedatives in the pre-anesthetic protocol will decrease the need for a high concentration of inhalation anesthetics. Providing anti-inflammatory drugs at the beginning or end of a procedure will reduce the local pain response due to tissue manipulation. Providing patients with postoperative pain relief aids in healing. Instructing clients to follow the suggested dosing schedule of postoperative oral medication helps to eliminate the chance of overdosing.

1 Preoperative

A wide variety of drugs exists for aiding in systemic pain control prior to anesthetizing a patient. These include hydromorphone, butorphanol, morphine, dexmedetomidine, and the like. All of these drugs work differently in the brain. The drug of choice is determined by many factors including:

○ Patient's condition: assess age, body score, underlying medical conditions, and so on.

○ Cost: some drugs are prohibitively expensive to use in large patients

○ Procedure: length and invasiveness, e.g. renal transplant versus bladder stone removal

○ Hospital policy: clinics "get in the habit" of using certain drug protocols

Assess each patient, in consultation with the surgeon, to determine the best choice of medication for its individual situation.

2 Perioperative

Regional and local anesthetic blocks are often used in veterinary dentistry to control pain at the site of the procedure. Local blocks, in combination with sedation, may be used for a minor laceration repair in general surgery. More commonly, using an epidural spinal block preoperatively maintains a patient's comfort at a lower anesthetic plane. Epidurals provide complete anesthesia to the caudal half of the body. They are contraindicated in patients with elevated intracranial pressure, clotting disorders (due to the chance of causing an epidural hematoma), decreased blood volume, as well as animals with pyoderma at the injection site or with abnormal anatomy creating difficulty locating the epidural landmarks (Egger and Love 2009).

3 Postoperative

Upon recovery from anesthesia, it is important to keep patients comfortable and slowly encourage return to normal habits as soon as they are awake and walking. The most commonly used medications are non-steroidal anti-inflammatory drugs (NSAIDS) and opioids.

NSAIDS: Treat pain and extreme sensitivity associated with inflammation. Most NSAIDS used in veterinary medicine are Cox-2 selective. The breakdown of arachidonic acid by cyclooxygenase (Cox) enzymes released at the site of surgery produces prostaglandins. Further production is created by the development of cytokines and growth factors at the site. Prostaglandins are a component of the inflammatory cascade and contribute to sensitize neurons to noxious stimuli. Inhibition of Cox enzymes will limit prostaglandin production and painful inflammation reduces (Figure 2.19).

The choice of anti-inflammatory medication is dependent upon the patient's current medication, general health, and condition to be treated as well as clinician and client preference (Table 2.4).

Opioids: Opioids provide consistent, effective pain management. Opioid receptors are found throughout the body, particularly in the central and peripheral nervous system. Desired effects and undesired side effects will vary depending upon the drug type and the particular receptor stimulated. Desired results are pain suppression through peripheral, spinal, and supraspinal analgesia with minimal sedation. Potential side effects include respiratory depression, bradycardia, ileus, urine retention, excitement, delirium, tachycardia, hypertension, and temperature reduction.

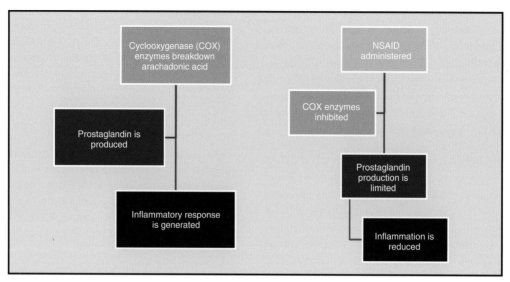

Figure 2.19 Simplified inflammatory cascade diagram.

Table 2.4 Non-steroidal anti-inflammatory drugs (NSAID) doses.

Drug	Route	Canine dose	Feline dose
Carprofen	Injectable/oral	4.4 mg/kg q 24 h or 2.2 mg/kg q 12 h	Not applicable
Deracoxib	Oral	1–4 mg/kg q 24 h, max 7 days	Not applicable
Firocoxib	Oral	5 mg/kg q 24 h prn for 3 days for postop pain or prn for osteoarthritis	Not applicable
Meloxicam	Injectable/oral	0.2 mg/kg once IV or SQ then 0.1 mg/kg q 24 h PO or mixed with food	0.3 mg/kg Single, one-time SQ dose
Robenacoxib	Oral	Not applicable	1 mg/kg Q 24 h for up to 3 days

Abbreviations: h = hours, IV = intravenous; SQ = subcutaneous, PO = per os, oral Dosing schedule taken from medication inserts provided by manufacturers.

Table 2.5 Narcotic drug doses.

Drug	Type	Route	Canine dose	Feline dose
Morphine	Agonist – Class II narcotic	IM or SQ	0.5–2.0 mg/kg q 3–4 h	0.1–0.2 mg/kg q 3–4h
Hydromorphone		IV, IM, SQ	0.1–0.2 mg/kg q 4–6 h	0.1–0.2 mg/kg q 4–6 h
Oxymorphone		IV,IM, SQ	0.1–0.2 mg/kg q 1–3 h	0.05–0.1 mg/kg q 1–3 h
Fentanyl		IV (CRI) of Transdermal Patch	CRI: 5–10 µg/kg/h Patch: 3–5 µg/kg/h for 3–5 days	CRI: 5–10 µg/kg/h Patch: 3–5 µg/kg/h for 3–5 days
Butorphanol	Partial Agonist/Antagonist Class IV narcotic	IV, IM, SQ	0.1–1 mg/kg q 1–3 h	0.1–1 mg/kg q 1–3 h
Buprenorphine	Partial Agonist Class IV narcotic	IV, IM, SQ,SL	Inj: 0.005–0.02 mg/kg q 6–12 h	Inj: 0.005–0.02 mg/kg q 6–12 h SL: 5–30 µg/kg q 12h
Naloxone	Antagonist	IV, IM, SQ	0.002–0.04 mg/kg given to effect for reversal of agonist	0.002–0.04 mg/kg given to effect for reversal of agonist

Plumb's Veterinary Drug Handbook, 7th Edition, Plumb Donald C. John Wiley & Sons (2011).

h, hours; IV, intravenous; IM, intramuscular; SQ, subcutaneous; PO, per os (oral); CRI, constant rate infusion; SL, sublingual.

The major classes of opioids are agonists, partial agonist/antagonists, partial agonists, and antagonists. Agonists produce the best effect by binding to a given receptor. Partial agonists bind to a receptor but give less effect than agonists give. Partial agonists/antagonists bind to more than one receptor but do <u>not</u> affect both receptors. Antagonists have no effect on opiate receptors and are often used to reverse the effects of agonist drugs (Table 2.5).

Patients must be monitored closely when using any controlled substance. All agonists are reversible if the patient displays undesirable side effects. A fentanyl constant rate infusion (CRI) can be stopped but its effects will continue for about 30 minutes. Fentanyl Patches will take effect within 12–24 hours of application. Fentanyl will remain in the body for 12–24 hours after patch removal.

Controlled substances are required to be stored in a secure location. Meticulous records must be kept following Drug Enforcement Agency (DEA) guidelines. Clients should be counseled regarding the proper disposal of any unused medication.

A multimodal approach to analgesia is desired. The duration and extent of a procedure will help to determine the desired drug protocol. The goal is to have a patient that is comfortable, eats well, returns to normal activity, and heals quickly.

References

Kahn, C.M. (2011) *The Merck Veterinary Manual*, 9th edn. Whitehouse Station, NJ, Merck, Sharp & dohme Corporation.

Piermattei, D.L., Flo, G.L. & DeCamp, C.E. (2006) *Handbook of Small Animal Orthopedics and Fracture Repair*, 4th edn. Saunders-Elsevier, St. Louis, MO.

Le Heron, J., Padovani, R., Smith, I. & Czarwinski, R. (2010) Radiation protection of medical staff European. Journal of Radiology, 76, 20–23.

United States Nuclear Regulatory Commission (2014) Regulations Title 10, Part 20c Code of Federal Regulations.

Lang, A.S. (2012) Proceedings, Orthopedic Workshop for Technicians, University of Wisconsin Madison

Thrall, D.E. (2007) Chapter 4. In: Tidwell, A.S. (ed), *Textbook of Veterinary Diagnostic Radiology*, 5th edn. Saunders-Elsevier, St. Louis, MO.

Lopchinsky, R.A., VanName, N.H. & Kattaron M. (2000) Physical Principles of Ultrasound UIC 2000, webinar

Johnson, A.L. (2007) Fundamentals of orthopedic surgery and fracture management. In: *Small Animal Surgery*, 3rd edn. St. Louis, MO, TW Fossum Mosby.

Holzman, G. (2009) *Pain Control in Dentistry and Oral Surgery*. Annual Veterinary Dental Forum, Phoenix, AZ.

Shaffran, N. (2011) Managing Difficult Pain Cases: Neuropathic Pain and Wind-Up Phenomenon on http://secure.aahanet.org/eweb/images/AAHAYC2011/pdfs/Advances_Animal_Pain_Management.pdf [accessed on 6 November 2014].

Egger, C. & Love, L. (2009) Local and regional anesthesia techniques, Part 4: Epidural anesthesia and analgesiaveterinarymedicine.dvm360.com.

CHAPTER 3
Asepsis and Infection Control

Surgical suite preparation

There are many factors that influence the outcome of any surgical procedure. The patient is an obvious contributor to the outcome. The patient's health status at the time of surgery, the ability of the patient to heal, and the invasiveness of the procedure will affect success. The personnel involved in the surgical procedure will also influence the outcome. Anesthesia personnel have the responsibility of keeping the animal alive while under anesthesia and guiding the patient through recovery with as little incident as possible. The surgeon and any member of the sterile surgical team have the potential for introducing pathogens that may compromise the success of the case. Finally, the environment of the operating room can contribute to potential contamination if not properly cared for.

Maintaining and controlling the operating room environment is a critical step in protecting the patient and personnel from contamination. Areas to be considered include: air handling; attire; traffic; air particles; cleaning products contaminants, and a standardization of operation room cleaning procedures.

Air exchanges

Currently the Center for Disease Control (CDC) recommends 15 air exchanges per hour for operating rooms (CDC 2008). In addition operating rooms should have a laminar air flow system. Studies have shown that laminar air flow significantly reduces the number of particles in the air. If a laminar air system is not possible, a positive air flow (air flows out when the door is opened) will aid in keeping irritants out of the operating suite. Incoming air should be at the ceiling level while outgoing air should be at the floor level. Whatever type of system is used, proper care and maintenance is critical in achieving optimal efficiency. Cleaning of the system (ducts, grates, filters, and drain pans) will increase the efficiency of the system. Annual assessment of air quality in the operating room should also occur.

Surgical attire

Proper surgical attire is critical in reducing the potential for the introduction of contaminants to the surgical suite. Facility-approved, freshly laundered scrub suits are most commonly used. According to AORN (Association of Operating Room Nurses) clothing to be worn in restricted areas of the hospital (operating rooms) should not be worn to the facility from outside areas (i.e., home). Tops must be tucked into pants to avoid skin cell shedding at surgical table height. Scrubs should not be laundered at home due to increased risk of cross contamination. Once soiled or at the end of the day, the scrubs should be put in a designated hamper for laundering by the facility. Street clothes must never be worn underneath scrubs. Undershirts or tank tops can be worn for added warmth, but no article of clothing should extend beyond the sleeves or pant legs of the scrubs. Other "attire" to be worn is some type of hair-coverage device. Most commonly used is a bouffant hat. It must be large enough to cover all hair for both men and women (Figure 3.1). There are surgeon's caps available for those individuals that can have very short hair that will be covered by this smaller type of cap (Figure 3.2).

Beard covers are also available for those with facial hair that needs to be covered. Beard covers have elastic loops on either end and those loops fit over the ears. A head covering must be worn in addition to the

Surgical Patient Care for Veterinary Technicians and Nurses, First Edition. Gerianne Holzman and Teri Raffel.
© 2015 John Wiley & Sons, Ltd. Published 2015 by John Wiley & Sons, Ltd.
Companion Website: wiley.com/go/holzman/surgical.

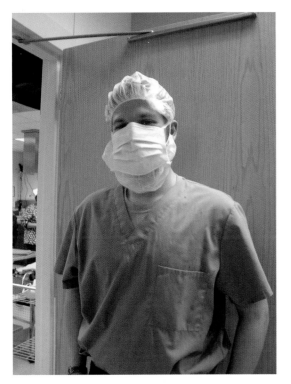

Figure 3.1 Bouffant hat.

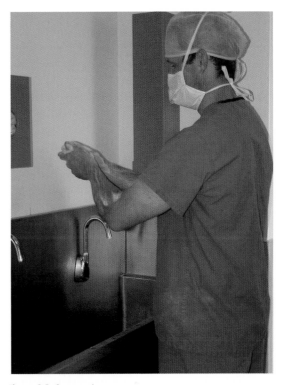

Figure 3.2 Surgeon's cap.

beard cover. There is the option of wearing a surgical hood if facial hair is present and a beard cover is not available. The surgical hood is designed to cover head hair as well as facial hair (Figure 3.3).

The use of shoe covers is still debated among facilities. Some require dedicated shoes for the operating rooms and that shoe covers be worn when *leaving* the restricted area of the operating rooms. Other facilities required shoe covers to be worn in order to enter the restricted area of the operating rooms. At any rate, the policy that is established by the facility must be adhered to and enforced by the veterinary technician in the operating room area. Surgical masks are the final piece of attire to be addressed. Masks should be worn whenever sterile packs are open or when there is a surgery in progress. Masks are designed to filter exhaled air, so it is imperative that they be worn correctly. Some manufacturers even print the work "inside" on the side that should be toward the face. Two styles of surgical face masks are available. First of all, the most common style is the double tie face mask. The ties are secured at the crown of the head and also at the back of the neck.

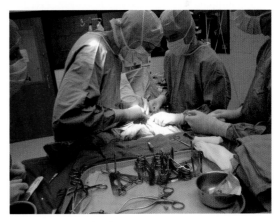

Figure 3.3 Surgical hood.

Ties should not be crossed behind the head (lower ties tied at the crown of the head and upper ties secured behind the neck) and then secured as this leaves too large a gap on the side of the face for particles to escape. Masks frequently have a malleable metal band that runs across the bridge of the nose if the mask is put on correctly. This band is intended to be molded to the bridge of the nose for a conforming fit – again in an effort to reduce the number of expired particles from escaping. Another style of face mask is a pre-formed cup style that doesn't cover as much of the face as the tie style. With the elastic strap instead of ties, it offers a speedier application and removal, but does not cover as much surface area of the face, therefore increasing the risk of aerosolized particles.

Traffic

Traffic in the operating room is an often overlooked situation. People just "sticking their head in" to ask a quick question, anesthesia personnel entering and exiting the room frequently, circulating technicians being unprepared for a case and having to leave and re-enter the room numerous times with equipment, are all examples of traffic that can be avoided. Minimal movement in and out of the operating room is obviously the ideal. Once the patient has been moved into the room, positioned on the table, and has received the final sterile prep, people moving around should be minimized. Especially true with joint arthroplasty, no opening of the operating room door should occur unless there is an emergency. Since joint replacement cases are extra sensitive to surgical site infections (SSI), every effort to reduce the introduction of potential pathogens needs to be observed.

Surgical suite cleaning

Before the first case of the day

Before the first case of the day, the furniture in the operating room needs to be arranged so a good traffic flow is possible. Back tables should be pushed up against the walls; cautery units and suction units should be plugged in and be ready for use, but pushed back away from the surgery table. The anesthesia machine should be placed from where it will be used. For most cases, it will be at the head of the table. For some cases however (i.e., ophthalmic procedures or other head/facial procedures), that may mean placing the anesthesia machine at the back of the table. The surgery table should be at the height of the transport table for ease of transferring the patient. The height of the surgery table for the surgeon can be adjusted after the patient is positioned. All flat surfaces including overhead lights should be damp dusted with a lint free rag and 70% isopropyl alcohol or commercially available disinfectant wipes.

In between cases

Gross debris (blood, fluids) should be cleaned up with paper towels or mopped up as soon as the case is finished. All flat surfaces should be disinfected. It is best to avoid applying disinfectants with a spray bottle as they aerosolize particles in the operating room. Either spray the cleaning rag outside of the operating room or use commercially available disinfectant wipes. The broadest spectrum disinfectant available would be a wise choice to reduce the exposure of potentially harmful bacteria to already compromised patients. If the surgery table has a split top, cleaning the drain tray under the split must be done. Elevate one side of the table to allow access to the drainage tray to remove any contaminants that may have fallen into the tray (i.e., blood, urine, hair, sutures, etc.) (Figure 3.4). When necessary, mopping the floor with a clean mop head may be done between cases, otherwise spot cleaning would be sufficient.

Terminal cleaning – end of day

After the last case of the day, the surgical suite should undergo a more vigorous cleaning. All furniture should have a physical scrubbing done. All surfaces, including wheels or casters should be freed of any debris (hair, suture ends, etc.). All shelves of equipment should be scrubbed as well. All equipment such as cautery, laser, and suction machines should be wiped down with a disinfectant. Linen hampers, kick buckets, sponge basin stands, and so on should be wiped down and disinfected as well. Floors should be wet vacuumed. Mopping should be avoided unless clean mop heads and fresh solution is used on each room to prevent the spread of

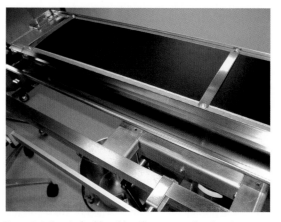

Figure 3.4 Surgical table with split top open for cleaning.

bacteria. Air intake grills, door handles, and window sills should be wiped down. Walls and ceilings should be checked and spot cleaned as needed.

Solutions to use for cleaning

There is no perfect disinfectant for use in the veterinary hospital, so facilities need to decide, based on their needs, what will work the best. Criteria to consider include cleaning versus disinfecting capabilities, spectrum of effect, time needed for optimum efficacy, method of application, efficacy in the presence of organic material, and of course, cost.

Sodium hypochlorite
A dilute bleach solution of 1:32 (1 oz. in 32 oz of tap water) is an effective disinfectant. Although this is inexpensive, the disadvantages may outweigh the cost effectiveness. Once mixed, it is highly unstable and light sensitive. So it needs to be made fresh every day and stored in an opaque spray bottle. The mechanism by which chlorine works is by a denaturing of proteins due to their electronegative nature. It is considered a broad spectrum disinfectant; however, it isn't a good cleaner. So areas need to be cleaned before being disinfected. Bleach does not perform well in the presence of a detergent or an organic material and so surfaces must be free of those products. Finally, as is true with many products, it requires a 10-minute contact time to reach full effectiveness.

Potassium peroxymonosulfate
Potassium peroxymonosulfate (Trifectant®) claims bacteriocidal, virucidal, and fungicidal capabilities. Its method of action is by the denaturation of proteins and lipids of organisms. Once mixed to the 0.5, 1 or 2% solution it is stable for 7 days. It also requires a 10-minute contact time, but is an effective cleaner as well as disinfectant. Some references claim unreliable performance against dermatophytes. At the time of writing, California allowed limited use of this product.

Quaternary ammonium compounds
Quaternary ammoniums (Roccal-D® or A-33) are commonly used due to their cleaning and disinfection properties. The mode of action for the quaternary ammonium compounds QACs on microorganisms is that they irreversibly bind to the phospholipids in the cell

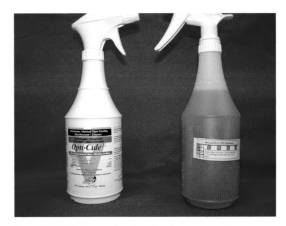

Figure 3.5 Disinfectants for cleaning the surgery suite.

membrane and then they denature proteins. They also require a 10-minute contact time and strict attention to dilution/mixing directions from the manufacturer (Figure 3.5). One common mistake is diluting the product with tap water when the manufacturer specifically indicates distilled water. Tap water generally contains too many minerals and contaminants that interfere with the product's performance. Some discussion has been had regarding the ineffectiveness of these types of chemicals against non-enveloped viruses (canine parvovirus, feline panleukopenia, and feline calici virus). The addition of diluted bleach to these cleaning products produces an effective cleaning/disinfecting combination, but with the instability of bleach may prove to be an inefficient and costly alternative.

Phenols
Phenols (One Stroke Environ®) are broad spectrum disinfectants that are formulated in soap solutions so as to improve cleaning potential. Phenols are known to maintain activity in the presence of organic material as well as hard water. While 5% concentrations are bacteriocidal, tuberculocidal, fungicidal, and virucidal for enveloped viruses, concentrations greater than 2% are highly toxic to all animals, especially cats. This contradiction requires the discussion/decision of the use of this product in veterinary hospital situations.

Oxidizing agents
Hydrogen peroxide is one example of an oxidizing agent found in some veterinary disinfectants. Accel® Disinfectant is one product for veterinary clinics.

With good effectiveness against 26 organisms including Trychophyton mentagrophytes, it also has good cleaning, sanitizing, and disinfecting properties. This agent is available in concentrate, ready-to-use spray bottles, and convenient saturated wipes.

Regardless of the type of disinfectant chosen, there are some very important things to remember. First and foremost is to read and follow the directions on the label! All too often in veterinary medicine, we inaccurately dilute chemicals based on shortage of time, no measuring device readily available, or historical visual assessment ("make it a light green color"). Improper dilution can affect the health and safety of both workers and patients as well as the overall efficacy of the products. Disinfectants will not act the way they are expected to act when improperly diluted. This inaccuracy can lead to the unintentional spread of potentially lethal organisms.

Application of the disinfectant must be done as directed by the manufacturer in order to achieve the expected action. Whether sprayed on, wiped on, mopped on, or foamed on, inappropriately applied products are ineffective.

To achieve microorganism kill/control, the chemical must also be left on the surface for the directed time. Spraying a table top and wiping it right away does practically nothing. Following the manufacturer's instructions is imperative. Many chemicals are required to be in contact with the surface 5–10 minutes, but reading instructions for use will identify the specific time. After the proper duration of contact, completely drying the surface is critical. Often this step is "short cutted" and the surface is left damp. Moisture can actually counteract the efficacy of the products as it promotes bacterial growth, therefore making sure that the surface is dry is essential.

Patient preparation

Proper preparation of the surgical patient is a critical step in the surgical case and is related to the outcome and subsequent potential infection of the surgical site. Improper patient preparation can have catastrophic consequences for the surgical procedure and incision integrity (Tear, M. 2012).

Clipping
Surgical prep of veterinary patients consists of two steps: clipping (removal) of the hair/fur and skin cleansing

with an antiseptic. Clipping and prepping of the patient must be done outside of the surgery room. Loose hair, dermal flora, and splashing solutions greatly increase the risk of contamination of the area. A smock must be worn over scrubs to protect the clothing underneath whenever clipping a patient. When clipping surgical patients, the use of a size 40 clipper blade with an electric clipper is a standard approach. Various other sizes of clipper blades are available but do not provide the close removal of hair that is achieved with the 40 blade. It is also imperative that the hair be shaven *against* the grain of the hair to ensure the closest cut of the hair that is possible. Even with long-haired patients, it is ill advised to clip with the grain (growth) of the hair. Helpful hints that insure a symmetric, neat, nontraumatic shave include: pulling the skin tight and moving the clipper blade away from the opposite hand; keeping the clipper blade level against the skin; Figures 3.6 and 3.7 using the toothed edge of the clipper blade – at a 90^0 angle to the hair – to create a straight edge for the margins of the clipped area; always using a clean, sharp clipper blade to provide the cleanest, shortest cut of the hair shaft. Clipper blades with missing teeth or that feel dull should not be used and should be replaced or repaired.

Knowing the anatomic landmarks and margins for clipping a patient for a surgical procedure is the responsibility of the technician. Having a skilled, knowledgeable person handling this task is an invaluable peace of mind for the surgeon. Good communication between the technician and the surgeon is critical for this step of the process. The technician should check with the surgeon to be sure the site of the incision is understood. Also, the technician should check with the surgeon to see if any

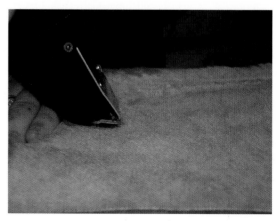

Figure 3.6 Proper angle of clipper blade to skin.

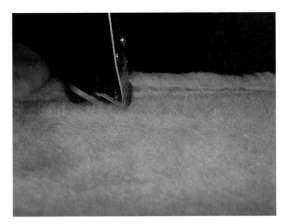

Figure 3.7 Improper (too steep) angle of clipper blade to skin.

additional areas need to be clipped for the procedure (i.e., graft site for a fracture repair or a chest tube exit site for a thoracic procedure). Technicians must have a thorough knowledge of the procedure being performed and possible intra-operative complications in order to adequately prepare the patient. The following guidelines for clipping of the surgical patient are merely guidelines. Each case must be treated individually in the event unusual circumstances are present.

Abdominal

In general, abdominal procedures for both male and female patients will be fairly standard. An abdominal clip will extend from the either mid sternum or the xyphoid to the pubis and laterally to the ventral edges of the ribs. Surgical procedures that are more focused on the cranial abdomen may necessitate a more cranial clipped margin to mid sternum. More caudal abdominal procedures may require the extension of the caudal margin back to the scrotum/vulva of the patient. It is recommended that when clipping an abdomen, the clipper blade always moves away from the umbilicus. That will create a cut against the grain of the hair and will provide as close a clip as possible. Short hair left on

the skin, from an inadequate clip, could potentially be incised by the blade and end up as foreign body in the abdomen. Infection could result from the presence of a foreign body. Table 3.1 shows recommended guidelines for clipping margins for abdominal procedures. Whether or not the prepuce of a male is to be included in the surgical field, the hair on the prepuce should be completely removed and the prepuce flushed with a weak Povidone-Iodine solution mixture. The most common exception to this rule is when prepping a canine patient for a castration. Adding 1 ml of full strength Povidone-Iodine solution to 20 ml of tap water will be adequate. After clipping is completed and vacuuming of the hair has occurred, the prepuce can be flushed. Insert the tip of the 35 ml syringe into the prepucial opening (Figure 3.8–3.10). Pinch the tissue around the tip of the syringe (to trap fluid within the prepuce) and dispense approximately 10 ml of the solution. Gently massage the prepuce. Place a towel on the abdomen and pull the prepuce to either lateral side, release the pinch grip on the prepuce, and allow the fluid to escape from the prepuce onto the towel. The entire procedure should be repeated until all the dilute solution has been

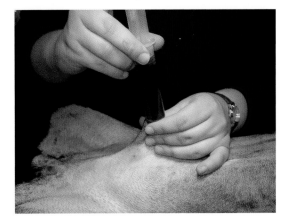

Figure 3.8 Infusing prepuce with dilute Povidone-Iodine solution.

Table 3.1 Abdominal procedure clipping guidelines.

Procedure	Cranial edge	Caudal edge	Lateral edge
Gastrotomy, gastropexy, splenectomy, liver biopsy/lobectomy, gall bladder, kidney	Mid sternum	Cranial edge of pubic bone	Ventral edge of ribs
Urinary bladder, duodenum, jejunum, pancreas	Xyphoid	Cranial edge of pubic bone	Ventral edge of ribs
Prostate, ileum, colon	Xyphoid	Scrotum/vulva	Ventral edge of ribs

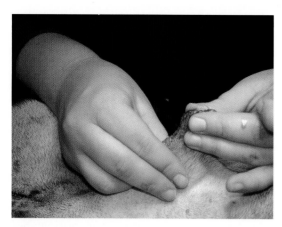

Figure 3.9 Gently massaging prepuce.

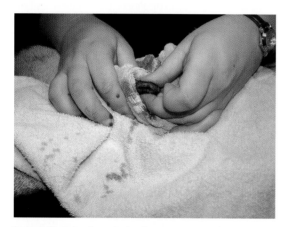

Figure 3.10 Releasing solution from prepuce.

used. Modifications of volume of dilute solution made and administered must be considered if the patient is either a very small or a very large dog.

Thoracic

Thoracic procedures require either the lateral side or the ventral side of the chest to be clipped (Figure 3.11). Depending on the surgical procedure and the approach the surgeon will use, clipping margins can vary greatly. Communication with the surgeon is imperative in order to ascertain that the correct area of the patient is clipped. An additional special circumstance is true with a thoracic case, which does not occur with any other type of surgical procedure; more often than not, a chest tube will be placed in patients that have undergone thoracic surgery. The exit site of the tube must be known by the technician clipping the patient

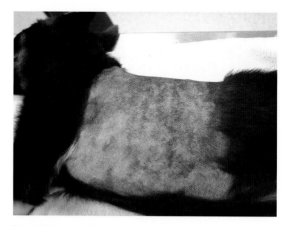

Figure 3.11 Lateral thoracotomy prep.

Table 3.2 Thoracic procedures clipping guidelines.

Procedure	Clipping guidelines
Ventral approach via sternotomy –(lung lobectomy, heart base tumor)	Cranially to the base of the ventral neck, caudally 2–3 clipper widths caudal to the xiphoid process, laterally to halfway between the dorsal and ventral midlines
Lateral approach (4–5 intercostal space usually)- (PDA ligation, lung mass, chylothorax)	Cranially to the base of the neck, caudally 2–3 clipper blade widths caudal to the last rib, dorsal, and ventral midline

in order to guarantee enough hair has been clipped to accommodate the surgeon's intentions for the chest tube. Again, communication with the surgeon, prior to clipping, is critically important. Table 3.2 identifies guidelines for clipping for thoracic procedures.

Orthopedic

Prepping a patient for an orthopedic procedure is generally quite extensive (Figure 3.12). Even if the procedure is a single joint arthroscopy, the potential of an arthrotomy being performed necessitates a wide clip. The standard rule of thumb when clipping for an orthopedic procedure is to clip from the joint proximal to the incision to the joint distal to the proposed incision site. In the event of a proximal joint surgery (hip or shoulder), the clip extends a minimum to two clipper blades beyond the ventral and dorsal midline. Especially with orthopedic procedures like an arthrodesis or fracture repair, the technician must be certain to communicate with the surgeon regarding the need for clipping for an

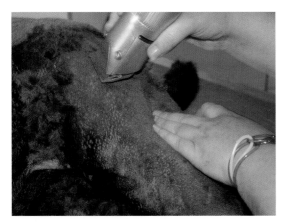

Figure 3.12 Clipping for an orthopedic procedure.

autogenous cancellous bone graft harvest. Procedures on the fore limb generally use the head of the humerus or the proximal tibia as a graft site, unless that bone is involved in the surgery. For hind limbs, the wing of the ilium is the most common bone graft harvesting site. Large margins should be clipped for the graft, and due to wide variations in animal size, exact measurements cannot be provided. A good rule of thumb is to clip 2–3 clipper blade widths in all directions from the graft site incision. Tables 3.3 and 3.4 show recommended guidelines for clipping margins for orthopedic procedures.

Neurologic

Patients having a neurologic procedure performed have one of the easiest clipping situations. The recommended margins are to clip 3–4 vertebral spaces cranial and caudal to the suspected space. This allows ample room for the surgeon to extend the incision should other vertebral spaces need to be explored. As with other clipping guidelines, the technician must communicate with the surgeon to be sure the appropriate area is clipped. Additionally, if a cervical procedure is being performed, be sure to ask the surgeon if a dorsal or ventral approach will be utilized. Much time can be wasted if the dorsal cervical area is clipped and prepped only to find out the surgeon planned on a ventral approach! Table 3.5 displays suggested clipping guidelines for neurologic cases.

Miscellaneous sites

Patients having a surgical procedure that involves the sensory organs – eyes, ears, tongue, or facial bones – are more challenging to prep. Special anatomic configurations as well as extra sensitive tissue require a special approach.

Ophthalmic

Ophthalmic procedures should never have a clipper involved in the surgical site prep, unless the procedure to be performed is an enucleation. This type of extra ocular procedures requires the removal of the entire eye and therefore, any accidental trauma to the eye from the clipper is a non issue because the eye is being removed anyway. Any intra-ocular procedure should have fine-bladed scissors (i.e., baby metzenbaum) used to remove eyelashes and/or any fine hair on the eyelid margins that needs to be removed. Applying

Table 3.3 Forelimb orthopedic procedures clipping guidelines.

Procedure/location of surgery	Proximal margin	Distal margin
Phalange, meta carpal procedures	Shoulder	Toenails – including hair in interdigital space
Carpal arthrodesis, distal radius/ulna fractures, angular limb deformity, mid-shaft radius/ulnar fracture	Shoulder	First phalanx
Elbow surgery, distal humeral fracture, ununited anconeal process repair, fractured coronoid process repair	Dorsal midline; ventral midline	Carpus
Proximal humeral fracture repair, Scapular fracture repair	Two clipper widths beyond dorsal midline; ventral midine	Mid radius
Forelimb amputation	Two clipper widths beyond dorsal midline; ventral midline; caudal to last rib; cranial to base of neck	Mid radius

In addition to proximal and distal margins, all hair should be removed circumferentially on the limb.

Table 3.4 Hindlimb orthopedic procedures clipping guidelines.

Procedure/Location of surgery	Proximal margin	Distal margin
Phalange, digits, metatarsal	Mid-femur	Toenails – including hair found in interdigit space
Tibia/fibula fracture repair	Hip	First phalanx
Stifle surgery (cruciate ligament repair, arthroscopy, medial patellar luxation repair)	Hip	Tarsus
Femur (distal fracture repair)	Hip	Tarsus
Femoral head osteotomy, proximal femoral fracture repair	Two clipper widths beyond dorsal midline	Tarsus
Total hip arthroplasty	Ventral midine; two clipper widths beyond dorsal midline; caudally to tuber ischii; cranial to last rib	Tarsus

In addition to proximal and distal margins, all hair should be removed circumferentially on the limb.

Table 3.5 Neurologic procedures clipping guidelines.

Procedure	Cranial/caudal margins
Cervical ventral slot*	Clip 3–4 vertebra cranial and caudal to suspected vertebral space.
Cervical dorsal laminectomy	On the dorsal midline – Clip 3–4 vertebra cranial and caudal to suspected vertebral space.
Cervical dorsal laminectomy – Suspect site C_1–C_2	Clip mid cranium to C_5
Thoracic laminectomy/hemi – laminectomy; lumbar laminectomy/hemi – laminectomy	On the dorsal midline; clip 3–4 vertebra cranial and caudal to suspected space. (i.e., if suspect space is T_{13}–L_1 , clip from T_{10} to L_4)

*Note: This clip occurs on the ventral neck.

Table 3.6 Ophthalmic procedures clipping guidelines.

Procedure	Margins
Ophthalmic cases – intra ocular – corneal laceration repair; foreign body removal	Using a fine bladed scissors with water soluble lubricant on blades – trim eyelashes and hair on eyelids near conjunctival margin
Ophthalmic cases – extra ocular – enucleation	A clipper blade width from eyelid margins (dorsal and ventral direction); a clipper blade width from medial and lateral canthus.

Note: eyelids should be sutured closed prior to beginning clipping for an enucleation.

a water-soluble lubricant to the blades of the scissors prior to trimming the hair will have the hair adhere to the blades rather than falling into the eye. The blades of the scissors should be wiped with clean gauze frequently and lubricant reapplied each time the blades are cleaned. Table 3.6 shows the recommended guidelines for ophthalmic procedure clipping.

Aural

Aural surgeries vary greatly in nature and so does the clipping. Procedures of the ear canal and inner ear require a much different clip than those just involving the pinna. As a word of caution, bulla osteotomy procedures also require the clipping of the ventral neck to facilitate the approach the surgeon will make to the surgical site. Table 3.7 describes recommended clipping margins for various aural procedures.

Head and mouth

Procedures of the mouth and head can be intra oral or extra oral. Intra-oral dental surgery is generally performed by veterinary dentists and will not be addressed in this text. Intra-oral procedures involving the removal of a mass may be performed by a soft tissue surgeon. Suffice to say, however, that intra-oral procedures generally require little to no clipping. If the mass is entirely within the mouth, there is no need to clip any hair. Procedures that are extra oral in nature do require some caution when clipping so as not to injure or traumatize either of the eyes, depending on where the incision is to be made. Table 3.7 describes the recommended clipping margins for cranio/facial procedures.

Table 3.7 Facial/aural procedures clipping guidelines.

Procedure/location of surgery	Margins
Mandibuar mass removal, mandibulectomy, fracture repair	Rostral edge of mandible caudally to ramus of mandible; dorsally to commissure of lip; ventrally to ventral midline
Maxillectomy, maxillary fracture repair	Rostral edge of maxilla caudally to ear; dorsally to lateral canthus of eye.
Aural procedures* – pinna hematoma lancing, mass removal, laceration repair	Clip entire pinna from tip to dorsal attachment to head.
Aural procedures – lateral ear canal resection; total ear canal ablation	Remove hair from medial and lateral sides of pinna; dorsally to dorsal midline; ventrally to ventral midline; rostrally to lateral canthus of the eye; caudally to base of neck
Aural procedure – ventral bulla osteotomy	Laterally to the base of the affected ear; entire ventral mandible from mandibular symphysis to the mid-cervical neck.

*Check with surgeon to find out if both medial and lateral sides of pinna need to be clipped.

Perineal

Perineal procedures are also a unique clipping situation. Whether a perineal hernia repair, an anal sacectomy, or a perianal tumor removal, the margins for clipping are fairly standard. One additional step in the patient prep that is unique to any perineal procedure is the placement of a purse string suture in the anus. The method of a purse string suture placement will be described in the patient prep section of this chapter. In most states, this should be considered a task that can be delegated to technicians as it is not a primary closure of a wound but rather a step in a nursing procedure. It is advisable to check with the Practice Act in the state to determine the eligibility to perform this task. Table 3.8 outlines the recommended hair removal margins for various perineal procedures.

Open wound clipping

Open wounds are considered contaminated but still require special attention when clipping. The main focus when prepping an open wound is to prevent any more contamination (hair) from entering the wound. A couple of options are available to achieve this goal. First of all, a saline soaked sponge can be placed over the wound. Be sure to leave all wound edges visible; so removal of hair can be accomplished on the edges. Any hair that may fly or fall into the wound will land on the sponge and will be much easier to remove than if it had landed on the tissue. Once clipping has been completed, simply fold the corners of the sponge(s) to the middle and lift it out of the wound.

Another option is to cover the open wound with a thick layer of water soluble lubricant. Once the wound is covered with a lubricant, clipping may begin. It is always best to clip away from the wound, but clipping against the grain of the hair must also be observed. Care should be taken to avoid, as much as possible, depositing any clipped hair in the wound. Once clipping is completed, the wound must be flushed well with sterile saline, before the prepping begins, to remove the lubricant and any hair that may have fallen into the wound.

After clipping for any surgical procedure, a complete vacuuming of all the removed hair must occur (Figure 3.13). Ensure stray clumps of hair under the patient or on the towel the patient is lying on are removed. If the technician's smock has large amounts of hair on it, don't forget to vacuum the smock as well. Holding the vacuum hose with one hand permits

Table 3.8 Perineal procedures clipping guidelines.

Procedure	Cranial edge	Caudal edge	Lateral edge
Anal sacectomy	Base of the tail	Ventral side of tail	To level of tuber ischii on both sides
Perineal urethrostomy	Base of tail	Ventral side of tail and ventrally on limbs to stifle. Only medial aspect of limbs need be clipped	To the level of the tuber ischii
Perineal hernia	Base of tail or cranially to lower sacral vertebra	Ventral side of tail and ventrally to level of abdomen	To level of tuber ischii

Amount of hair to be clipped is dependent on the size of hernia.

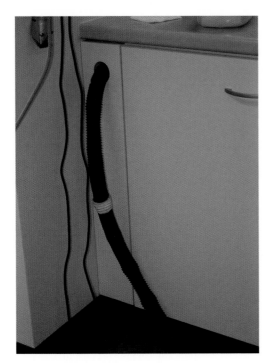

Figure 3.13 Central vacuuming system.

the other hand to be free to manipulate the animal's skin or the towel to avoid having those items sucked into the hose. Placing one finger (of the hand holding the vacuum hose) over the end of the hose will cut the suction to aid in avoiding traumatizing tissue with excessive suction power.

Clipper care

After each patient has been clipped, the blade should be evaluated. If any teeth are missing from the blade, the blade should be removed and thrown away. If the blade appears to be intact, it needs to be cleaned and lubricated. After each use, clipper blades must be disengaged from the clipper head, removed, and cleaned. Using a stiff plastic (not metal) bristle brush, remove the hair from the blade, the teeth and the clipper head. Re-attach the blade, but do not snap the blade into place until the clipper is running. Once the clipper has been turned on, snap the blade into position being certain to properly engage the blade. If the teeth are not moving or there is a knocking or rattling sound, the blade is not properly positioned. Once the blade

is running smoothly, spray a commercially available clipper blade lubricant on the teeth and allow it to run for at least 1 minute. After a minute of running, take a paper towel or gauze and blot away any excess lubricant. Blades should also be greased according to manufacturer's recommendations. If a new clipper blade is placed on the clipper head, before it is used on a patient, it must be cleaned with a commercial blade wash. With the clipper running, submerge just the teeth in the blade wash for a minute or so. Remove the blade from the solution, turn off the clipper and blot away any excess solution on the blade. This step will remove oils from the factory and will improve the longevity of the blade.

Patient skin preparation

Preparation of the skin of the surgical patient has been a long debated issue. Information used as a guideline for human surgical patients doesn't translate exactly for veterinary patients. Efficacy of products on animal skin differs from human skin due to the different thickness (i.e., bovine skin vs. human skin), fat content (i.e., porcine skin vs., human skin) and that fact that animal skin, for the most part, is covered by fur. Nonetheless, often references with a human surgical patient base are utilized as standards of care with veterinary patients. Smocks worn while clipping should be removed for the prep. A surgical head cover, mask, and exam gloves should be worn to decrease the risk of cross contamination of the surgical site.

Surgical scrub products

There are two basic options of surgical scrub products available for use for surgical patient preparation. Each has redeeming qualities of its own, but overall one is superior when all categories are considered (Figure 3.14).

Chlorhexidine

Chlorhexidine scrub is a 2% or 4% detergent-based product that can be used to cleanse the surgical site of veterinary surgical patients. It has a rapid onset of action, persistent effectiveness in the presence of bodily fluids and has excellent residual effect. Chlorhexidine requires a 3-minute contact time to maximize the benefits of the product. It can be rinsed with sterile water

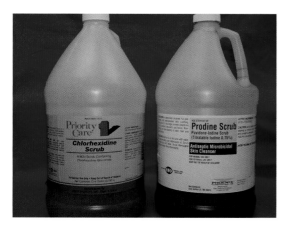

Figure 3.14 Scrub products available for patient prep.

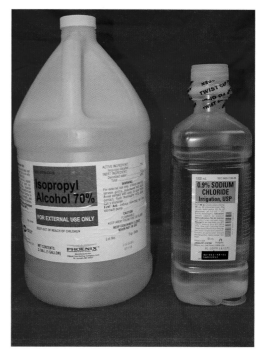

Figure 3.15 Rinsing products available for patient prep.

or 70% isopropyl alcohol. Generally, the 2% product is rinsed with 70% isopropyl alcohol and the 4% product is rinsed with sterile water. Care should be taken to supplement body heat with an external device as much as possible because rinsing agents can cause hypothermia.

Povidone-iodine

The other option for patient prep is povidone-iodine. Although less expensive than chlorhexidine, it is inactivated in the presence of organic material, has significantly lower residual activity, and when rinsed with isopropyl alcohol, has lower effectiveness. Because it is an iodine-based product, the orangish/brown color is appreciated by some as an indicator of what area has been covered.

Although there have been a few studies comparing Chlorhexidine and Povidone-Iodine as patient prep materials, there is a recent study with human surgical patients, comparing the rate of SSI (surgical site infections) and the skin preparation product used, that proves helpful. The patients were either prepped with 2% Chlorhexidine gluconate and rinsed with 70% isopropyl alcohol or 10% Povidone-Iodine scrub and painted with 10% aqueous Povidone-Iodine solution. The study showed that those patients prepped with 2% Chlorhexidine had a significantly lower rate of SSI 30 days post operatively. The findings concluded that due to Chlorhexidine's many redeeming qualities, the skin flora of the patient was reduced, thus lowering SSI (www.thedoctorschannel.com). It would seem reasonable to translate this same application to veterinary medicine and veterinary surgical patients.

Rinsing agents

Rinsing agents have traditionally been either 70% Isopropyl Alcohol or sterile water/saline (Figure 3.15). While alcohol does add some antiseptic qualities, some feel the hypothermia caused by evaporating alcohol outweighs any antiseptic benefit. Using sterile water/saline to rinse the detergent product from the animal's skin has less of a hypothermic effect and offers no additional antiseptic value. Additionally, sterile water/saline may increase the sudsing action of the scrub product, which means special attention must be paid to ensure that complete removal of the scrub agent is attained. Determining which product to use may be based on the size of the patient having surgery, the product used to cleanse the skin, the type of surgery being performed, and the estimated length of the anesthetic episode. All these factors can contribute to hypothermia and the benefits must be compared to the consequences.

Final paint solutions

Final painting of the clipped and scrubbed area needs to happen as a final step in the skin preparation process. Which ever chemical base (Chlorhexidine or

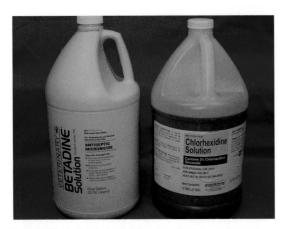

Figure 3.16 Final solution products available for patient prep.

Povidone-Iodine) is used for the scrub, the same solution should also be used for the final paint (Figure 3.16). Povidone-Iodine is used full strength as it comes from the manufacturer. Chlorhexidine however is diluted according to the manufacturer's direction, which is generally one ounce Chlorhexidine solution in one gallon of tap water.

Patient prep patterns

Target pattern

Depending on the proposed incision site, there are various methods or patterns for cleansing the skin that can be utilized. For abdominal, thoracic, neurologic, or lump/mass removals, a target pattern should be used. It is aptly named the target pattern because when properly executed, it resembles a target or bulls eye. Starting at the center of the clipped area (which should be the proposed incision site), the skin is cleansed with surgical scrub applied in a linear, back-and-forth movement. When using a sponge, it is advantageous to fold the corners of the sponge to the center to better control the surface area of the sponge touching the patient. There need not be excessive pressure placed on the skin. In fact, too much pressure can result in abrading the skin which can create a breeding ground for bacteria and actually compromise the incision. If redness or capillary oozing appears, the amount of pressure being exerted by the person prepping must be greatly reduced to the point of barely touching the skin. Contact time with the surgical scrub is what affects the effectiveness, not

the amount of pressure used to apply the product. After constant contact with the proposed incision site (about 15 seconds), the sponge continues to be moved in a small back-and-forth motion while moving outward from the center to the periphery of the clipped area. If the sponge becomes contaminated (by hair or other organic material), it should be discarded and a new sponge obtained. The new sponge should begin where the old one ended and continue moving in an outward motion toward the hairline. Once the sponge touches the hair, it may continue to be used if only touching hair (Fossum, T. 2007). The entire area that is clipped should be scrubbed. After the initial scrub is completed, a decision needs to be made. Some surgeons prefer to have the site scrubbed two more times with the surgical scrub before rinsing with a rinsing agent. This approach provides a constant contact time. Other surgeons prefer to have the site scrubbed once, rinse with either 70% Isopropyl alcohol or sterile water/saline, then scrub again, then rinse, then repeat the cycle one more time. This approach has interrupted contact time, but it is easier to remove all the scrub detergent from the skin. There has been no proof that one method is more beneficial than the other as long as the recommended contact time is achieved.

The rinsing agent should be applied to the shaven area using the same target pattern. If using sterile water/saline to rinse, a good squeeze of the sponge, to remove excess fluid, will be helpful. This will help decrease excessive sudsing as mentioned previously, which can hinder complete removal of the scrub agent. It is important that all detergent be removed from the skin as it can cause tissue irritation if transferred to internal tissues. The clipped area needs to be cleansed at least three times to meet the essential contact time without excessive drying or abrading of the skin. If however, after checking the rinse sponge of the third cycle of cleansing, there is still dirt being removed, cleansing should continue until the rinse sponge is clean. Most small animals will be clean after the three cycles, but animals that live in an area where they are exposed to more dirt (outside kennel, farm) or those involved in a trauma (hit by car, penetrating wound) may need the additional cleansing. In an ideal situation, at this point the patient would be transported to the surgery room, positioned on the surgery table, and then have a sterile prep performed. However, quite frequently this doesn't occur. If no sterile prep is performed, a final application of paint solution is applied, using the same target pattern. Paint solution may be applied with a spray bottle instead of with a sponge, although the disadvantages outweigh the advantages. Application with a spray bottle results in the solution falling on surfaces not intended to be sprayed (patient's fur, table top, and floor) and causes a mess. Also, application with a spray bottle may mean the solution is sprayed in uneven amounts on the animal's skin, which may mean not all solution is dry before surgery begins. Although spray application is accomplished quickly, this is the only advantage. Application of the final solution with a sponge allows for a controlled, even application of solution. However applied, the solution must be allowed to fully dry prior to draping and the incision is made to allow the product to perform to its full potential. The patient can then be moved into the surgery room, taking special care not to contaminate the prepped area. At a minimum, another final paint solution application should occur after final positioning on the surgery table.

Orthopedic prep

Patients having surgery on any limb will most likely need an orthopedic prep. This method of skin preparation offers the surgeon the ability to have full circumferential access to the limb as well as having the ability to handle and maneuver the limb as needed during the procedure.

First of all, the distal end of the surgical limb, if available, must be covered to the carpus/tarsus with an exam glove or a nonadhesive elastic type bandage material (Figure 3.17). Once the distal limb is covered, a stirrup (for suspending the limb) must be made. Using 1″ or 2″ tape, rip a piece approximately 30″ long to be used to create the stirrup, which will elevate the limb (Figure 3.18). Large breed dogs or dogs with long legs may need a slightly shorter piece, while small dogs or shorter legs will need a longer piece of tape. Regardless of the length, leave the last 1–2″ on either end as a regular-width tape. The tape in between needs to be folded on itself lengthwise, with the sticky sides facing each other, to form a nonsticky surface. The ends are then adhered to the covered paw, on either the medial and lateral surfaces or the dorsal/palmar or plantar surfaces, leaving the loop visible. The tape is then used to cover the tape ends on the paw to secure the stirrup so it doesn't slip (Figure 3.19). If the distal portion of the limb is the surgical site, a Backhaus penetrating towel clamp

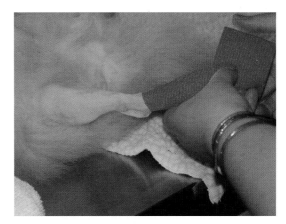

Figure 3.17 Covering the distal end of the limb.

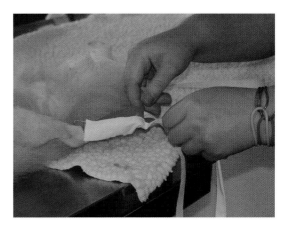

Figure 3.18 Applying a hanging stirrup.

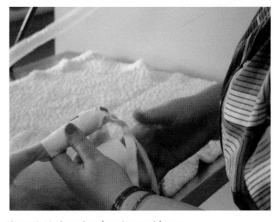

Figure 3.19 Securing the stirrup with tape.

can be clamped onto a toenail for limb suspension. The tape stirrup is then passed through the ring handles of the towel clamp, the free ends of the stirrup are secured to one another and the limb is ready for suspension. Providing support to the limb, lift the leg and place the loop over an IV pole hook. Elevate the pole so the leg is straight, but not lifting the animal off the table. In the case of a fracture, providing support to the limb is imperative to avoid bone fragment ends from causing more trauma to the tissues. Once elevated, the traction on the limb tissues will stretch and fatigue the muscles. This action may help the surgeon with reduction of the fracture, due to the muscles being more relaxed.

The orthopedic prep begins at the center of the clipped hanging limb, at the proposed incision site. Fold the corners of the prep sponge into the middle and hold all four corners to better control the sponge. Holding the limb by the taped, suspended foot, begin scrubbing the skin, moving the hand in short vertical strokes, circumferentially (all the way around) on the limb. Once one complete circling of the limb has been completed, the sponge is moved just proximally on the limb and the pattern is continued. Due to the larger surface that needs to be covered with this prep, subsequent sponges may be needed as the pattern moves proximally on the limb. When starting with another sponge, the prep should begin where the previous sponge ended. As with the target pattern, once the sponge touches hair, it can only continue to touch hair and may never return to the clipped skin. With a new scrub sponge, the prep is again started at the center of the suspended limb. Begin scrubbing the skin, moving the hand in the same short vertical motion, circumferentially on the limb. Once one complete circling of the limb has occurred, the prep continues moving the sponge distally toward the foot. Once the taped foot is reached, the sponge is discarded. Care should be taken to avoid over saturation of the tape as that may loosen the adhesive and the limb may fall down. After scrubbing the entire clipped area, the pattern can be repeated either with another scrub sponge or with a rinse sponge, as previously discussed. After the limb is sufficiently cleansed (at least three scrubs/rinses or until the rinse sponge is free of dirt and minimal contact time has occurred) a clean (not sterile) towel needs to be laid over the down limb. The surgical limb is then carefully lowered and laid on the towel. The patient is transported to the surgical suite and positioned on the surgery table. The leg is then carefully

re-suspended and the towel removed in preparation for the final prep. ALL orthopedic procedures should always have a sterile prep performed following final positioning of the patient on the surgery table.

Perineal

Perianal/perineal procedures are generally prepped utilizing a modified target pattern. Once the clipping and vacuuming is complete, the next step is the placement of a purse string suture in the anus. This is done to help eliminate the leakage of fecal material onto the surgical field. Unless the surgeon requests that this need not be done, it is a standard inclusion in the patient preparation. Depending on the type of surgery being performed, the anal sac openings may or may not be contained within the purse string suture. Anal sacectomy surgery generally requires the anal gland openings be left outside of the suture, or within the surgical field. However, some perineal surgery (i.e., perineal herniorraphy) will require anal sac opening inclusion within the suture pattern. Most urinary related procedures such as episioplasty or perineal urethrostomy surgeries will also encourage anal gland openings within the purse string. In the case of anal sac carcinoma, no purse string pattern may be placed at all in order to provide the surgeon with full access to the entire gland. It is best to check with the surgeon prior to placement of the purse string if there is any doubt. Some people find it easier to place this suture with a straight needle, although a curved needle certainly can be used, as long as the suture is 2–0 or 3–0 in size. Since it is a limited term suture, whether the suture is absorbable or non-absorbable is not an issue, but a monofilament is preferred. In this situation, placement of this stitch is not a primary wound closure, nor a curative measure, so it should be allowed by most jurisdiction's Practice Acts. If any doubt arises regarding the legality of a credentialed veterinary technician performing this procedure, the Practice Act should be consulted. To place the suture pattern, start first by looking at the anus and imagining it as a clock face. With the needle at the 11 o'clock position take a superficial bite and have the needle exit at the 1 o'clock position. Starting the next bite where the previous one exited the skin, drive the needle superficially and exit at the 5 o'clock position. For the ventral placement, enter the skin at 5 o'clock, drive the needle superficially and exit at the 7 o'clock point. The final bite begins at 7 o'clock and moves in a dorsal direction, superficially and exits at the 11 o'clock point. Superficial placement is imperative for all the bites, but especially for the lateral stitches to avoid inadvertently penetrating the anal glands. In essence a "box" has been placed around the anus. Pull the suture tight to cinch down the anal opening and tie the suture. A simple square knot is sufficient. Cut the suture tails long enough to be able to find them, but not so long they interfere with the procedure. A bold note should be made on the anesthesia sheet or the surgical report indicating the placement of the purse string. This note will act as a reminder to remove the suture post procedure, but before recovery.

After the purse string stitch has been completed, the prep can begin. Working from clean to dirty areas, the clipped area lateral to the anus should be scrubbed with the target pattern. Using a new sponge for each side, perform the target pattern until hair is touched. Use a new sponge and scrub just the anus, then discard that sponge. This modified pattern is repeated until the rinse sponge is free of dirt, with a minimum of three repetitions. The appropriate contact time must also be met. The final solution is applied using the same pattern.

Patient positioning

Once the patient has received the initial prep, they are ready to be transported to the operating room. There are many devices available for assisting with positioning the patient on the surgery table. Proper positioning of the patient is a critical step in the patient prep process. Surgeons require the patient be positioned in a straight and anatomically correct fashion. Once patients are positioned to the surgeon's liking, they must not shift or move from that position until the end of the surgery. Some surgery tables have a split top, which allows either one or both sides of the table top to be adjusted. Options from a flat surface to a full "V" position are available. For patients in dorsal recumbency this may be all that is required to maintain the patient in the surgical position required. For deep chested dogs, long sandbags will be an effective method for maintaining dorsal recumbency in addition to the table "V". Foam wedges may also be used but may slip and if contaminated by blood or other fluids may be difficult to clean. Also available for use, if the table top is solid and cannot be adapted to the animal's shape, is a thoracic positioner (Figure 3.20).

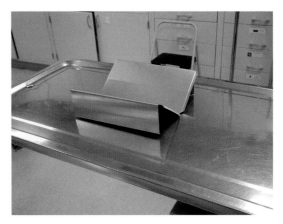

Figure 3.20   Thoracic positioner for maintaining dorsal recumbency.

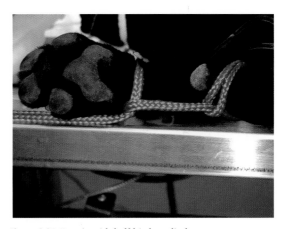

Figure 3.21   Leg tie with half hitch on limb.

Additionally patients in dorsal recumbency will need to have their limbs restrained away from the surgical field. Soft ropes or "leg ties" are available and work well. Roll gauze, IV tubing or elastic bands are not recommended as they may apply too much pressure to the soft tissue and impede distal limb circulation. Leg ties should be placed just proximal to the carpus and tarsus, with a half hitch placed just distal to those joints (Figure 3.21). Double placement aids in better distribution of pressure to reduce circulation issues. Most surgery tables have either brackets or rubber rollers on the sides of the table near each corner. Brackets require a figure 8 method of securing of the leg tie with a half hitch on the last loop to hold the rope (Figure 3.22). Rubber rollers are easier to use and simply require the leg tie be passed

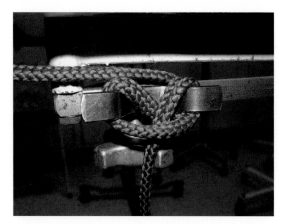

Figure 3.22 Table bracket with figure 8 leg tie.

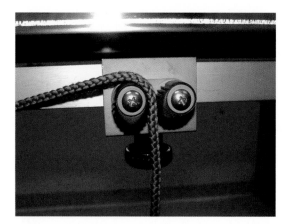

Figure 3.23 Table roller for securing leg tie.

between the two rubber rollers to securely hold the rope (Figure 3.23). Care should be taken to avoid excessively extending the limbs. The forelimbs should have the leg ties brought over the head of the table, not the sides, to help maintain normal joint anatomy. Hind limbs should be extended to full range of motion, although not excessively stretched, and the ropes should be brought over the end of the table, not the sides. Normal anatomy of the hind leg joints can be maintained with this approach. Rear limb leg ties brought over the side of the table force the hips into a frog leg position and for lengthy procedures, this is not recommended. Additionally, the limbs will be closer to the animal's body and not impede the surgeons work. There is a special type of positioning aid for dogs having arthroscopic surgery on the stifle. The brace holds the limb in a flexed position to assist the

surgeon. The brace must be covered by a sterile drape before the limb can be placed on it.

Patients in lateral recumbency may be maintained in the desired position by the use of sand bags or vacuum positioning aids. Hug-U-Vac® and Vac-Pac® are both positioning devices that conform to the patient to maintain the position; then a vacuum process is used to evacuate the air from the device. As the positioning aid hardens as the air is removed, the patient is held in the desired position. These devices help with thermostasis as well as they are insulated and protect the patient from the cold surface of the surgery table. Vacuum aids are especially helpful when positioning patients for ophthalmic procedures or thoracic cases that necessitate the patient be positioned in an oblique state rather than a level lateral position. Patients in lateral recumbency will also require the limbs to be restrained by leg ties. Larger breed dogs may have sandbags, foam, or some other type of "spacer" placed between the upper and lower limb to help alleviate stress on the upper limb joints.

Patients undergoing spinal surgery are generally placed in ventral recumbency. The use of sand bags and/or vacuum aids is required in order to achieve and maintain proper positioning of the patient. Patients in this position must be monitored for adequate respiratory capability. The vacuum positions aids are quite stiff and hard following evacuation of the air and are therefore not very good at allowing expansion of the chest wall if conformed too tightly to the patient. Positioning aids should not be "wrapped around" the chest of the patient, but rather gathered or formed along the sides of the chest.

Patient warming

Normal body thermoregulatory systems are compromised by anesthesia, so maintaining an appropriate body temperature for the patient is very challenging. Surgical complications can often be linked to patient surgical/post-surgical hypothermia, so external supplementary means must be used. In addition to peripheral vasoconstriction, hypothermia can compromise the immune system and elevate both blood pressure and heart rate, thus affecting wound healing.

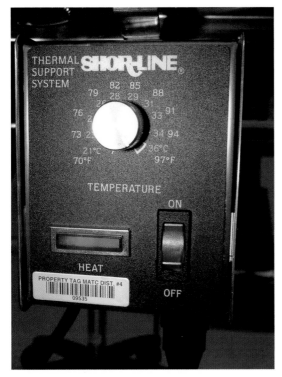

Figure 3.24 Control box for heated surgery table.

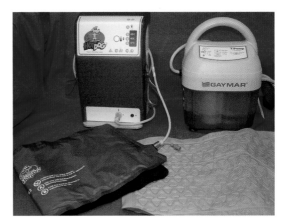

Figure 3.25 Supplemental heating devices.

Heated surgery tables

One method of supplemental heat is the use of a heated surgery table top. Some surgery tables are constructed with heating elements enclosed with in the table top and a control box to adjust the temperature setting (Figure 3.24). As there is a constant source of heat, there is the potential for a thermal burn; so placing a towel between the table and the patient is advised. Care should be taken not to use a towel that is too thick as then the benefit from the heated top may be compromised by the density of the towel.

Circulating water blankets

Other types of supplemental heating generally revolve around the use of a pad of some sort and a control unit or box (Figure 3.25). Circulating water blankets have been employed for a long time and are now available with hard plexiglass pads as well as the traditional softer vinyl pads. A claw or tooth that punctures a vinyl pad will result in a soaking wet patient due to the water escaping form the pad. A plexiglass pad eliminates the possibility of this occurring due to the durability of the plexiglass. Returning to the recovery area to check on a patient only to find a flood and a soaking wet patient is very frustrating. As with any constant heat source, a towel should be placed between the pad and the patient.

Convection warming systems

The use of forced warm air enveloping the patient has increased in recent years. A light weight disposable paper pad with many small holes is positioned to cover as much of the patient as possible. Once the patient is positioned on the surgical table, but before the drapes are placed, the pad is placed over the patient (Figure 3.26). After the surgical drapes have been placed, the unit is turned on. While the drapes do assist in keeping the warm air close to the patient, there is some concern with increased air particles and potentially compromising aseptic technique with the addition of the warm forced air. This type of warming device is effective at quickly warming hypothermic patients in recovery.

Solid warming pads

Multiple styles of solid warming pads that can be used are also available. Many of the pads deliver a low voltage current to the solid pad. Internal sensors regulate the temperature of the pad and greatly reduce the risk of hot spots or uneven heating. The highest setting on these pads should not be used unless there is a towel between the patient and the pad. Some models have an automatic shut off which inhibits thermal burns as well. Some of the styles of solid pads can be wrapped around (envelope) the patient, which in turn results in less hypothermia.

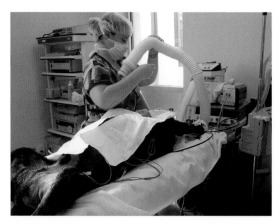

Figure 3.26 Hot air warming system.

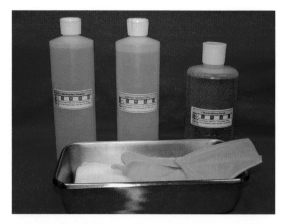

Figure 3.28 Sterile prep set with squeeze bottles of solutions.

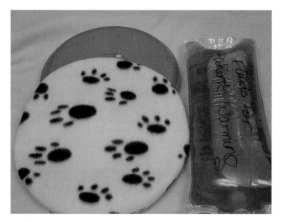

Figure 3.27 Alternative warming devices.

Alternative methods

Alternative methods of supplementary heat include warmed bags of fluids, rice socks, warming discs, and hot water gloves (Figure 3.27). These devices, while warm, can certainly provide external heat for the patient. They are readily available, relatively inexpensive, and reusable, but the disadvantages must be considered. First of all, smaller warming devices will provide supplemental heat to only an isolated area of the body. Other methods previously discussed have a much greater body surface contact area, therefore increasing heat absorption. Secondly, the warmed devices only provided warmth for a limited period of time and then they start to cool. As the rice socks or any other such device cools, it will also cool the patient, therefore making these choices contraindicated for procedures longer than 30 minutes.

Patient sterile prep

Following positioning of the patient, the sterile prep may begin. A sterile patient prep is done in exactly the same way as the initial prep, with the major difference being the use of sterile products. Prep sets can be made a couple of ways, depending on clinic choice. A small instrument pan (3″ × 8″) or a kidney basin (emesis basin) can be used as the pan. Two stacks of ten 4″ × 4″ gauze sponges are placed side by side in the pan. An indicator strip should be placed in the middle of the sponges. A right hand glove (size 7–7 1/2) can then be laid on top of the sponges (Figure 3.28). The pan is double wrapped using the envelope style of wrapping and is steam sterilized. Some clinics prefer to use sterile packaged gauze and a fresh pair of sterile gloves, which is an acceptable adaptation.

In addition to the prep set, squeeze bottles of the prep solutions are needed. The solutions and prep set should be set up in the surgery room when the rest of the packs and equipment are placed in the room. Once the patient is placed on the table and positioned, the prep set can be opened. Both wraps are aseptically opened to reveal the sterile contents. Before proceeding, the caps of the solution bottles should be opened. If a glove was not included in the sterile prep set, a pair of gloves should now be aseptically opened and using the open gloving technique, put on one glove on the dominant hand. If a glove was included, it is now aseptically placed on the dominant hand. Having one sterile and one non-sterile hand allows the technician the versatility to perform the sterile prep without assistance. The non-sterile hand is available to pick up the solution bottles to apply the product as well as to stabilize the suspended limb in the event of an orthopedic case.

With the sterile gloved hand, two sponges are picked up. The non-sterile hand picks up the surgical scrub bottle and aseptically applies some scrub solution to the sterile sponges. Care must be taken to ensure the cap of the bottle does not touch the sponges. The prep now continues using the same pattern as was used with the initial prep. New prep sponges should be retrieved as needed. The rinsing agent is aseptically applied to the sponges as needed. Be sure to save a few dry sponges to be used for the application of the final paint solution.

Once the final paint is applied, the draping may begin. Every effort should be made to allow the final solution to dry prior to draping to encourage optimal efficacy.

Personnel preparation

Attire
Any person entering the surgery room must have on the appropriate attire. Clean scrubs, with the top tucked into the pants, an appropriate head covering and shoe covers or facility dictated footwear should be a minimal dress code. Personnel in the operating room, whether they are scrubbed in or not, must also adhere to several personal hygiene rules. Bathing or showering should occur every-day. The use of fragrance or cologne should be minimal if at all. With increased sensitivity to fragrance by many people, it is a simple consideration not to heavily apply a fragrance. More importantly, if the room or area is filled with the odor of cologne, the anesthetist will have a difficult time detecting any odor of inhalant gas, which may indicate a leak in the anesthetic system. Finally, due to the increased sensitivity of the smelling sense of animals, heavy odors may be irritating to the patients.

Jewelry worn should be minimal and simple. If acting as the surgical assistant, no rings, watches, or bracelets can be worn. Even necklaces such as a simple chain are discouraged. Earrings should be removed or not worn at all. Some facilities allow small post-style earrings to be left in the ear lobes, but never should hoops or large dan-gling earrings be worn. Circulating technicians may have simple band style rings and watches left on. Rings with large precious gem stones risk damage from chemicals or getting caught on equipment and would best be left at home. Earrings may be left in and should be a small post-style earring. Simple single chain necklaces may be left on.

Fingernails of all surgical team members should be short, well groomed, and clean. Nails should not be longer than the pad of the finger. Long fingernails can cause pain to feline patients while scruffing them and can puncture surgical gloves. Artificial nails and/or nail polish are strictly prohibited. Chipped or flaking nail polish may contaminate the field, or worse, harbor bacteria that may infect the patient.

Surgeons hand scrub
Members of the surgical team that are scrubbing in need to perform a surgeons hand scrub or rub. A hand rub can be employed for subsequent surgical cases, after a hand scrub has been performed for the first surgery of the day. Details regarding the hand rub are discussed later in this section. A surgical scrub or hand rub is performed in addition to the use of the sterile gown and gloves. The hand scrub is a specific method of cleansing the hands, wrists, and forearms of a person who will be wearing a sterile gown and gloves. A surgical scrub, or cleansing, is performed in addition to the use of the sterile gown and gloves. It has been reported that the overall incidence of glove defects is 23% and glove defects increase as the duration of the procedure increases. Since the presence of glove defects can often be undetected, the surgical hand scrub is an essential step. Products used for a hand scrub must be rapid acting, should be effective against a broad spectrum of bacteria, and should be nonirritating as well as effective at inhibiting bacterial growth. There are three products that may be used for this procedure – Povidone-Iodine, Chlorhexidine and Chloroxylenol (PCMX).Other newer products are available, but will be discussed under the hand rub (brushless scrub) section. Povidone-Iodine has a broad spectrum of activity but it is inactivated by organic material. Additionally, it requires a minimum 2-minute contact time, which can be easily achieved using either method of surgical hand scrub patterns. Chlorhexidine also has a broad spectrum of activity and has the best residual effect due to it binding to keratin. It is not inactivated by organic material and causes less skin irritation than Povidone-Iodine (Sigler, M. 2001). Chloroxylenol is available as scrub impregnated sponges and traditionally has been outperformed by chlorhexidine.

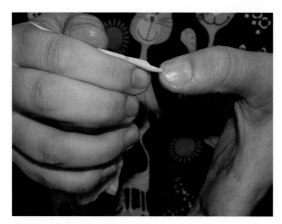

Figure 3.29 Cleaning nails.

Before a surgical scrub can begin, all jewelry must be removed from the hands and arms. Nails should be inspected and if too long, they must be trimmed. Neither nail polish nor artificial nails are permitted. Appropriate head and face attire must be put on and the surgical scrub top must be tucked into the scrub pants. If shoe covers are used, they must be placed on the footwear prior to the scrub beginning.

There are two options of procedure for performing the surgeons hand scrub. One method is the anatomical timed method and the other is the counted stroke method. Both the methods start with a thorough washing of the hands and arms with an antimicrobial product. While leaving the lather on the hands and arms, the nails can be cleaned (Figure 3.29). Nail cleaners can be found in either the package of a disposable scrub brush or purchased commercially and left in a receptacle near the scrub sink. In either case, the nail cleaner is disposable and should be used only once and then thrown away. After cleaning under the nails, the hands and arms can be rinsed. If an antiseptic-impregnated disposable sponge is used, it can be saturated with water and squeezed to produce lather. If a reuseable brush is used, it is aseptically removed from the sterilized brush dispenser. The foot-operated pedal for dispensing the soap is then depressed and the scrub brush is saturated with the scrub product. The surgical scrub should be approached systematically and always performed the same way to avoid missing any of the steps. As the scrub begins, the elbows must remain bent, with the fingers pointing toward the ceiling. Not only does this allow the water to run from the finger

tips to the elbows, (clean to dirty) but it also insures that the hands and arms do not touch the scrub top. The anatomic timed method usually lasts 3–5 minutes, depending on the facility policy. As soon as the sub-ungual area of the nails is cleaned, timing is started. Scrub each finger, in between the fingers, and both the front and back portions of the hand for 2 minutes. Then each side of the arm is scrubbed for 1 minute. The arm is rinsed by passing the bent arm under the running water moving from finger tips to elbow. The other hand and arm are scrubbed using the same timed method. The second arm is rinsed in the same fashion as the first and then the hands are aseptically dried with a sterile hand towel. For the counted stroke method, as soon as the nails are cleaned, the scrub begins with the nails. Starting with either hand, the scrub brush is moved back and forth (which equals one stroke) on the nails for 30 strokes. Care should be taken to ensure that the brush reaches under the nails as well as the nails themselves (Figure 3.30). Once the nails are done, the fingers are scrubbed next. It really doesn't matter if the scrub starts with the thumb or the little finger, as long as the same process is always used to avoid mistakes. The little finger is divided into four sides. Start the scrub on the lateral side moving from the tip of the finger to the base of the finger, counting as one stroke (Figure 3.31). Scrub the lateral side of the finger for 20 strokes. Move onto the palmar side of the finger for 20 strokes. The medial surface is scrubbed for 20 strokes next and finally the dorsal surface of the little finger is scrubbed for 20 strokes. That completes the scrub for one finger, so now the ring finger can be scrubbed

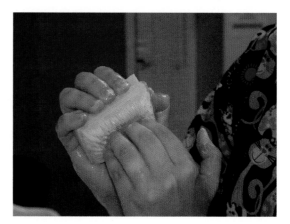

Figure 3.30 Scrubbing the nails.

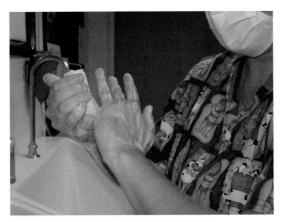

Figure 3.31 Scrubbing fingers start at the little finger and divide each finger into four sides.

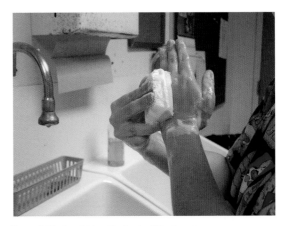

Figure 3.33 Scrubbing the back of the hand.

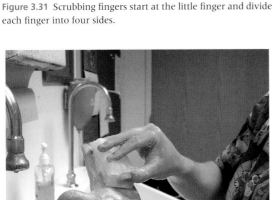

Figure 3.32 Scrubbing the palmar surface.

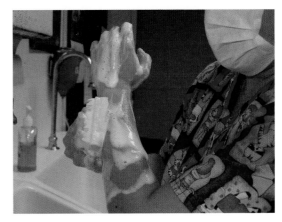

Figure 3.34 Scrubbing the arm divide the arm into four sides.

using the same approach. Be sure to cleanse and scrub the webbing between each finger as well. After the ring finger is completed the scrub follows the same pattern on the middle finger, index finger and finally the thumb. Following the scrub of the fingers, the entire palmar surface of the hand is scrubbed for 20 strokes (Figure 3.32). Following the palm, the dorsal surface of the hand is also scrubbed for 20 strokes (Figure 3.33). Completing the scrub of the hand allows progression to the arm. Dividing the arm into four equal sides, each side is scrubbed for 15 strokes, from the wrist to two inches distal to the elbow (Figure 3.34).

Leaving the antimicrobial detergent on the first arm, the sponge is transferred to the scrubbed hand and the same process is followed to scrub the second hand and arm. At any time, more water may be added to the sponge to generate more lather or more soap may be added as needed (Figure 3.35). When the second hand and arm are completed, the first hand and arm is then rinsed. Being careful to not touch the faucet, the rinsing begins at the finger tips (Figure 3.36). With the elbows bent and the fingers pointing toward the ceiling, the rinse is continued down the hand, wrist, and arm. Care needs to be taken to keep the elbow bent so the water always runs from the fingers to the elbow. After completely rinsing the first arm, the second arm is rinsed in the same fashion. A slight bend forward at the waist will help avoid splashing water onto the scrubs (Figure 3.37). After rinsing both arms, 15–30 seconds should be spent at the scrub sink allowing the water to run off the arms (Figure 3.38).

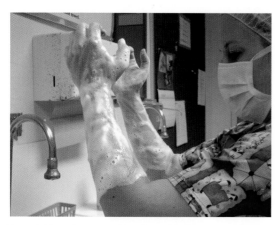

Figure 3.35 Both arms and hands scrubbed.

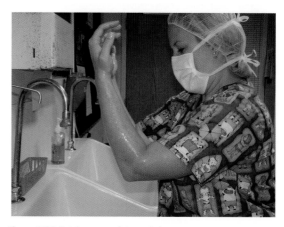

Figure 3.38 Letting arms drip at sink.

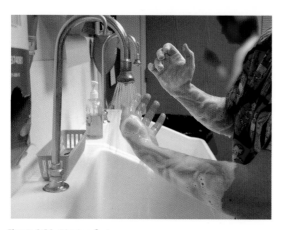

Figure 3.36 Rinsing first arm.

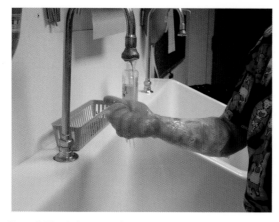

Figure 3.37 Rinsing second arm.

Surgical hand Rub

One of the most recent advances in veterinary surgery is the introduction of the hand rub. This procedure, performed with designated products, is intended to replace the surgical scrub. For surgeons and assistants that regularly scrub for multiple procedures as day, this is a welcome alternative. There are various products available (Avagard®, etc.) but the base chemical in most of the options is isopropyl alcohol. It is imperative that manufacturer's recommendations be followed. It is advised to perform a traditional surgical scrub for the first case of the day and then subsequent cases can have a surgical hand rub used. If there is a lot of patient contact or time spent outside the operating room between cases, then a traditional hand scrub may be a better choice. As stated earlier, specific manufacturer instructions for use of the hand rub should be followed. First of all the hands are washed with an antiseptic soap, being sure to clean under the finger nails with a nail cleaner. After rinsing the hands and forearms, they are dried with a paper towel. The recommended amount of product is dispensed into one hand. The nails and finger tips of the opposite hand are kept submerged in the solution. The remaining product is then rubbed into the hand and forearm, to the elbow. Another dose of product is dispensed into the other hand and the procedure is repeated. Continuous rubbing will thoroughly dry the arms and hands prior to gloving (CDC 1999). Proper exposure time to the product, as recommended by the manufacturer, must also be adhered to.

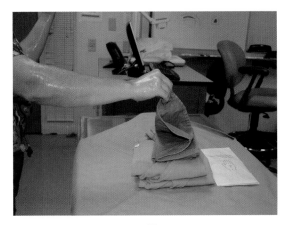

Figure 3.39 Picking up the towel by just one corner.

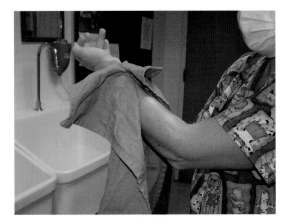

Figure 3.41 Drying the arm by pushing the arm through the towel.

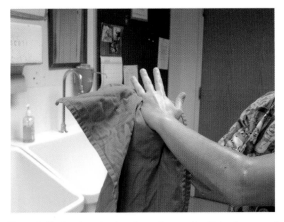

Figure 3.40 Drying the hand starting at the little finger and working through all the fingers.

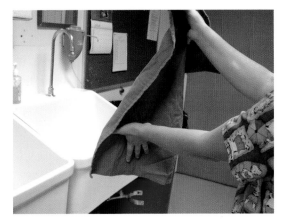

Figure 3.42 Place the dry hand on the underside of the towel. Drop the wet side to reveal the dry side for use on the other hand of the arm.

Drying the hands and arms

While the surgeon or assistant is performing the hand scrub, the circulating nurse should at the same time open the sterile gown pack. Both wrappers need to be opened in an aseptic fashion to permit access to the sterile hand towel. After performing a traditional hand scrub, the hands and arms need to be dried before gowning and gloving. The sterile hand towel must be picked up with either hand, by holding one corner (Figure 3.39). The hand that picked up the towel holds the towel as it is allowed to fully unfold. The hand holding the towel then gathers the towel into that hand. Starting with the little finger of the opposite hand, dry all surfaces of that finger (Figure 3.40). Move sequentially through the rest of the fingers and thumb,

drying all surfaces as well as in between the fingers. It is important to remember that once an area has been dried, it **cannot** be revisited. Upon completion of drying the fingers, the palm of the hand and then the back of the hand are dried. Extending arms in front as well as slightly bending forward at the waist will assist with keeping the sterile towel from touching the non-sterile scrub suit. To dry the arms, the hand holding the towel is wrapped around the wrist to be dried (Figure 3.41). Push the wrist and arm *away* from the body while the towel twists around the arm until the elbow is reached. Never dry the arm using a back-and-forth motion from the wrist to the elbow. Once the elbow has been reached, the dry hand is placed on the opposite end of the towel, on the underside (Figure 3.42). The wet

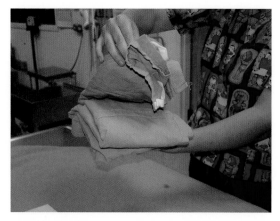

Figure 3.43 Picking up the gown holding the arm sleeve seams, just down from the neck. The other hand is slid under the gown.

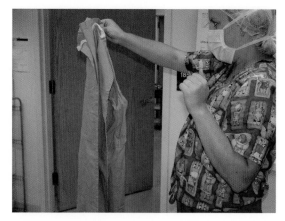

Figure 3.44 Let the gown unfold.

end of the towel is dropped, leaving a clean dry surface with which to dry the second arm and hand. Upon completion of drying the second hand and arm, the towel is dropped onto the floor without having either hand drop below the waist level.

Gowning

It is important to be familiar with how the gown is folded in order to aseptically pick up the gown and properly put it on. Whether a paper (disposable) gown or a cloth gown is used, proper donning of the gown is critical. Often the gown is folded with the seams of the sleeves on the top of the pack; so if the arm sleeves seams are visible, the person putting on the gown should use one hand to grasp the seams. The other hand is slid under the folded gown. The gown is then lifted off the wrapper and a step is taken back from the table (Figure 3.43). The hand under the gown is removed and the gown is allowed to unfold. At this point it should be possible to identify both sleeves (Figure 3.44). One arm is advanced into the corresponding sleeve but stopped before the fingers come out of the sleeve cuff. As the gown is put on, it is important to permit the arms to move only to the side – never up above the shoulders nor down below the waist (Figure 3.45). After one arm is in the sleeve, the other arm is advanced into its corresponding sleeve. Again care must be taken not to allow the gown to fall down or touch the floor as the second arm is advanced into the sleeve (Figure 3.46). At this point, the non-sterile circulating nurse needs to "tie in" the sterile person. Without touching any area

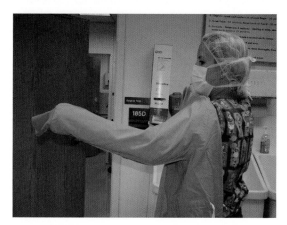

Figure 3.45 Slide one arm into the sleeve.

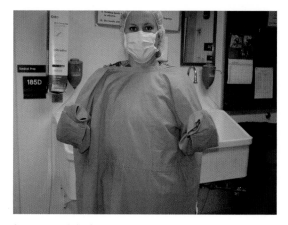

Figure 3.46 Slide the other arm into the other sleeve, keeping both hands inside the sleeve.

of the gown that is considered sterile, the circulating nurse must get access to the neck ties. Placing the hands on the underside of the gown (that which is touching the person) allows the circulating nurse to "flip" back the neck ties to the back of the person. A simple bow is made to secure the ties at the neck. Depending on the type of gown that is used, the next step can be accomplished in one of two ways. Since the back of the gown is not considered sterile, the circulating nurse may touch anywhere on the backside to retrieve the ties. If the gown is a non-sterile back style, then the two waist ties are tied in a bow at the waist. If the gown is a wrap around or sterile back style, the circulating nurse must be carful to touch only those ties that are considered non-sterile. One tie will be on the edge of the left flap of the back of the gown. The other tie will be on the inside of the gown on the right side seam (Figure 3.47). These two ties are tied into a snug bow. The ties on the edge of the right side, which may be tied to a front tie or attached to a paper card, are not touched. Standing behind the gowned person, the circulating nurse bends his/her knees to get to the floor level. Reaching around to the front of the gown, a gentle tug is given to the bottom edge of the gown to alleviate any bunching of the gown. If a wraparound gown is used, the tying process will need to be completed after the gloves have been put on. Once gloved, the sterile person detaches the tie attached to the gown from the card. The card is handed to the circulating nurse and the sterile person slowly spins in a circle to wrap the gown around them (Figure 3.48). The sterile person then grabs the **tie** from the card without touching the card and pulls the tie of the card. Now the sterile person has both ties and they can secure the gown with a bowtie.

Gloving

Closed gloving

The preferred method of donning sterile gloves when a sterile surgical gown has been put on is with a technique called closed gloving. The intention of closed gloving is that by keeping the hands within the sterile sleeves, there is little risk of contaminating the sterile gloves during application. Closed gloving can *only* be performed while wearing a sterile gown. After the ties of the neck and waist of the gown have been secured, gloving may begin. Sterile gloves should have been opened onto a sterile field by the circulating nurse. With hands and fingers staying within the gown sleeves, open

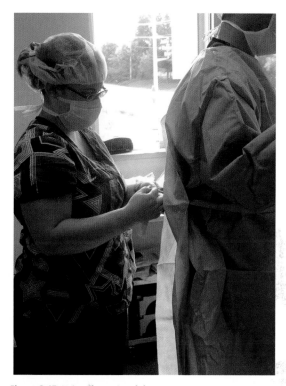

Figure 3.47 Tying the waist of the gown.

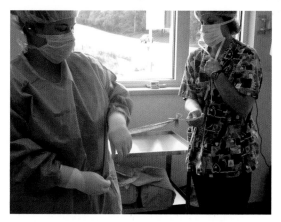

Figure 3.48 The sterile person spins slowly to wrap the gown around them while the circulating nurse holds the card.

the glove wrapper so the gloves appear with the palms up, fingers pointing away. Fold the bottom edge of the wrapper under to avoid the paper wrapper from spring back to original shape (Figure 3.49). The folded cuff of each glove should be closest to the person putting

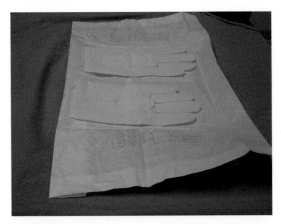

Figure 3.49 Glove wrapper edge folded under.

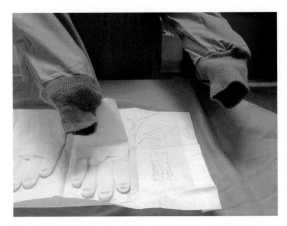

Figure 3.50 Right hand grabs the folded edge of the cuff.

the gloves on. Remember, before touching the gloves, all areas of the gloves are considered sterile, but once the gloving process begins, the inside of the glove is considered non-sterile because it will eventually touch the non-sterile hands. Use the following technique to aseptically perform closed gloving:

1 Until one glove is successfully and correctly placed on the hand, all contact with the gloves and glove wrapper is done with the hands inside the gown sleeves.
2 Keeping the hands within in the sleeves, turn the left hand so the palm is facing up. The right hand grabs the left glove on the top folded edge of the cuff (Figure 3.50).
3 Pick up the left glove and hold it vertically so the fingers are facing the floor (Figure 3.51).
4 Gently flip the glove and place it on the waiting left hand. The thumb of the glove should be facing the thumb of the hand and the fingers of the glove should be facing the forearm and elbow of the left arm (Figure 3.52).
5 Working through the sleeve, the fingers of the left hand grab the bottom folded edge of the glove, while the right hand (through the right sleeve) grabs the upper fold of the glove cuff (Figure 3.53).
6 With each hand securely holding the folded edge of the glove, stretch the glove to create a larger opening (Figure 3.54).
7 Pull the glove over the left hand. The entire knit cuff of the gown sleeve must be covered at this point (Figure 3.55).
8 Unroll the cuff of the glove completely to keep the gown sleeve secure (Figure 3.56).

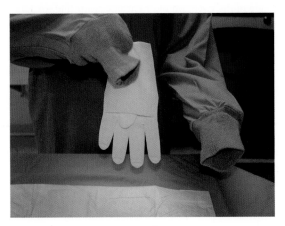

Figure 3.51 Hold the glove vertically.

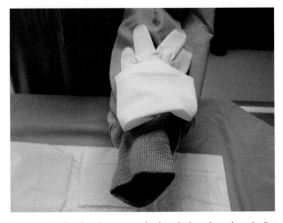

Figure 3.52 Flip the glove onto the hand, thumb to thumb, fingers pointing toward the operator.

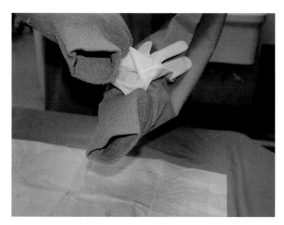

Figure 3.53 Each hand grabs a folded edge of the cuff – through the gown sleeve.

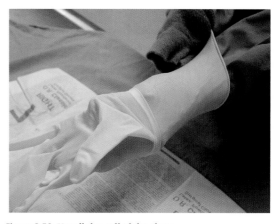

Figure 3.56 Unroll the cuff of the glove.

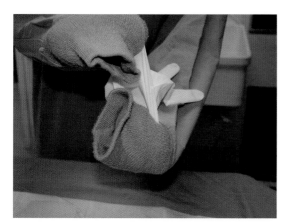

Figure 3.54 Stretch the glove to insert the hand.

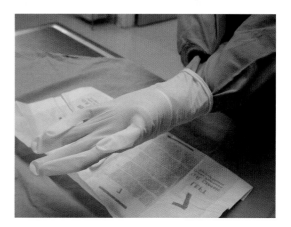

Figure 3.57 Pull sleeve to get fingers into finger holes.

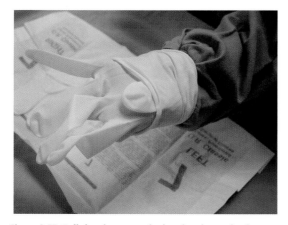

Figure 3.55 Pull the glove over the hand and completely cover the cuff of the sleeve.

9 Unroll the left hand fingers to match up with the finger holes on the glove.

10 Any adjustment of the glove fingers must be done with the right hand still within the right gown sleeve.

11 The sleeve of the gown may be pulled to get the cuff of the sleeve off the hand (Figure 3.57). The knit cuff of the gown sleeve must never extend beyond the glove cuff so excessive pulling of the sleeve is not recommended. Care should be taken to avoid wrinkles of the gown sleeve cuff in order to avoid compromising circulation to the hand.

12 The process is repeated with the right hand. After both gloves are in place, final adjustments to the gloves may be made to ensure the best possible fit.

Open gloving

The open gloving technique is used when a sterile gown has not been put on but sterile gloves are still required (i.e., urinary catheterization, jugular catheter placement, etc.). Open gloving may also be performed if a glove was contaminated during surgery and a replaced glove must be put on. Use the following technique to properly perform open gloving:

1. One of the most important things to remember when open gloving is being aware of what is considered sterile versus non-sterile. Even though all surfaces of the gloves have been sterilized, some surfaces are considered non-sterile once open gloving begins.

2. The glove wrapper is carefully opened revealing the gloves in a palm-up position in the wrapper. The folded cuff of the gloves should be closest to the person putting on the gloves. Fold the long edge of the wrapper under to keep it from springing closed (Figure 3.58).

3. The entire inner surface of the glove wrapper is considered sterile, but can be touched only from the edge to within 1″ of the edge of the wrapper.

4. The right hand picks up the top folded edge of the cuff of the left glove. Do not touch the wrapper underneath or any other part of the glove (Figure 3.59).

5. The left hand fingers are cupped together and the hand is slid into the glove, palm up. Fingers should be aligned with the glove fingers (Figure 3.60).

6. Leave the cuff of the glove folded until the other hand is gloved (Figure 3.61).

7. The sterile left hand is slid between the cuff and the sterile glove of the right hand. This position allows the sterile left hand to contact the outside of the sterile right glove (Figure 3.62).

8. Bring the thumb of the left hand down to hold the cuff against the left hand.

9. Keeping the palm of the right hand up, cup the fingers and slide that hand into the glove. DO NOT allow the sterile left thumb to touch any part of the non-sterile right hand (Figure 3.63).

10. The cuff of the right glove may be carefully unrolled as long as the sterile left hand does not touch anything non-sterile (Figure 3.64).

11. The now sterile right hand may slide under the cuff of the sterile left glove and carefully unfold the cuff (Figure 3.65). No part of the sterile right hand may touch a non-sterile surface.

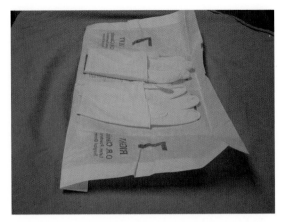

Figure 3.58 Glove wrapper edge folded under.

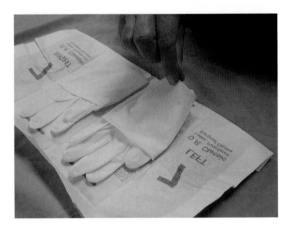

Figure 3.59 Right hand picks up the top fold of the cuff.

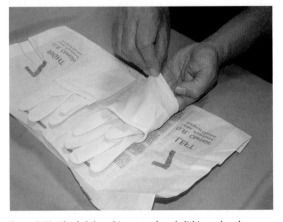

Figure 3.60 The left hand is cupped and slid into the glove.

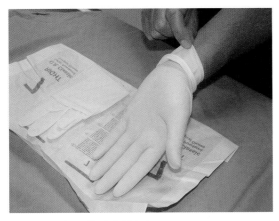

Figure 3.61 The cuff is left folded.

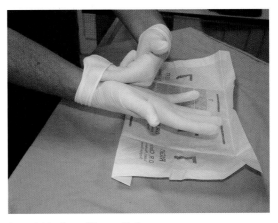

Figure 3.64 The cuff is unrolled.

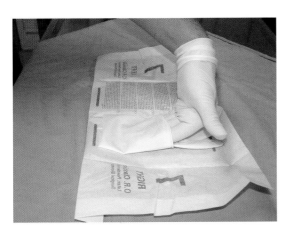

Figure 3.62 The left hand is slid under the cuff of the right hand glove.

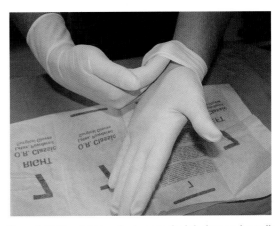

Figure 3.65 The right hand returns to the left glove and unrolls the cuff.

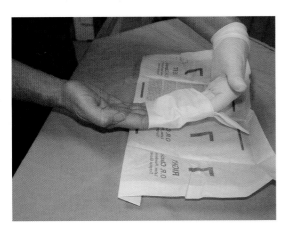

Figure 3.63 The right hand is cupped and slid into the glove.

Assisted gloving

Although infrequently used in veterinary surgery, this is the preferred method of re-gloving once a sterile gown has been put on. This method does require at least two sterile members of the surgical team, hence its limited use in veterinary surgery. To appropriately perform the assisted gloving technique, the following steps must be done.

1 A non-sterile person aseptically removes the contaminated glove (see the following section).
2 The sterile person that will be assisting with the gloving receives the gloves from the circulating nurse and opens the glove wrapper on a sterile surface.

3 The assisting sterile person picks up the glove that will be used and places both hands under the cuff of the glove.

4 They then spread the opening of the glove wide to accept the hand needing the glove. The person receiving the glove may also place their other sterile hand under the cuff to assist with stretching the glove.

5 Orient the glove so the palm of the glove is facing the person receiving the glove.

6 The team member needing the glove then inserts his/her hand into the glove. Be sure the fingers of the accepting hand are pointing downwards prior to insertion.

7 Pull the cuff of the glove over as much of the gown cuff as possible.

8 The person who received the glove may now make minor adjustments to the fit of the new glove.

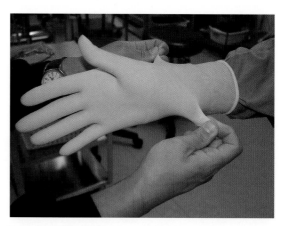

Figure 3.67 The circulating nurse grabs *only the glove* and pulls the glove off inside out.

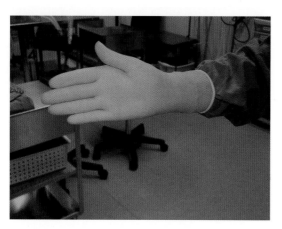

Figure 3.66 Present contaminate gloved hand for glove removal.

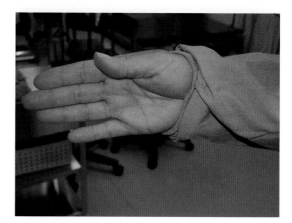

Figure 3.68 The open hand is left to re-glove.

Removing a contaminate glove

For various reasons, a glove may become contaminated during a procedure. The glove must be changed immediately to avoid further contamination of the surgical field. The following is the procedure for removing a contaminated glove during a procedure:

1 A non-sterile person must remove the contaminated glove.

2 The person having the glove removed presents the contaminated hand in a sideways orientation, as if shaking hands (Figure 3.66).

3 Care should be taken to ensure that the non-sterile person does not touch any part of the gown sleeve.

4 The non-sterile person grasps the glove at the level of the hand and pulls the glove off inside out Figure 3.67. The cuff of the gown should not be pulled over the hand as the inside of the gown has touched skin and would therefore contaminate the hand if they came in contact with one another (Figure 3.68).

5 The sterile member must now either open the glove to replace the contaminated glove (if working alone) or be re-gloved using the assisted gloving techniques if another sterile member is available.

Double gloving

Some surgeons will elect to double glove when draping a patient, and then remove the outer gloves once draping is completed. This will greatly reduce the risk of introducing contaminates from draping into the surgical

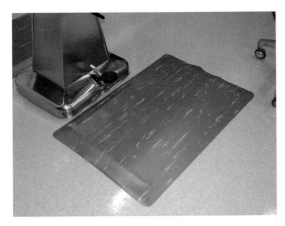

Figure 3.69 Stress mat in surgical suite.

field. Some surgeons, especially those performing a joint replacement procedure, will require all team members to wear double gloves for the entire procedure. Glove integrity has been show to fail as often as 51% of the time. Double gloving can reduce that failure rate to 7%. When double gloving, the second (outer) pair of gloves is generally a half size larger than the first pair of gloves.

Stress mats

Once properly gowned and gloved, the surgeon and/or assistant should proceed immediately to the surgery room, if they are not already there. Gaining interest in the surgery room is the use of stress mats for people standing still for long periods of time. Designed to help relieve stress and fatigue of legs and feet, stress mats can be positioned on the floor so the surgeon and assistant will stand on them during the procedure. When purchasing the mats, it must be noted that mats with a protective covering on all sides are desired. Mats that only have a vinyl top may have blood, solutions, or other fluids soak into the bottom of the mat and potentially harbor harmful bacteria. Mats are available commercially from office supply stores or medical supply distributors (Figure 3.69).

Instrumentation

Surgical instrumentation is an expensive and valuable asset of any hospital. Access to the correct, functioning instrument may determine the outcome of a surgical procedure. There may be one best instrument needed for a case and if it is not available something of lesser quality and unequalled function will have to be substituted. Efficient use of specialize veterinary surgical instrumentation requires those using it to understand proper application, handling, care, and troubleshooting. Often the surgeon relies on the veterinary technician for such knowledge.

Instrument manufacturing

The production of surgical instruments is a fine art and their proper functioning and longevity depend upon the end product. Surgical grade instruments are generally made from stainless steel and other metal alloys such as carbon and chromium. (Hempel, M. 1998) These metals are chosen due to their resistance to marring, pitting, scratching, and dulling. Floor grade instruments, while less expensive, are made from inferior quality metals and will rust within two to three steam sterilization cycles. Floor grade instruments are generally referred to as single-use items such as suture-removal scissors and disposable suture kits.

Finishes on surgical grade instruments can be a bright/mirror finish, a satin/dull finish or an ebony finish. The bright/mirror finish is a highly polished shine that reflects light. Due to the reflection, it may cause a glare and be annoying or interfering to some surgeons. The dull/satin finish is as the name implies. A nonreflective finish that doesn't glare is often preferred by many surgeons. The ebony finish is a black chromium finish for instruments used in laser surgery. The black finish deters the laser from bouncing off a shiny finish and damaging nearby tissues.

The instrument composition is either a martensitic stainless steel or an austenitic stainless steel. Martensitic stainless steel has higher carbon content and is used more often in cutting instruments for increased hardness and increased sharpness on the cutting edges. Austenitic stainless steel has higher chromium content and is usually used for hemostats and needle holders. Needle holders can also have tungsten carbide inserts in the tips of the instrument (Figure 3.70). The inserts are used to increase the durability of the needle holder. Although initially more expensive, the inserts can be replaced as they wear out. Needle holders that wear out and don't have the inserts, must simply have the entire instrument thrown away, therefore, in the long run being more expensive for the clinic. Tungsten carbide

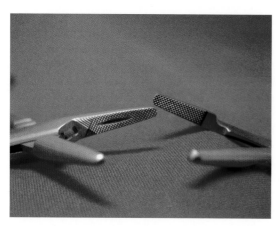

Figure 3.70 Tungsten carbide insert (right) in a needleholder jaw.

inserts can also be used on the cutting edges of scissors. Any instrument having a tungsten insert will have gold ring handles as the industry standard for quick identification of those instruments.

A five-step process is used in the creation of any surgical instrument. The first step is that of forging. Forging is the shaping or forming of the instrument through hammering and the use of heat. Second, the instrument undergoes a milling process. Milling is the cutting of a forged piece to create the final instrument. Tempering is the third step. By slowly heating the instrument in a salt bath and then immersing it in oil completes the tempering stage. Tempering may also be referenced as quenching. The fourth step is that of passivation. A chemical bath to remove any particles from the grinding process as well as strengthen the instrument is the passivation stage. This step also helps in rust prevention. The final step is polishing. Either a shiny or matte finish is the end result of the polishing step.

There are several basic components of surgical instruments that must be understood by all who use and care for the instruments. The working parts may vary slightly between ring-handled instruments and non-ring handled, but some similarities do exist. For ring-handled instruments the area of the instrument used on or near tissue is the jaw. The jaw may have horizontal, vertical, or cross-hatched serrations on the tip. The serrations can vary in depth, length, and closeness to one another, depending on the intended function of the instrument. Occasionally, a ring-handled instrument will have teeth on the tip, as with the Rochester-Kocher, but those

instruments are infrequently used. The shape of the jaw will be straight or curved depending on the intended use of the instrument. Non-ring handled instruments (thumb tissue forceps, handheld retractors) may have varying styles of tips or ends. Thumb tissue forceps that have teeth on either side of the jaw are named to identify the number of teeth on each side. For example, a thumb tissue forceps may be a 1 × 2, 2 × 3, or 3 × 4 style. Teeth can also be arranged in rows, which are recessed or projected from the tip (i.e., Adson Brown).

The next part of the ring-handled instrument is the box lock. The box lock is the hinged portion of the instrument. Excessive force on the jaw can cause misalignment of the box lock, resulting in rubbing of the metal when the instrument is opened or closed. Another trauma to the box lock is cracking of the metal, making the instrument useless. Even when the instrument is used for its intended purpose, this area of the instrument absorbs a lot of stress. Box locks must be carefully inspected following each use for any resulting damage. Some instruments, especially scissors, do not have a box lock, but rather a screw hinge. This area of the instrument continually is exposed to large amounts of stress, so evaluating the integrity of the hinge as well as the presence of any cracks is very important.

The longest part of the instrument is known as the shank. When an instrument is available in varying lengths, the shank is the variable. Some instruments (i.e., needle holders) may be available in size from 3″ to 12″ in length depending on the shank length. The next component is the ratchet. The ratchet is the locking portion of the ring handled instrument. Few non-ring-handled instruments have ratchets (i.e., Mathieu needle holders). Ratchets have interlocking teeth that lock the jaws of the instrument closed. The more the ratchet teeth is locked, the tighter the closure of the jaw. The interlocking teeth will wear down after time and the inability of the instrument to remain locked is a first indicator that the instrument is not functioning optimally. Finally, as previously mentioned, those ring-handled instruments that have tungsten carbide inserts in the tip will have gold ring handles for easy identification within the pack.

Non-ring-handled instruments will have no box lock or ratchet. The tips and shaft are still there, but the two separate sides are joined at the end. This type of instrument that has a tungsten carbide insert in the tip will have a gold identifier at the joined end.

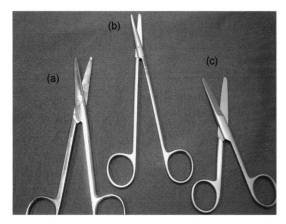

Figure 3.71 Scissors : (a) Mayo Dissecting, (b) Metzenbaum Dissecting, (c) Operating.

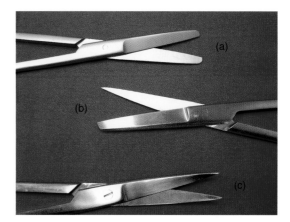

Figure 3.72   Operating scissors: (a) Blunt/Blunt, (b) Sharp/Blunt, (c) Sharp/Sharp.

General surgery instruments

Many resources are available for learning surgical instruments. While this text is intended to show the basic instruments, many company websites offer pictures of instruments. Some companies also offer flashcards for sale for easier studying.

There are many standard or general instruments that will be used in all surgeries. Thumb tissue forceps, scissors, needle holders, and hemostats do have some case specificity, but some styles will be used in every surgical procedure.

Scissors

Many types of scissors are available ranging from ophthalmic to orthopedic uses. As with all instruments, it is imperative that scissors be used only for their intended purpose (Figure 3.71).

Operating scissors

Operating scissors are a general-use scissors for cutting inanimate objects such as suture, paper drape material, sponges, and drains. The blade tips of the operating scissors can be blunt or sharp and the overall blade shape can be straight or curved. The style of scissors is usually included in the name of the scissors (i.e., sharp/blunt curved operating scissors). The length of the blade is about 1/2 of the overall length of the instrument (Figure 3.72).

Mayo dissecting scissors

Mayo dissecting scissors generally have a thicker, heavier blade than other scissors. The tips are rounded but are not classified as sharp or blunt. The blades may be curved or straight. Mayo dissecting scissors as the name implies, are used for cutting large muscle mass, dissecting non-delicate tissue, or cutting tougher tissue such as cartilage or tendons. The blade length is approximately 1/3 the length of the entire instrument.

Metzenbaum dissecting scissors

Metzenbaum dissecting scissors are designed for the dissection of delicate tissue. The blades are fine, delicate, and only about 1/4 of the length of the entire instruments. Delicate tissue and vessels are often dissected with this type of scissors, so keeping the blade tips fully functionally and extremely sharp is very important.

Miscellaneous scissors

Ophthalmic scissors often have a spring-loaded handle instead of ring handles to permit cutting with less overall instrument movement. Intraocular scissors such as Castroviejo scissors are extremely delicate and usually have sharp-tipped blades. Extraocular scissors such as Stevens Tenotomy scissors or Iris scissors have ring handles as motion with cutting isn't as much of an issue with extraocular procedures (Figure 3.73).

Bandage scissors

Bandage scissors are not considered a general surgery instrument, but deserve comment. Bandage scissors are designed to be used to cut off bandages. The longer blade has a blunt probe at the tip of the blade to assist with cutting through the bandage material (Figure 3.74).

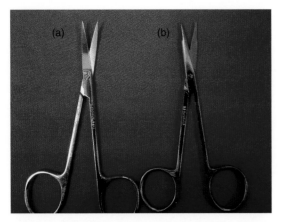

Figure 3.73 Ophthalmic scissors – Iris (a); Stevens Tenotomy (b).

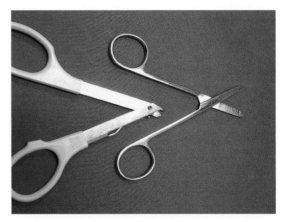

Figure 3.75 Suture removal scissors and staple remover.

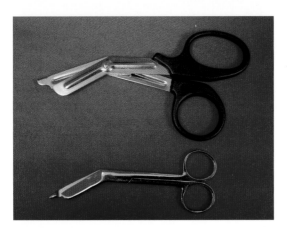

Figure 3.74 Bandage Scissors.

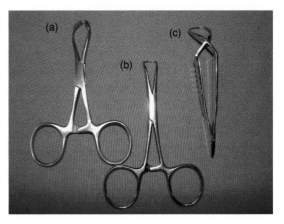

Figure 3.76 Towel Clamps: (a) Lorna Non-Penetrating, (b) Backhaus Penetrating, (c) Jones.

Orthopedic scissors

Orthopedic scissors such as wire cutting scissors and cartilage scissors have a very specific function. As the name implies, wire cutting scissors are used for cutting orthopedic wire. Wire can be very damaging to the cutting edge of a scissors, but this instrument is designed with short sturdy blades to be used exclusively with wire. Cartilage scissors have a serrated cutting edge to grip cartilaginous type tissue while cutting, instead of having smooth cutting edges, which would slide on the tissue and create a more uneven cut edge.

Suture removal scissors

Suture removal scissors have a short blunt tip blade on one side and the other blade has a hooked tip. By its name it is designed to aid in the removal of skin sutures. The hooked blade is slid underneath the suture circle

on one side of the knot and then the suture is cut. The staple remover is not a scissors, but a required piece of equipment for removing skin staples. The two-prong tip is placed under the staple and the handle is squeezed. The squeezing action closes the single-prong tip to bend the staple to allow removal (Figure 3.75).

Towel clamps

Towel clamps are instruments designed to hold drapes in place when draping a patient for surgery. Penetrating style towel clamps hold the sterile drapes to the patient by piercing the skin and holding the drape securely. Nonpenetrating styles are designed to hold sterile drapes to other sterile drapes (Figure 3.76).

Backhaus penetrating towel clamps

Backhaus towel clamps are the most common penetrating clamps used and are available in 3 1/2″ or 5″ sizes. When draping a patient this type of towel clamp is used to secure the drapes to the patient.

Roeder towel clamps

Roeder towel clamps are a penetrating style with balls about 1/2″ from the tip of the jaw. The balls are in place to avoid penetrating the skin too deeply. This type of towel clamp is often used in large animal surgery.

Jones towel clamp

The Jones towel clamp is a spring loaded, squeeze handle type of clamp. It is smaller in size and more light weight than other penetrating clamps. They are best suited for small drape placement in delicate tissue.

Lorna (Edna) non-penetrating towel clamp

Lorna towel clamps – sometimes called Edna towel clamps – are a non-penetrating style of towel clamp. They are used on a second layer of draping and attach the top layer of drape material to the underlying first layer of drapes. They are available in 3 1/2″ and 5″ sizes.

Scalpel handles and scalpel blades

Scalpel handles have the function of holding the scalpel blade to allow the surgeon to make a skin incision, or other types of incisions, in a safer manner (Figure 3.77). Number 3 scalpel handles are used with scalpel blades numbered 10–19. Number 4 scalpel blade handles are

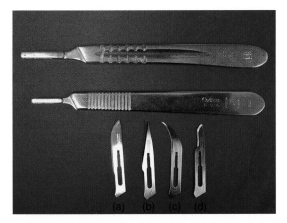

Figure 3.77 Scalpel Handles (number 3 & number 4); and Scalpel Blades (a–d) number 10,11,12,15.

used with scalpel blades numbered 20–29. Number 7 scalpel handles are a slender, longer style that fits blades 10–19. A Beaver handle is a short cylindrical handle designed to work with Beaver Blades. Scalpel blades are designed for very specific applications. Number 10 blades are the most common type of blade for skin incisions. With a full blade belly, it is great at creating a swift, clean incising of the skin. The number 11 blade has a very sharp point and a straight cutting edge. This blade is often used for stab incisions such as for an arthrotomy or abscess. A number 12 blade is in the shape of a hook with the cutting edge on the inside curve of the hook. A number 12 blade is often used for feline declaw dissection. The final blade most frequently seen in veterinary surgery is the number 15 blade. This blade has a cutting surface the same shape as a number 10 blade, but the cutting edge is only half as long as a number 10. The blade can be used for a feline declaw procedure or in other situations where a small delicate blade is needed. A number 20 blade on a number 4 blade handle is sometimes used in large animal surgery. The initial skin incision is made with the number 20 blade; then a number 10 blade is used for deeper tissue. The number 4 handle and 20 series blades have limited use and application in small animal surgery. The Beaver handle used with Beaver blades is most frequently used in ophthalmic or neurologic cases.

Hemostatic forceps

Hemostatic forceps are available in a variety of sizes and styles. As the name implies, the function of a hemostatic forceps is to occlude flow from a vessel or tissue mass. The tips of a hemostat can be straight or curved, but the style used is often the surgeon's preference. The serrations on the tips can be horizontal, vertical, or a combination of the two. When placing a hemostatic forceps on tissue, if a curved style, the curve should always be placed facing up. The smallest amount of tissue possible should be clamped to avoid excessive tissue damage (Figure 3.78).

Mosquito hemostatic forceps

The mosquito hemostat is the smallest forceps of the most commonly used instruments. It is available in both 3 1/2″ to 5″ sizes with the shank length being the only difference. The fine, closely positioned, transverse serration extends from the tip of the jaw to the box lock. Mosquito hemostats are used to occlude flow from

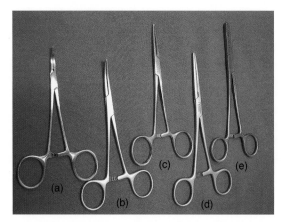

Figure 3.78 Hemostatic Forceps: (a) Mosquito, (b) Kelly, (c) Crile, (d) Rochester-Carmalt, (e) Ferguson Angiotribe.

small vessels. Both the Hartmann and Halsted variety are available with very little discernable difference between the two.

Kelly hemostatic forceps

Kelly hemostats are a larger clamp usually 5 ½″ in size. The horizontal serrations are wider than the mosquito serrations and most significantly extend from the tip of the jaw to only half way down. Kelly hemostats are used on larger vessels or tissue bundles that can be best accommodated by the larger jaw (Figure 3.79).

Crile hemostatic forceps

Crile hemostats are very similar to Kelly hemostats in size, design, and intended function. The primary difference is the transverse serrations on the Crile extend the entire length of the jaw, from the tip to the box lock. Like the Kelly hemostat, the Crile is used for larger vessels or tissue bundles.

Rochester-Carmalt hemostatic forceps

The Rochester-Carmalt is a large instrument with a jaw length approximately twice as long as the Kelly or Crile. The Rochester-Carmalt has longitudinal serrations the entire length of the jaw and horizontal cross serrations at the distal tip of the jaw. This larger instrument ranges in size from 7 ½″ to 9 ½″. The larger jaw enables this clamp to be used to occlude larger tissue bundles such as during an ovariohysterectomy.

Rochester-Oschner hemostatic forceps

A Rochester-Oschner forceps is a large clamp like the Carmalt. It has widely spaced horizontal serrations on the entire jaw and there is one large traumatic tooth at the tip of the jaw.

Rochester pean hemostatic forceps

The Rochester-Pean is a forceps that is exactly the same in appearance as the Oschner, without the toothed tip. Wide horizontal serrations on the entire jaw and a long instrument overall make it useful for large muscle or tissue masses.

Thumb tissue forceps

Thumb tissue forceps are tweezers like instruments that are used as an extension of the surgeon's fingers. Many different styles are available for many situations (Figure 3.80).

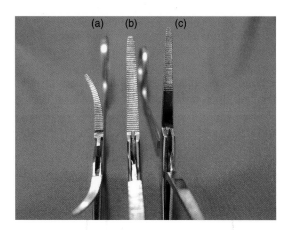

Figure 3.79 Hemostatic forcep tips: (a) Mosquito, (b) Crile, (c) Kelly.

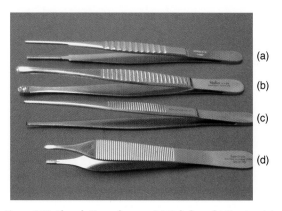

Figure 3.80 Thumb Tissue forceps: (a) Debakey, (b) Russian, (c) Rat Tooth, (d) Adson.

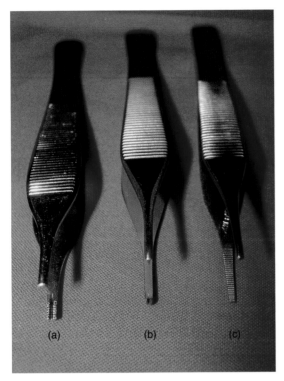

Figure 3.81 Adson tips: (a) Brown, (b) 1 × 2, (c) Dressing.

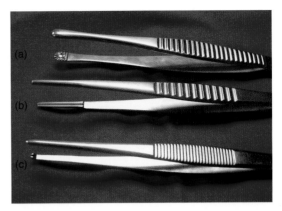

Figure 3.82 Thumb tissue forcep tips: (a) Debakey, (b) Russian, (c) 1 × 2.

Adson

Adson forceps can be recognized by a very distinctive shape. A broad shank that narrows to a small tip describes its classic appearance. The Adson Brown has two rows of teeth on either side of the tip. The Adson 1 × 2 has one tooth on one tip and two teeth on the opposite tip. The teeth interdigitate for secure grasping. There is also an Adson 2 × 3 style that has the same purpose. The Adson Dressing forceps has the standard Adson shank, but the tips are smooth with horizontal serrations. This forceps is atraumatic but was designed for the use with wound dressings (Figure 3.81).

Rat tooth

Rat toothed thumb tissue forceps have toothed tips, and they have straight shanks. The 1 × 2 and the 2 × 3 styles are most frequently used. They are very good general, all-purpose thumb tissue forceps.

Russian

Russian thumb tissue forceps are a broad-tipped, straight shank forceps. The tip is circular in shape with a

very traumatic toothed end. This forceps is usually used on inanimate objects or tissue being removed from the patient (Figure 3.82).

Debakey

The Debakey thumb tissue forceps was originally designed for vascular surgery. Its slender shank and fine tip make it easy to use. The tip has either a groove with two vertical rows of fine teeth or a ridge. This atraumatic instrument is used primarily for handling delicate tissue during general, thoracic, and neurologic surgical procedures.

Needle holders

Needle holders were designed to hold suture needles when closing wounds. They are also the instrument of choice when placing a scalpel blade on a scalpel blade handle. They are not intended to handle tissue of any sort. Sometimes after a needle holder is no longer useful for the intended purpose due to worn tips, it will be "converted" to use as a wire twister. If this happens, the instrument must be very clearly marked as a wire twister rather than a needle holder so as to avoid any accidental misuse.

Needle holders have very short tips that can either be stainless or have tungsten carbide inserts. As previously discussed, the tungsten carbide inserts can be replaced when they get worn. Regardless of the type of tip, the instrument will have serrations or cross hatching to better grip the suture needle. It also helps grip the scalpel blade as it is placed on the scalpel blade handle. Needle holders are available in lengths from 4″ to 12″.

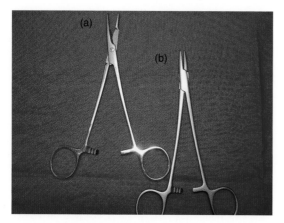

Figure 3.83 Needle holders: (a) Mayo Hegar, (b) Olsen-Hegar (note gold rings indicating tungsten carbide inserts).

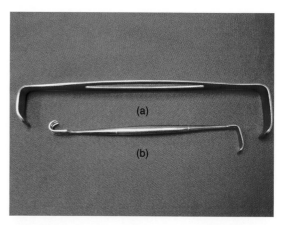

Figure 3.84 Hand held retractors: (a) U.S. Army, (b) Senn double ended

Mayo hegar

A Mayo Hegar needle holder is one of the most common styles of needle holder used by surgeons. The tips of this instrument connect directly to the box lock of the instrument. This instrument has ring handles at the end of the each shank, which allows the surgeon to use either the traditional ring finger/thumb grip or the palmed grip. This needle holder most often is used with larger, heavier needles due to the wider jaw of the instrument.

Olsen-Hegar

The Olsen-Hegar needle holder looks identical to the Mayo Hegar with only one major difference. With this instrument, scissor blades are found between the tips and the box lock. This feature allows the surgeon to cut the suture without having to use an additional instrument. A word of caution however to the less-experienced surgeon: careful placement of the needle in the tips of the instrument must be observed. Poor placement can result in the inadvertent cutting of the suture before it should be cut (Figure 3.83).

Crile-Wood

The Crile-Wood needle holder also looks very similar to the Mayo Hegar. The defining characteristic of this instrument is the much narrower, more delicate jaw. This instrument may be chosen by the surgeon when working in a smaller more confining surgical field or when using smaller needles.

Derf

The Derf needle holder is a cross between the Mayo Hegar and the Crile Wood. The jaw shape is smaller than a Mayo Hegar but is larger than a Crile Wood. Derf needle holders are limited to shorter lengths (4″–5″) and are often chosen for smaller mammal or exotic patients or extraocular procedures.

Mathieu

The Mathieu needle holder is very different from all other needle holders described thus far. The tips and jaw are most similar to the Mayo Hegar, but at the end of the shanks there are curved corners that form a ratchet lock mechanism. The absence of rings makes this instrument easiest to use by surgeons who prefer the palmed grip.

Hand-held retractors

This type of retractor requires an assistant to physically use this instrument to retract tissue for the surgeon. Unless there is another sterile person scrubbed in for the procedure, these instruments have limited applicability. The advantage to the use of hand-held retractors is that the pressure exerted on the tissue can be monitored and regulated by the person holding the instrument (Figure 3.84).

Senn

The Senn double-ended, hand-held retractor has one end with a blade and the other end has a rake. The rake end has three separate prongs that can have either blunt or sharp tips (Figure 3.85). The tissue being retracted will

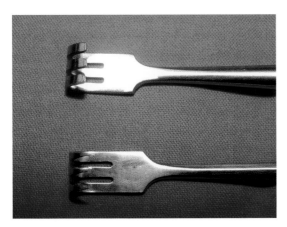

Figure 3.85 Senn double ended retractor ends: sharp and blunt.

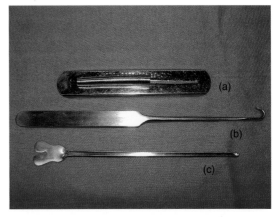

Figure 3.86 (a) Needle rack , (b) Snook Spay Hook, (c) Groove Director.

determine whether a sharp or blunt style is used. The narrow blunt blade is only about 1″ in length, so use is limited to small muscle masses or superficial tissues. The two ends of the Senn retractor point in opposite direction from one another.

Army–Navy

The Army–Navy retractor (sometimes called the U.S. Army retractor) has blunt, wide blades on either end. Both blades point in the same direction. One blade is about 2″ in length while the other blade is about 1″ in length. The wider, sturdier blade allows for deeper/larger tissue retraction.

Miscellaneous instruments

Snook spay hook

This instrument has a long (~8″) handle with a blunt hook at the end. Some surgeons use this instrument to exteriorize the uterine horns when performing an ovariohysterectomy on either a canine or feline patient.

Dowling spay retractor

The Dowling retractor was designed for the veterinary surgeon that must often work alone. The instrument allows better visualization and stabilization by isolating the uterine horn.

Groove director

The Groove director is a useful instrument when making an abdominal incision. It is approximately 5″ in length

with a deep groove on one side. After the surgeon makes the initial puncture on the linea alba, the grooved director is slipped under the created incision with the grooved side facing up. Keeping the instrument parallel to the linea, this instrument provides a "channel" for the surgeon to follow with the scalpel blade so as to avoid deviating from the linea as well as protecting the abdominal viscera from accidental incising (Figure 3.86).

Alligator forceps

This instrument has ring handles, a long delicate shank and a jaw that opens just at the very end of the shank. It is designed for narrow, deep cavities such as the ear canal or nasal passages. The tips have horizontal serrations for more secure grasping of tissue (Figure 3.87).

Allis tissue forceps

The Allis tissue forceps is a very traumatic, ring-handled instrument. At the end of the shanks, the tips have interdigitating rows of 3 × 4 or 4 × 5 teeth. The large traumatic teeth are intended to grasp tissue that is very durable (i.e., linea alba, tendons, etc.) or tissue that is being removed from the patient. This instrument is useful for retracting tissue that is to be removed (i.e., tumor) (Figure 3.88).

Needle rack

The needle rack is a spring mounted on a flat platform. This instrument is intended to hold free suture needles within the pack so they don't get misplaced. Needles are merely pushed down between the coils of the spring to be held securely.

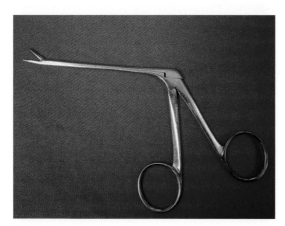

Figure 3.87 Alligator Forcep.

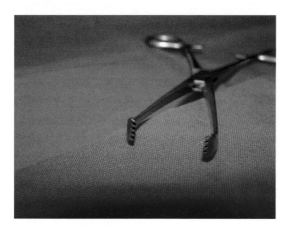

Figure 3.88 Allis Tissue Forcep.

Abdominal intestinal forceps

Babcock intestinal forcep

The Babcock is a noncrushing forceps with a tip that has horizontal serrations. The appearance resembles an allis tissue forceps, but the function is much less traumatic.

Doyen intestinal forceps

The Doyen is a large, long forceps with longitudinal serrations in the jaw. The jaw length is approximately 1/2 the length of the entire instrument. It is a noncrushing instrument for use with the intestines.

Thoracic instruments

Retractors
Finochetto

Probably the most frequently used self-retaining retractor for thoracic surgery is the Finiochetto retractor (Figure 3.89). Available in two different sizes, it can be used with adult or pediatric patients. The smooth unserrated blades can efficiently retract ribs and delicate pleural tissue without trauma. Blades may have a window to decrease pressure. This retractor should be used with moistened laparotomy pads positioned between the blades and the tissue to avoid unnecessary pressure necrosis.

Malleable

Malleable retractors (also known as ribbon retractors) are sometimes requested by surgeons to retract delicate lung tissue. A variety of widths from 1″ to 3″ allow the most efficient size to be chosen. As the name indicates, this type of retractor can be bent into the desired shape to achieve the desired effect. Solid blades allow for even pressure distribution. Assistants must take care to avoid excessive pressure when using this retractor.

Thoracic scissors
Potts Smith scissors

Thoracic scissors such as the Potts-Smith scissors have very short, sharp-tipped blade. The blades are angled approximately 45° from the shank. This construction allows for easy use in a deep thoracic cavity where minimal movement is desired.

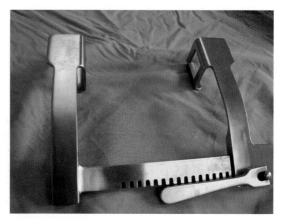

Figure 3.89 Finiochetto Retractor.

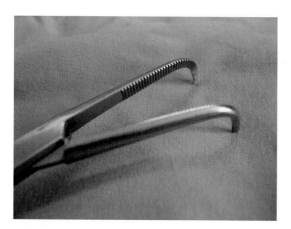

Figure 3.90 Right Angle Mixter forcep.

Vascular clamps

Mixter

Vascular clamps have a unique design when designed specifically for use in cardiovascular procedures. One such clamp is the Mixter forceps. With serrations in a horizontal fashion, extending the length of the jaw, the tip of this forceps can form either a 90° or a 45° angle (Figure 3.90). This unique design facilitates vessel ligation with minimal disruption or manipulation of the vessel. When working with an especially friable or stressed vessel, this instrument can be invaluable.

Satinsky/Cooley

Other clamps often found in thoracic instrument packs are the Satinsky and/or the Cooley clamp. These specialized vascular clamps are used for clamping cardiac vessels. Due to their design, they are especially helpful in situations where traditional hemostatic forceps are not an option. The Satinsky clamps has a tip that can be straight, angled, curved, or tangential. A Cooley clamp has a semi-circular jaw. Satinsky clamps have a jaw with horizontal serrations the length of the tip, and a concave channel in the middle of the jaw (Figure 3.91). Vascular clamps are used to provide temporary occlusion of pulmonary and cardiovascular structures such as vessels or bronchi.

Abdominal instrumentation

Retractors

Balfour retractor

The self-retaining retractor of choice for abdomens is the Balfour retractor (Figure 3.92). This instrument has deep cut out blades, which allow spreading of the abdominal wall to provide adequate visualization. This retractor also has a third blade option that can be placed on the cranial end of the incision to provide the surgeon better visualization. Balfour retractors are also available in a small version for use with pediatric or smaller patients. The retraction is maintained by the use of a tension mechanism as opposed to a box lock or hand crank (as seen with the Finiochetto retractor).

Orthopedic instruments

Orthopedic surgeries require the most intricate and mechanical instrumentation. Advanced training on the use and care of this instrumentation is highly advised due to its complexity and value.

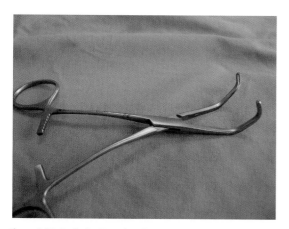

Figure 3.91 Satinsky Vascular clamp.

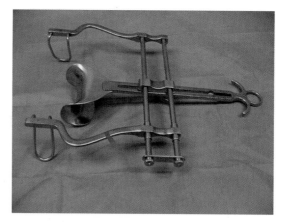

Figure 3.92 Balfour retractor.

Retractors

Retractors used in orthopedic surgery can be either self-retaining or hand-held in style. Often the surgeon is working alone, so the self-retaining styles are popular.

Gelpi self-retaining

Gelpi retractors are self-retaining and have two arms that end with sharp points. They are available in small or large sizes and deep or shallow angles. The smaller retractors are seen used during joint surgeries or fracture repairs of small (~ < 15 kg) patients. The larger shallow style is commonly used for canine stifle surgery, fracture repairs, femoral procedures, humeral procedures, and so on. The large deep-angled retractors are generally reserved for large breed hip surgeries or procedures where retraction of large deep muscles is required. Deep Gelpi retractors can also be used during neurologic/spinal surgeries, especially cervical cases.

Weitlaner self-retaining

Another type of self-retaining retractor is the Weitlaner. The Weitlaner also has two arms, but at the end of the arms are multi-pronged blades. The pronged blades can be either a sharp or blunt tip style. This retractor can be used in almost all of the same situations as a Gelpi retractor; however, larger surgical incisions are better suited for the Weitlaner. Also, if nerves or large blood vessels are present in the dissected area, a blunt Weitlaner is a better choice as any sharp retractor may damage the nerve or vessel (Figure 3.93).

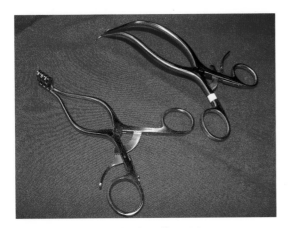

Figure 3.93 Weitlaner and Gelpi Self-Retaining retractors.

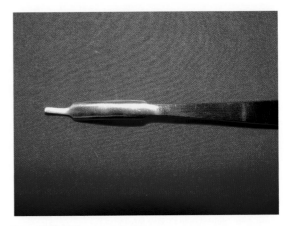

Figure 3.94 Hohmann retractor.

Meyerding

Other hand-held retractors previously discussed may be a better choice in certain orthopedic procedures. If the procedure involves the large muscle masses in the caudal pelvic area, Meyerding retractors may be used. The Meyerding is a retractor with a wide blade that is positioned 90° to the handle. The end of the blade has teeth from side to side to better grip the muscle. Pressure must be monitored to avoid damage to the muscles and nerves. The Langenbeck retractor has the same style as the Meyerding with the exception of the teeth on the blade. The Langenbeck had a smooth blade tip and therefore, may prove more challenging to retract large muscle masses without the tissue slipping.

Hohmann

Hohmann retractors are specific orthopedic hand-held retractors that are not used in any other situation. The Hohmann has a curved tip, with a broad plate just after the tip. The handle narrows a little after the plate to better fit into the hand of the person using it. The plates can be of various widths, from 1/2″ to 2″(Figure 3.94).

Ronguers

There are multiple styles of ronguers that the surgeon may use during an orthopedic surgery, depending on the procedure being done. The ronguer is an instrument that has squeeze handles with cupped tips having cutting edges. A single-action ronguer allows the tips to close as the handles are squeezed (Figure 3.95). Generally with a finer tip than other types of ronguers,

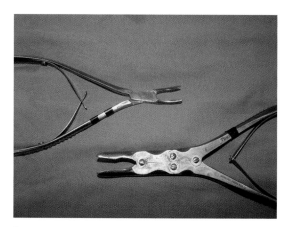

Figure 3.95 Single- and double-action ronguers.

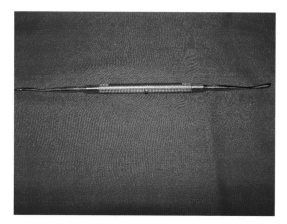

Figure 3.96 Freer periosteal elevator.

the single action can be used for crushing bone pieces for autogenous bone graft implantation. It can also be used for removing small projections of hyperplastic bone. The double-action ronguer had a joint that bends out as the tips come together when the handles are squeezed. This ronguer has a larger cupped tip and is more appropriate for removing larger pieces of bone. In addition to the standard construction, there is also a duck-billed style that is a double-action ronguer with a body style that resembles the alligator forceps.

Periosteal elevators

Periosteal elevators are designed to elevate the periosteum from the bone. They are often used during internal fixation of fractures and other orthopedic surgeries. The look of a periosteal elevator can have the tip being rounded or squared, narrow, or wide (Figure 3.96). Some of the more commonly used elevators are the Freer, ASIF®, and Adson (Figure 3.97). The edge of the tip is sharp in order to easily remove the periosteum.

Osteotomes

Osteotomes are long-handled instruments used for cutting bone. They can be 1/2″–2″ wide and have a beveled side on either side of the tip. Osteotomes can be used to shave off smaller pieces of bone or remove larger pieces (i.e., femoral head during a femoral head and neck osteotomy). They can also be used to remove bone for cortical bone autographs or for creating access for

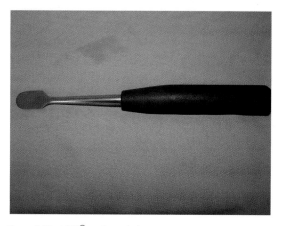

Figure 3.97 ASIF® periosteal elevator.

cancellous bone autograph collection. Osteotomes are non-electric and must be used with some type of mallet. Some osteotome handles are flat, whereas others are octagonal in shape to better fit into the hand of the user.

Chisels

Chisels are very similar looking to osteotomes with the exception of having only one beveled side. Chisels are generally used in similar situations as osteotomes.

Mallet

A Mallet is an orthopedic hammer used to advance osteotomes and/or chisels. Most are two headed having either metal or replaceable plastic heads.

Bone holding forceps

Bone holding forceps are instruments used to internally stabilize bone fragments until permanent stabilization of the fracture is achieved. Bone holders can have ratchet locks or speedlocks to secure the instrument to the bone. The tips may be pointed or blunt and have teeth or serrations. Often the bone holder used is determined by the type of fracture, the location of the fracture, and the surgeon's preference. Many of the bone holders are available in both small and large sizes. Some types of bone holders commonly used are Kern, blunt reduction, sharp speedlock, and Verbrugge (Figure 3.98).

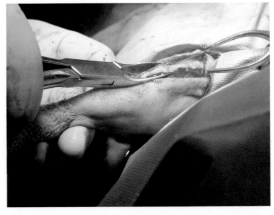

Figure 3.99 Bone cutter being used for tibial crest osteotomy.

Bone cutters

Bone cutters are double-action, squeeze handle designed instruments with cutting edges on the inside of the blades on the tip. Bone cutters are used with the same hand motion as ronguers but have flat tips as opposed to the cupped tips of ronguers (Figure 3.99). Removal of small pieces of bone is the most common use.

Jacob's chuck

A Jacob's chuck is a hand held "drill" that is used for simple IM pin placement or K-Wire placement (Figure 3.100).

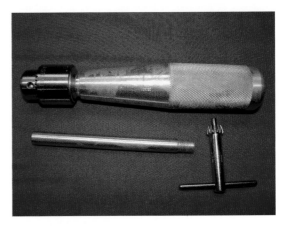

Figure 3.100 Jacob's chuck.

Drills

Many styles of drills are available for use by the orthopedic surgeon. Some are electric, some are pneumatic, and others are battery operated. Electric drills obviously must be sterilized with ethylene oxide (EtO) and therefore have limited feasibility in practice. Pneumatic drills are run by connecting a hose to a nitrogen tank and can be steam sterilized. Battery-operated drills can be steam sterilized, but the battery is generally inserted post-sterilization and covered by a sterile wrap once introduced into the sterile field. If the hose of the drill cannot be sterilized, a sterile clear plastic sleeve can be placed over the hose to allow manipulation by the surgeon (Figure 3.101). Regardless of the brand of drill,

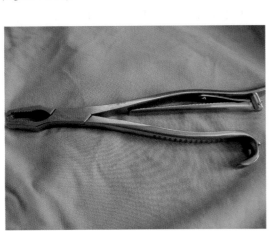

Figure 3.98 Large Kerns bone holding forcep.

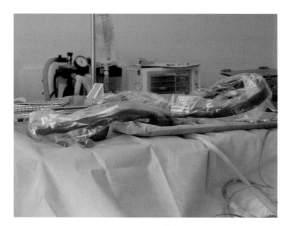

Figure 3.101 Protective sleeve over drill hose.

almost all are equipped with multiple accessories. Drill bit adapters, either quick connect or chuck style drill bit attachments and mini wire drivers are common extras. Some also include a saggital saw adapter (Figure 3.102). Some of the more common drills are the Synthes® drill, 3 m Mini® or Maxi® driver, Stryker®, and Kirschner®. Power equipment is necessary for almost every orthopedic case, whether it is used to place bone screws, perform osteotomies, or secure intramedullary (IM) pins.

Internal fixation implants

There are many types of internal implants available for use by veterinary surgeons. Some implants are used for fracture stabilization and repair, some are for stabilizing bones post lengthening or corrective osteotomy for deformity repair. Bone plates, bone screws, interlocking nails, IM pins, and orthopedic wire are the most common implants. Bone plates, screws, and interlocking nails will be shown in Chapter 5.

Intramedullary pins

IM pins are implants often used for repair of diaphyseal fractures in many bones except the radius. Surgeons may choose an IM pin due to the advantage of the ability of the implant to resist bending loads. Conversely, they have the disadvantage of no resistance to rotational loads and do not have an interlocking fixation with the bone. Pins are available in many sizes from $1/16''$ to $1/4''$ width. They are made of 316L stainless steel and are round in appearance. The ends can both be pointed (double armed) or have one end blunt (single armed). The most common style of points is either a trocar point with three cutting edges for easy movement through cancellous bone. The other style of point is the chisel point, which is a double-cutting edge better for use with cortical bone. The ends of the pin may be smooth or threaded. The use of threaded pins was originally to increase the holding power of the pin in the cancellous bone; however, that theory is controversial. Kirschner wires are small ($0.035''$–$0.062''$) pins that are smooth and generally have a trocar point. Too small to stabilize a fracture when used alone, they are often used to cross wire fractures to supplement stabilization by another means (Figure 3.103).

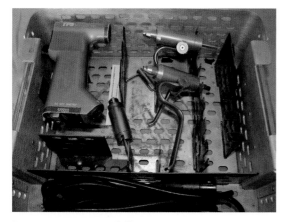

Figure 3.102 Pnuematic drill.

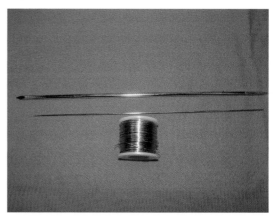

Figure 3.103 Intramedullary (IM) pin, K-wire, orthopedic wire.

Orthopedic wire

Orthopedic wire used in the repair of fractures can be used alone or in addition to other internal implants. Wire is available on spools that can be autoclaved or in pre-cut lengths with a preformed loop on one end. Orthopedic wire is available in sizes from 18 ga to 32 ga and is made of a pliable form of 316L stainless steel material. Cerclage wire is the term used for wire placed around the entire circumference of the bone, while hemi-cerclage is the term for wire passed through holes drilled in the bone. Spiral fractures or reconstructed oblique fractures are the most common procedures where wire is used. However, mandibular symphyseal fractures of the feline are often repaired with wire alone.

Interlocking nails

Interlocking nails are implants placed in the medullary canal of a fractured bone. This implant has a design that allows resistance to all forces that may be placed on a fracture. It is primarily indicated for use in femoral, humeral, and tibial mid-diaphyseal fracture stabilization. The implant is design with screw holes at either end of the nail to allow screw placement for additional support. A variety of sizes, 4.0, 4.7, 6.0, 8.0, and 10.0 mm are available to permit use in many animals. There are also multiple lengths for each diameter size. Each size pin has a specific size screw that accompanies that pin. The 4.0 and 4.7 pin use 2.0 mm screws. The 6.0 mm pin uses a 2.7 or 3.5 mm screw. The 8.0 mm pin uses a 3.5 or 4.5 mm screw, while the 10 mm pin uses only the 4.5 mm screw. In addition to the implant itself and the screws, there are multiple pieces of equipment needed for proper placement of the nail. The drill guide jig is used to align the drill bit with holes in the nail. The extension piece is used to attach the drill guide jig to the nail. Drill guides are used to protect the surrounding tissue from the rotation of the drill bit. The drill bits are used to drill a hole in the bone for placement of the bone screw and the reamer is used to prepare the medullary canal for the placement of the nail.

Bone plates

A wide variety of bone plates are available for use in veterinary surgery. The plates are very specific to the needs of the fracture or surgical case. Although the ultimate decision for the size and type of plate to be used in a procedure is determined by the surgeon, it is critical that technicians understand the various types of plates and all the accompanying equipment. Sizing of bone plates includes two different characteristics of the plate. First of all the width of the plate is expressed in millimeters or the size of the screw that will be used with that plate. Plates are available in the following sizes: 2.0, 2.7, 3.5, 3.5 broad, 4.5, and 4.5 broad. The number on the plate refers to the size screw that will be used with the plate. In the case of the "broad" labeled plates, that merely means that the screw size is the plate size; however, it is a "wider" version of the original plate and hence the addition to the name of the term "broad". Also involved in the sizing of the plate is the length of the plates. The length of the plate is determined by the number of holes in the plate: a 7 hole plate has 7 screw holes, a 10 hole plate has 10 holes, and so on. Therefore, the complete name of a bone plate would be a 9 hole 3.5 plate meaning there are 9 holes, each sized to accept a 3.5 mm screw, in the plate.

Plates may also have the type of screw hole configuration included in the name. Screw holes can be DCP, which stands for dynamic compression plate (DCP); LC-DCP which means limited-contact dynamic compression plate or LCP, which means locking compression plate. Depending on the type of screw hole, a different function of the plate will occur. In the DCP hole, the principle is that an oblong hole with beveled edges to accept a conical head-shaped screw will allow compression on the fracture site. In the LC-DCP hole, the same principle of the DCP hole is true, but the plate construction has a cut out area of the plate on the underside, therefore allowing less contact with the bone. The LCP hole also has threads in addition to the beveled hole edges. The threads allow for use of either a traditional bone screw or a locking head screw.

Other types of plates that are available are reconstructive plates, Veterinary cuttable plates (VCP), acetabular plates, distal tibial fracture plates (also known as T plates), step plates and TPLO plates. The reconstructive plates have areas of the plate cut out along the edge between the holes to allow for three-dimensional bending and manipulation to fit the bone. Not only can they be bent up or down, but they can also be bent sideways. The cuttable plates are available in lengths up to 50 holes and can be custom designed in length for each case. VCP are available in two sizes – 1.5/2.0 and 2.0/2.7 mm. Cuttable plates are the only plates used in a stacking fashion when bridging a comminuted fracture to provide additional stability. Acetabular plates are specifically designed to match the varied configuration of the acetabular bone. Distal tibial fracture plates or "T" plates are also specific to use in canine distal tibial fracture repair, although originally they were designed for carpal arthrodesis. Step plates are used when a TPO/DPO (Triple Pelvic Osteotomy/Double Pelvic Osteotomy) is performed. TPLO plates are designed for use during the TPLO procedure to stabilize the canine stifle in which the cranial cruciate ligament has ruptured.

The function of the plate can be determined by appearance, as already discussed, or by application. Depending on how the plate is applied to the bone, it may be a compression plate, a neutralizing plate, or a buttress plate. Any plate can serve any function, depending on how it is applied by the surgeon.

Bone screws

There are two types of bone screws. One is a cortical bone screw and the other is a cancellous bone screw. The name indicates the placement of the threads of the screw, either in cortical bone or cancellous bone. Cortical bone screws are fully threaded, meaning the threads of the screw are present the entire length of the screw. The pitch, or the number of threads per inch, is greater that the cancellous screw, thereby allowing a greater number of threads to contact the cortical bone. Cancellous bone screws have a greater thread height than the cortical screw. The thread height is determined by the difference between core diameter and the outer diameter of the screw. A larger thread height means the threads are allowed to go deeper into the cancellous bone to hold the screw stable. Cancellous screws can be fully threaded or partially threaded, which means there are threads on only about 1/3 of the length of the screw at the most distal end. As with plates, screws are generally made of 316L stainless steel or titanium. Bone screws can be either self-tapping or not. The self-tapping style has threads that tap the bone on its own and has a flute (a channel along the threads) on the screw to accept bone debris. A non-self tapping screw obviously is not capable of that action and requires the surgeon to use a hand tap. Screws can be used by themselves, along with pins or orthopedic wire or with a plate. Regardless of the function of the screw, the placement requires basically the same equipment. First of all, the surgeon will use a drill bit and drill guide to create the screw hole. The size of drill bit used is determined by the screw size

being implanted. The inner core of the screw is the determining factor of drill bit sized (i.e., a 3.5 mm screw has a 2.5 inner core diameter so a 2.5 mm drill bit is used). Along with the drill bit, a drill guide is used to protect the drill bit from becoming wrapped up in the surrounding tissue. The drill guides may have either a neutral or a load end. Depending on the intended function of the screw, the surgeon will choose the appropriate end to use. For a cortical screw being used with a plate or by itself or for a cancellous screw being alone, the drill bit is passed through one cortice and then the other. There is a bit of a "give" in the resistance of the drill when the far cortice has been passed through. The drill bit is removed and the depth gauge is then used to determine the length of the screw needed. The hook end of the depth gauge is hooked on the far cortice and the sliding sleeve of the depth gauge is slid down until contact with the bone is achieved. The length in millimeters is then read from the scale on the instrument. After determining the length, the surgeon will use a tap sleeve and tap to prepare the hole for the screw. The size of the tap used is determined by the outer diameter of the screw being implanted (i.e., a 3.5 mm screw had a 3.5 mm outer diameter so a 3.5 mm tap is used). A tap handle is attached to the tap quick coupling end and the surgeon then taps the drilled hole. The tap makes small cuts in the bone to make it easier for the screw to grab onto the bone. A tap sleeve is used to keep the tap in alignment with the drilled hole as well as protect the surrounding tissue from becoming wound up in the tap (self-tapping screws do not need this step performed). Once the tap is removed, the screw hole can be flushed with sterile saline to remove bone debris and then the screw is placed. The screw is inserted by using a screwdriver and is tightened to a "finger tip" tightness to avoid stripping the screw hole.

Lag screws are placed using the same equipment; however, multiple drill bit sizes will be needed by the surgeon to place the screw properly to act as a lag screw is intended (to compress a fracture line between two fragments). Another additional piece of equipment needed for lag screws is a countersink. The countersink will be used after the drill bit but before the depth gauge. The countersink creates a bevel at the screw hole opening to allow the screw to sit deeper in the screw hole.

Although technicians are not routinely responsible for placing screws, it is quite frequent that they will be involved in the drilling of the holes or stabilization of the bone while the surgeon drills the hole. Technicians assisting in orthopedic surgery must be very comfortable with the equipment and the order in which the instruments will be used to place the screw to be of the most use to the surgeon.

Other implants and equipment that is needed for specific orthopedic procedures (i.e., TPLO, TTA, Joint arthroplasty) will be discussed in Chapter 5.

Wire twisters

Wire twisters are instruments used to twist the orthopedic wire to secure its placement. Wire twisters can be as simple as an old needle holder or pliers, or they may be specifically designed wire twisters. Generally, when looped cerclage wires are employed, a specifically designed wire twister is used to attain appropriate tightness and placement. If using an old needle holder, it is imperative that the instrument be identified as a wire twister to avoid placement in a general surgery pack. The tips of the needle holder get quite damaged when used as a wire twister and could prove to be a very frustrating situation if it was used as a true needle holder.

Pin/bolt cutters

Pin cutters are handled instruments designed for cutting small intramedullarry pins or K-wires (Figure 3.104). Generally these are squeeze handle designed instruments that require the sharpness on the tips of the instrument be maintained. A fair amount of hand strength is required for operation of a pin cutter, so dull cutting edges will further impede proper use. Pin cutters are designed to cut IM pins, which are

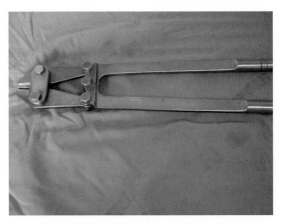

Figure 3.105 Bolt cutter.

fairly small in diameter. A bolt cutter, sterilized by EtO methods so it does not rust, will be needed for larger pins (Figure 3.105).

Arthroscopic instrumentation

Arthroscopy in small animal surgery is a very common procedure. It often will be done in an attempt to forego the need for a more invasive procedure. For multiple advantages including faster patient recovery time, less patient discomfort, better visualization and assessment of the joint, and earlier diagnosis of joint disorders, the arthroscopic procedure is being performed more frequently. The care of this delicate and expensive instrumentation is a critical skill that the veterinary surgical technician must possess.

The arthroscope itself can be varied depending on the length, angle, and diameter. Arthroscopes are available in both short and long lengths. Most surgeons will choose the short length. The angles of arthroscopes available are 0°, 30°, and 70°. (Sessum, J.D. 2003) Most often a scope with an angled tip will be used for better visualization of the joint. Most frequently that will be the 30° scope. The diameters used most frequently in small animal veterinary arthroscopy are 1.9, 2.3, and 2.7 mm. The size used for the procedure will ultimately depend on the size of the patient and the size of the joint. In addition to the scope, usually a camera, which attaches to the scope is also utilized. Cameras can have one chip or multiple chips, with the major difference being found in the resolution of the picture. One end of the camera

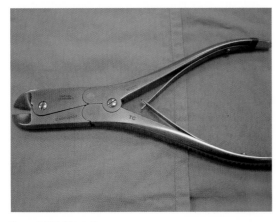

Figure 3.104 Pin cutter.

attaches to the scope eyepiece on the sterile field and the other end attaches to a control box, which transmits the image to a monitor for all in the room to see. The control box will allow modification of focus, white balance, and so on. Another accessory for the arthroscope that is a necessity is the light source. A fiber optic cable attaches the light source to the scope and provides light via either a tungsten-halogen bulb or a Xenon bulb. A brighter light is provided by the Xenon bulb, but it is also the more expensive bulb. Cannulas and obturators are also needed for placement and use of the arthroscope. Obturators are used to create a path into the joint to allow placement of the cannula. Various hand instruments such as probes, graspers, and curettes can also be inserted through the cannulas for use within the joint. Some procedures will require the use of a motorized shaver in the joint. Most shavers have the option of three modes of operation: oscillating, forward/reverse, and variable speed. A control box for the shaver allows selection of the desired mode. There are three types of tips available for use with a motorized shaver: a full radius blade, an aggressive cutter blade, or a bur. The blades are generally used for soft-tissue removal with the shaver in the oscillating mode. The bur is used most frequently for bone removal with the shaver in the forward/reverse mode. Finally, a fluid source is required to allow free flow of fluid into the joint. The fluid infusion provides lubrication, flush, and will improve visualization. A gravity-assisted system may be used (with the assistance of a fluid compression bag) but does have its disadvantages. Foremost is the inability to provide high pressure flushing when needed. Additionally, the lack of constant fluid pressures and additionally attention by surgical staff, make this system less desirable. More often, a fluid pump is used to alleviate the aforementioned issues. A fluid pump maintains a constant pressure of delivery but does allow for variation of pressure when necessary. The initial cost of the unit, the specific tubing required, and the learning curve for mastering the set of the system are disadvantages worth considering.

Laparoscopic instruments

Much like the arthroscopic instruments, the laparoscopic instruments are very expensive and require extreme care when being handled. Although the visualization tool is called a telescope, much of the other equipment and instrumentation is very similar to arthroscopic equipment. Either a 0° or a 30° rigid telescope is used; however, preference is for the 30° scope as it allows more evaluation of the cavity being scoped with less manipulation (Radlinsky, M. 2007). A variety of lengths and sizes are available with patient size being the determining factor for use. In small dogs and cats a 2.7 mm, 18 cm scope is often recommended. With larger dogs a 5.0 mm telescope is best used. As with the arthroscopic equipment, laparoscopes require a light source that attaches to the scope via a fiber optic cable and then the cable is connected to a light source. Again either a halogen or a Xenon bulb is available commercially. A camera and monitor are a necessity in order for all members of the surgical team to view the procedure. Trocars and cannulae are also needed for placement of the scope and accompanying instruments. The trocar can be either sharp or blunt and is used to create path for placement of the cannula. Sometimes the surgeon may make a small incision to facilitate the placement of the trocar. The instruments and scope are then inserted into the cavity through the cannula to decrease irritation to soft tissue. Soft or flexible cannula are recommended for thoracic endoscopy as they may decrease postoperative pain due to less rib nerve pressure associated with rigid cannulas. For abdominal laparoscopy, an insufflator is also required. CO_2 insufflation, via a Veress (insufflation) needle is necessary to inflate the abdomen to allow visualization for the surgeon as well as provide distension of the abdominal wall to minimize tissue trauma. (Monnet, E., 2011) A valved cannula should be used with the insufflator to control the infusion of the CO_2. An insufflator is not needed with thoracic endoscopy or the ribs provide adequate distension of the thoracic cavity without the need for any additional distension. Additional instruments such as biopsy forceps or punches, grasping forceps or scissors are similar for both abdominal as well as thoracic endoscopy. Many of the instruments used are capable of being connected to an electrocautery or radiosurgical unit. This type of instrumentation is advantageous as it minimizes the passage of different instruments in and out of the patient as well as providing hemostasis in the surgical field.

Neurologic instrumentation

Equipment needed for neurologic procedures is quite varied. An air-powered drill is needed to make the approach. Other air powered drill styles are used in orthopedic surgery. Once the roof of the spinal cord has been removed or the craniotomy completed, the delicate instruments for used in manipulating the spinal cord or brain are often the same instruments that may be used on an ophthalmic procedure.

Large, double-action rongeurs, single-action rongeurs, and periosteal elevators may be used to remove large quantities of bone prior to the use of the pneumatic drill. Kerrison ronguers may be used to assist with bone removal as well.

The pneumatic drill is a cylindrical unit that is held like a pencil when being used. The trigger for the control of power is conveniently located on the side of the main piece (Figure 3.106). The drill bits available are either short or long in design and both require the use of a burr guard before being inserted into the drill. Tips can be broad in shape, often called a pineapple burr, or very fine and small. The broader tips are used for larger gross bone removal, whereas the finer tips are reserved for delicate bone removal when close to the spinal cord or brain. Instruments used for neurologic procedures are micro instruments such as an iris spatula, Stevens tenotomy scissors, Iris scissors, Bishop-Harmon thumb tissue forceps, and Colibri thumb tissue forceps. Nerve retractors, ear curettes, and dural hooks may also be needed.

Retractors used in neurologic cases can be Gelpi self-retaining retractors or Weitlaner self-retaining

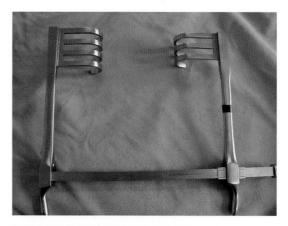

Figure 3.107 Frasier laminectomy retractor.

retractors. Another type of self-retaining retractor limited to spinal surgery is a Frasier retractor (Figure 3.107). Similar in design to a Balfour retractor, the blades are similar to a Weitlaner with multiple blunt prongs fairly long and circular in shape.

Ophthalmic magnifying head loops are also beneficial to the surgeon during neurologic surgery. Simple minimal magnification loops are easily available, but lighted, more powerful eye loops may be the surgeon's choice.

Instrument cleaning and care

Proper maintenance of surgical instrumentation falls exclusively to the veterinary surgical technician. The value of the surgical instrument and implant inventory is a significant investment by the practice and requires the utmost care and attention. Knowledge of acceptable cleaning methods, inspection procedures, and required preventative maintenance will significantly affect the performance of the instrument and well as prolong longevity.

Manual cleaning

Cleaning of surgical instruments should occur immediately after the procedure is finished. Allowing instruments to sit unattended, with blood, saline, and other fluids drying on them will cause great damage to the instruments. The presence of chloride ions from blood, pus, or other secretions will contribute to the corrosion of the instrument. (Reuss-Lamky, H., 2011) If blood is allowed to sit on an instrument for longer

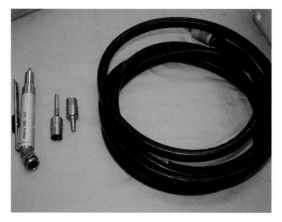

Figure 3.106 Pnuematic drill for neurologic surgeries.

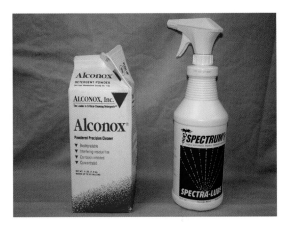

Figure 3.108 Instrument cleaning product and lubricant.

than 20 minutes, the residue will mark and stain the instrument. Manual cleaning is performed with a soft wire bristle brush, designed for instrument cleaning and a cleaning product approved for surgical instrument use. Nylon bristle brushes and commercial toothbrushes should not be used for most instruments; however, they may be used for general cleaning of retractors, scissors, and so on. The bristles are not stiff enough to clean the serrations and tight spaces found on instruments such as hemostats and needle holder tips. Cleaning agents, such as dishwashing soap, are alkaline based and will damage the instrument by pitting or corrosion. Other products commonly used in veterinary practices are chlorhexidine-based solutions or detergents, quaternary ammonium products, and surgeons hand-scrub products. These are examples of agents that will cause spotting and corrosion of the instruments; therefore, they *should not be used*! Cleaning products should be neutral in pH (7–8 pH) and be designed with the specific use of cleaning surgical instruments (Figure 3.108). Products can be a powder formulation or liquid. When cleaning instruments manually, first rinse the instruments to remove the gross debris, then proceed with cleaning. If using a powder, dip the soft bristle brush in the powder and proceed to scrub all surfaces of the instrument including the jaws, serrations, box lock, and ratchet. After thoroughly cleaning, place the instrument in the basket of the ultrasonic cleaner that will be used. The basket should not be in the ultrasonic, but rather sitting in the sink where the instruments are being cleaned. Remaining instruments are cleaned in the same fashion until all are done. Instruments with

multiple pieces must be disassembled prior to cleaning to ensure thorough cleaning. Equipment with a lumen (suction tips, biopsy instruments, cannulas, etc.) should have a long brush run through the lumen to remove all gross debris.

Ultrasonic cleaning

After manual cleaning, it is essential to follow with cleaning the instruments in an ultrasonic cleaner. An ultrasonic cleaner is a device that is used to remove fine particles of debris that may be missed by other methods of cleaning and is 16 times more effective at cleaning that manual cleaning alone. The use of cavitation – the physical vibration created by sound waves in a solution – is the premise of ultrasonic cleaning. Minute bubbles are created by the sound waves and as those bubbles come in contact with debris, they implode and remove the debris from its attachment. The debris is suspended in the solution, thereby rendering the instrument clean. The solution in the ultrasonic cleaning should be a neutral pH ultrasonic specific agent that has been properly diluted according to manufacturer's instructions. After changing the solution, the machine should be run for 5 minutes to "degas" the solution. When placing instruments in the ultrasonic, there are a few things to remember:

* Take care to place heaviest instruments in the ultrasonic basket first, with lighter instruments on top.
* Instruments made of different metals (stainless, copper, chrome plated, etc.) should not be put in the same cleaning cycle.
* Instruments should be fully opened when placed in ultrasonic cleaner – box locks open and ratchets open.
* Don't overload the cleaner – instruments need plenty of room and should be completely submerged in the cleaning solution (Figure 3.109).

Once loaded, the ultrasonic should be run for no longer than 10 minutes. Cycles longer than 10 minutes have not shown increased efficacy and may result in increased loosening of screws in some instruments. Also, the addition of heat to the ultrasonic tank has not shown additional benefit. Ultrasonic tanks should always be filled to within 1/2″ from the top and a basket must always be used when the ultrasonic cleaner is running. Solutions should be changed daily, or upon appearance of cloudiness. Frequency of refreshing the solutions will depend on surgical case load. Upon completion of the cycle, the instruments should be

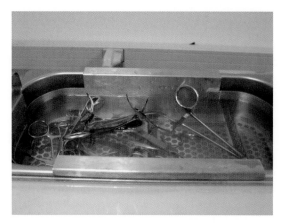

Figure 3.109 Ultrasonic cleaning unit overloaded.

removed from the solution immediately and rinsed with distilled water. After being rinsed, the instruments need to be lubricated.

Instruments that cannot be cleaned with water or ultrasonic submersion still must be cleansed before sterilization. Power drills and accessories cannot be submerged in any solution but must rather be wiped down with a cloth dampened with an instrument cleaning solution. Accompanying hoses must have the full length of the hose wiped down with the cloth as well. Large table top plate benders and other big pieces of equipment will also need to be processed only with manual cleaning. Any instrument containing optic fibers (endoscopes, arthroscopes, fiberoptic cables, etc.) must also be manually cleaned very carefully. Delicate handling of the instrument to avoid bumping or hitting the light end on a hard surface is imperative. Flexible scopes and light cables must be treated very gingerly and carefully. No bending of the item or abrupt trauma to the casing should occur.

Delicate ophthalmic or neurologic instruments can be manually cleaned and then processed in the ultrasonic cleaner, but should always be washed separately from other heavier instruments. The delicate nature of the instruments may necessitate reducing the ultrasonic time to 5 minutes.

Instrument lubrication

Instrument lubrication, often referred to as "instrument milk" should be used after every cleaning. Instruments need to have all moving parts lubricated after every cleaning to keep them moving freely and to help eliminate rubbing and scraping against each other. Especially

important are the box lock and ratchets. If the box lock is sticky while the surgeon is using it, after the instrument is cleaned, spray the box lock with lubricant and move the shafts of the instrument back and forth to aid in having the lubricant penetrate deeply into the joint. Only water-base lubricants, intended for surgical instruments should be used. Mineral oil, WD-40, or other industrial lubricants are NOT to be used on surgical instruments. Current recommendation for lubricant application is to spray it on rather than submersion in a bath. Lubricant baths may have been contaminated with bacteria from other instruments and may be left unchanged long after the recommended expiration of the solution. Spray on lubricant is less expensive, easier to apply and requires less storage/use space.

Instrument maintenance

After cleaning and lubricating, but before packaging, each instrument must be inspected for appropriate function and condition. Certain types of instruments require more attention and maintenance than others. Scissors, for instance, are designed to be resharpened. After each use, the scissors should be opened and closed to insure a smooth, gliding action between the blades. (Schultz, R. 2011, How to test & inspect scissors) Any catching or rubbing indicates the need for repair. Scissor blade tips should be inspected for burrs or corrosion. Blades should be evaluated for chips, burrs, or cracks on the cutting edge. Screws in the hinge of the scissors should be inspected for retained debris and for cracks near the screw head. Ring handles should be inspected for cracks as well. Testing for sharpness may be accomplished by using commercially available test material for various lengths of scissors. Regardless of the size, after multiple cuts are made in the test material, the scissors are extracted. If there is no pinching or grabbing of the material, the scissors are sharp. If the scissors are not sharp, they will need to be sent in to a qualified instrument repair company for sharpening. Stainless steel scissors will have the entire blade sharpened. Scissors that have a tungsten carbide insert cannot have the insert replaced nor sharpened, but are sharper and stronger to begin with so that it will ultimately last longer than stainless blades.

Needle holders are another type of instrument that needs special attention. The jaws need to be inspected for worn, cracking, or missing inserts and chipped or worn edges. (Schultz, R., 2011, How to inspect needle holders) If the jaws are smooth, close the ratchets all the way and look at a light through the jaw of the instrument. If light can be seen between the jaws, the instrument needs to be repaired. Jaws will wear out with normal suturing, so accessing the degree of wear is required after every use. The box lock should be looked at for cracking. Shanks should be straight and not bowed or angled. The ratchet action should be smooth and tight. Once closed, the teeth should not become disengaged until intentionally done.

Thumb tissue forceps should have the tips evaluated for proper teeth alignment if it is a toothed design. Edges of the tips should also be properly aligned. Hemostatic forceps must have the tips evaluated for wear, edge alignment, and ratchet security.

Penetrating towel clamps may have the tips damaged, bent, or barbed so checking for alignment and damage should happen after each use.

Pack preparation

Assembling packs for wrapping and subsequent sterilization is a detailed and important process that must be done meticulously to guarantee that the equipment the surgeon is expecting to be in the pack is actually there. When packing an instrument pack, it is often very helpful to have a check list of items that belong in the pack. As the instruments are placed in the pack they can be checked off on the sheet to show that the assembler did place the item in the pack. The check list can be folded and placed inside the pack for use by the sterile person for an instrument count when the pack is opened. All instruments in a pack must have the ratchets open, the box locks open and packed with enough room to allow circulation of the steam, gas or plasma to touch all the surfaces of the instruments. This requires 3 mm of space between each instrument. Instrument racks are the best option for achieving these requirements, but they can sometimes be difficult to find for purchase. Instrument brackets are designed to have a rod pass through each ring handle. Instrument rings can also be used, but because they only pass through one ring handle, the instruments are left hanging open with little support (Figure 3.110). When placing instruments on the instrument rack, it is best to stack them longest to shortest with the straight instruments first, followed

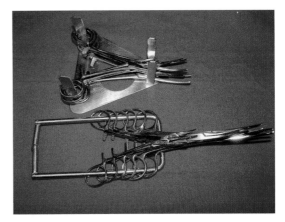

Figure 3.110 Holders for instruments in packs.

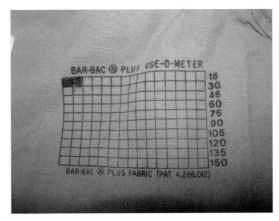

Figure 3.111 Washing grid on gown.

by the curved instruments, with the curves up. If there are enough racks available using two racks (one for straight instruments, one for curved instruments) is a nice option. Towel clamps should be placed on a separate rack, with the nonpenetrating towel clamps on the bottom and the penetrating towel clamps on top, since they will be used first.

Folding linens for placement in a pack is a very important skill. All cloth gowns and drapes need to be inspected before being used in a pack. The technician should check to see if there are any holes or worn spots on the gown or drape. Defective items are not allowed to be placed in surgical packs. Items should be inspected for lint, stray threads, or hair and have any debris removed before they are placed in a pack. If the items have a water-resistant property, there should be a grid in one of the corners of the item (Figure 3.111).

This grid is intended to track the number of uses of the items to ensure maximum water-resistant properties. Each time the item is used in a pack, one of the grid squares must be filled in with permanent marker. Once the grid is full, the item should be removed from use. Items must be folded in the same manner consistently so that those using the items in the pack will be familiar with what to expect. There are many ways to fold a gown but the simpler the better. It is important to fold the gown so that the person putting the gown on will be able to recognize where their hands may or may not go so as to avoid contaminating the gown. Non-sterile back, or standard gowns, are used frequently in veterinary clinics. While providing a sterile field when facing the surgical table, the biggest disadvantage to this type of gown is that the back is not sterile. This significantly impacts the potential for movement of the sterile personnel in the room and well as limits the surgeon to only having surgical instrumentation on the instrument table. In the case of a fracture or other involved case, back tables are often draped and used for placement of sterile items. Without a sterile back gown, this scenario is impossible. Figures 3.112–3.118 shows the method for folding a non-sterile back gown. Figures 3.119–3.124 shows the method for folding a hand towel for a gown pack. Wraparound gowns are a much better choice for all surgeries, but especially for procedures that will involve a lot of equipment because of the sterile back. The design of the gown allows the person wearing it to cover their back with a sterile part of the gown. When folding a wraparound gown, the steps are essentially the same with the exception of the first step. Lay the gown out on a solid surface with the "right" side of the gown facing the ceiling, just as with a standard gown. With a wraparound gown, the next thing that must be done it to secure the tie of the wraparound section to the tie on the front of the gown. This will allow the sterile person to handle the ties without contaminating themselves once the gown has been put on. After these two ties have been tied together, the folding of the gown is the same as for a standard surgical gown.

Whether a hospital chooses to use cloth or paper surgical drapes, a process for folding must be established. It is important that the drapes are easy to unfold and aseptically place on the patient. If paper drapes are used, it must not be a challenge for the surgeon to identify the area of the drape that will need to be cut to create the

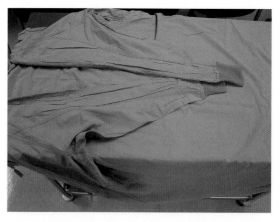

Figure 3.112 Lay the gown out on the table with the outside of the gown facing the ceiling and the neck of the own to the left. Sleeves should be folded into the center of the gown.

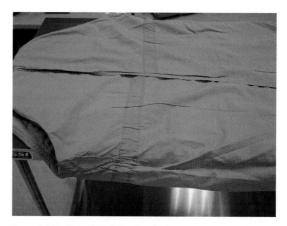

Figure 3.113 Grasping the seamed edge of the gown closest to the folder, fold the body of the gown up over the sleeves to the center of the gown. Reach over the gown and fold the opposite side in the same fashion.

fenestration. Often surgeons will use "huck" towels or ground drapes. These drapes are used first on the patient as a primary layer and must be folded in a manner that facilitates easy opening and placement. Whether ground drapes, large paper drapes or large cloth drapes, all folding should be identical. Drapes, whether cloth or paper, should be folded using the hand towel folding described earlier. The one exception is that the last step does not require the formation of a dog ear. The dog ear is present only on the hand towel in the gown pack.

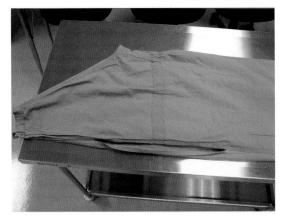

Figure 3.114 Pick up all layers of the neck with the left hand and all layers of the hem of the gown with the right hand and lift the gown into the air. The gown will fold in half. Lay the gown down on the table with the neck to the left and the raw edges of the gown facing the folder.

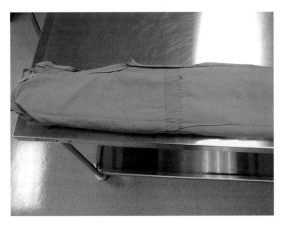

Figure 3.115 Picking up the edges closest to the folder, fold the gown in half lengthwise with the raw edges winding up away from the folder.

Pack wrapping and instrument packaging

Unless being flash sterilized or chemically sterilized, all instruments and equipment required for surgery must be wrapped prior to sterilization. Instrument packs should be wrapped with either cloth or paper surgical wraps. Cloth wrappers should be a minimum of 140 thread count, which means there are 140 threads per square inch. Any cloth with a lower thread count may allow dust and bacteria to penetrate into

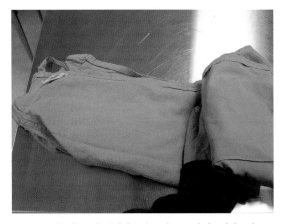

Figure 3.116 Place the left hand at the armhole of the sleeve, slide the right hand under the body of the gown, and fold the gown body up over the left hand.

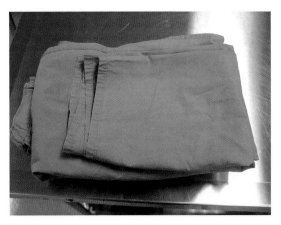

Figure 3.117 Continue the accordion folding until all of the body of the gown is folded.

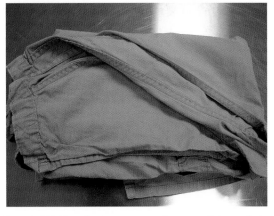

Figure 3.118 Turn the gown over so the seams of the armholes are found diagonally across the gown.

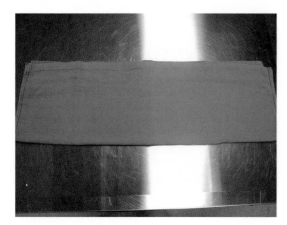

Figure 3.119 Folding the hand towel starts with laying the towel out on the table horizontally with the finished seam facing the ceiling.

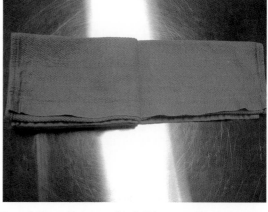

Figure 3.122 Fold the towel in half horizontally. Grasp the top two layers of the towel and fold it back on itself.

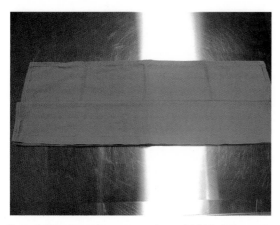

Figure 3.120 Grasp the top raw edge and fold it down so the towel is folded in half.

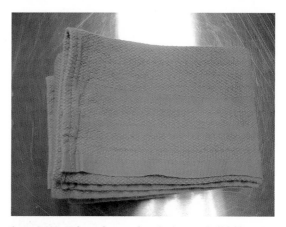

Figure 3.123 Pick up the towel so the bottom half folds underneath.

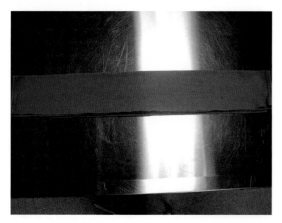

Figure 3.121 Pick up the towel on either short side to allow the bottom half of the towel to fold underneath.

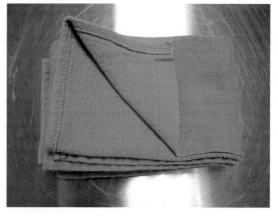

Figure 3.124 Fold the top corner of the towel back on itself to form a dog ear.

the pack, therefore contaminating it. Cloth wrappers may be a greater initial cost to the hospital, but with life expectancies of around 75 autoclaving cycles, it will be more economical in the long run. Currently, cloth wrappers cost approximately one quarter of the price of a comparable size paper wrapper. Cloth wraps are more durable than paper wrappers and are not subject to the minute tears or trauma that can happen so easily with paper. Some manufacturers provide a use grid near a seam, which allows for one square to be filled in each time the wrapper is washed. Once the grid is filled, the wrapper should not be used any further. Wrappers should be washed after every use to rehydrate the material. Minimal soap and an additional rinse cycle are encouraged when washing surgical linens. Wrappers should be inspected after each washing to check for holes, areas of thinness, or other imperfections that would compromise the sterility of the item. Small holes in cloth wrappers can be repaired using iron on patches, but care should be taken to not use a wrapper that has more patches than the original material. Paper wrappers are also available to be used to wrap surgery packs. Paper wrappers are designed to be a disposable item and therefore should be used only once due to the high risk of trauma and subsequent sub-par performance. Paper may be less expensive initially, but using them only once will increase the overall cost. Paper wrappers may be appropriate in situations where controlled handling can be monitored and the risk of trauma to the pack is minimal. Peel packs are available for single instrument or small pack packaging and sterilization. Peel packs are plastic on one side and paper on the other. Peel packaging is available in pre-cut sizes as well as on the roll for more custom packaging (Figure 3.125). Peel packs were designed for use with single, light-weight instruments. Manufacturing recommendations do not include using them for heavy instruments. If using the pre-cut sizes, it is important to use a package large enough to comfortably hold the item without giving it too much room to move around. There should be about 1″ of space between the end of the instrument and the peel pack seal. Whenever placing an item in a peel pack the ratchets should be open, box lock open and the handle end of the instrument should be placed in the package first so the handles are by the end that is opened. If sharp tips are present on the instrument or piece of equipment, protective tips should be placed over the sharp end (Figure 3.126). Vinyl protective tips can be fenestrated or need not be. Items such as spinal needles, IM pins, Gelpi self-retaining retractors, and so on are all examples of the types of instruments that should have a protective tip. When writing on the peel pack, information should be written only on the plastic side. Writing on the back paper side of the package permits migration of bacteria as the paper is a porous surface. If using the roll product, a heat sealer will also be needed. Peel packages should *never* be sealed with paper clips, staples, tape, or other closure devices. A heat sealer will melt the plastic side into the paper side, thereby creating a seal. If the heat sealer creates a very thin seal, multiple seals will be needed to insure the integrity of the package is maintained. If multiple items are to be

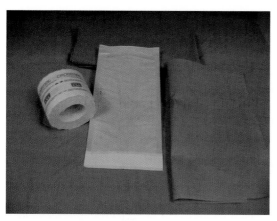

Figure 3.125 Peel Packing options.

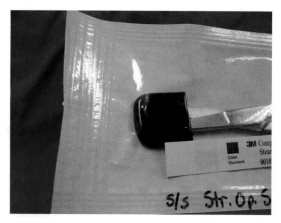

Figure 3.126 Protective end cap over sharp instrument; notice multiple seals on end due to thin sealing line.

packaged in the peel pack, double packing is indicated. Foremost it makes it easier for the sterile person to grab a single package as opposed to multiple pieces. Second, it provides greater barriers for contamination and provides a stronger package for the items. The inside package should be placed film (plastic) side to film side to allow proper sterilization and visualization of the item inside. Extremely heavy items (i.e., osteotomes, mallets, curettes, etc.) should not be packaged in peel pack material as they will break through the paper. These types of items should be double wrapped in muslin wrappers.

Methods of wrapping packs

There are two main methods that can be employed when wrapping instrument packs or equipment for sterilization – the envelope style and the horizontal (or square) style. The envelope style is better suited for packs that will be held while being opened or when placed on a surface to be opened, it is not important to cover the entire surface with a sterile field (i.e., gown packs). Wrapping packs using the horizontal style is generally reserved for packs that are very large, heavy, or long (plate sets, large instrument packs, etc.). When unwrapping horizontally wrapped packs, the packs are usually placed on a surface or table and then as the packs are unwrapped a sterile field that completely covers the table is created. Assembly and wrapping of gown packs and drapes packs are shown in Figures 3.127–3.135.

The horizontal wrapping style starts with the drape opened fully and lying on the table. The item to be wrapped in placed in the middle of the wrapper. The farthest edge of the wrapper is brought over the item and folded back on to itself for a dog ear. The closest edge of the wrapper is then folded over the item and then back on to itself to form a dog ear. Either side is brought over the item and folded back on itself. The final side edge is folded over the item and folded back on itself. If the last folded side edge is the last fold of an outside wrap, no dog ear is needed. Tape is then placed as two parallel pieces, tabs on top, and the same information is applicable as for any sterilized pack.

Any pack that is to be sterilized (using any method of sterilization) must have the correct information on the label. Using a black permanent marker is best when writing on the packs because pencil and ball point pen tend to fade drastically when steam sterilized, thereby making the label unreadable. Information on

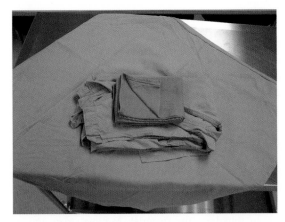

Figure 3.127 Lay the wrapper out on the table in a diamond formation to wrap a pack in the envelope style. Place the items for pack, on the wrapper in this order: gown first, then sterilization indicator then hand towel.

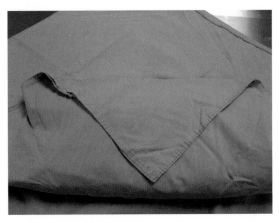

Figure 3.128 Grasp the point of the wrapper closest to the folder and fold it over the pack, then back on itself to form a "dog ear".

the pack label should include the date of sterilization, the size of the item wrapped (i.e., large), the name of the item wrapped, the autoclave, and load numbers and finally the initials of the person making the pack (Figure 3.136).

Sterilization

Sterilization is the process of using either physical or chemical means to kill all microorganisms on an item. There are a variety of options for sterilizing instruments

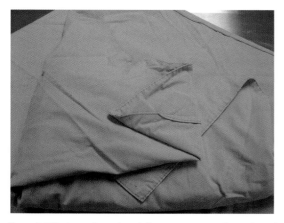

Figure 3.129 Grasp the point of the wrapper on either side and fold it over the items, and then back on itself to form another "dog ear".

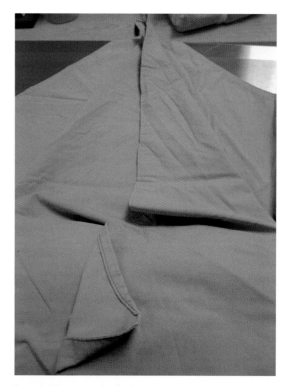

Figure 3.131 Grasp the final point of the wrapper, fold in the extra material, fold it over the pack and tuck it into the pack.

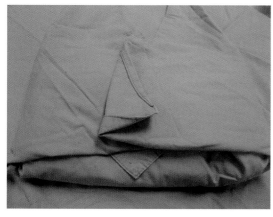

Figure 3.130 Grasp the point of the wrapper on the opposite side. Fold the wrapper over the pack and then again back on to itself to form a "dog ear".

and equipment for use in surgical cases. The method chosen will depend on the availability, the operator's familiarity with the method of sterilization, the window of time available to sterilize the equipment and the type of equipment that needs to be sterilized.

Chemical

Gluteraldehyde is classified as a high-level disinfectant, but when used appropriately it can provide sterilization of items. Effective sterilization depends not only on the age of the solution but also on the dilution and the amount of organic material present. Solutions greater than 2% and buffered to a pH solution of 7.5–8.5 have

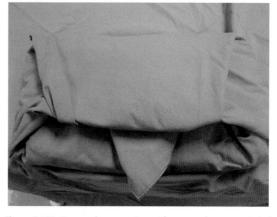

Figure 3.132 Repeat the wrapping with a second wrapper. Label the pack with the required information.

been shown to kill vegetative bacteria in less than 2 minutes. Fungi and viruses have been killed in less than 10 minutes and certain spores are killed in 3 hours.

Gluteraldehyde is an effective product for high-level disinfection or sterilization of devices and lensed

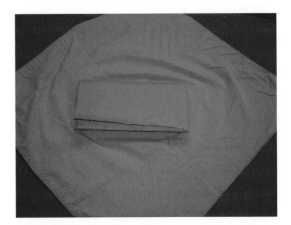

Figure 3.133 For drape pack assembly, begin with the wrapper in a diamond formation. Place the paper drape on the wrapper in a horizontal orientation.

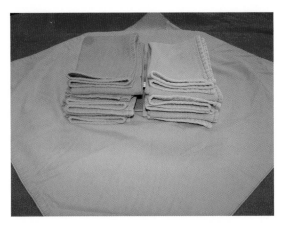

Figure 3.135 Place two more ground drapes on top of the sterilization indicator. Proceed to wrap exactly the same as the gown pack.

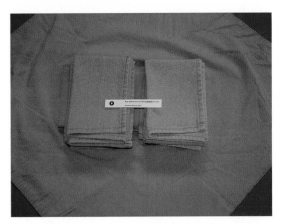

Figure 3.134 Next place two ground drapes on top of the paper drape. Be sure short open sides are facing the folder and all long open sides are facing in the same direction. Place sterilization indicator on top of ground drapes.

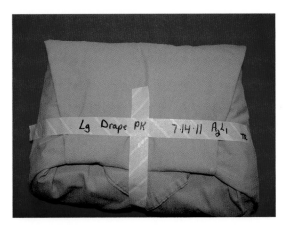

Figure 3.136 Properly labeled drape pack.

equipment such as endoscopes, arthroscopes, and cameras when other options are not available. Any items immersed in gluteraldehyde-based products must be rinsed with sterile water before contacting viable tissue. Gluteraldehyde is a potential irritant to the eyes, nose, and skin; so protective gloves (nitrile not latex), eye protection, and a respirator should be worn when working with this chemical. Disposal of the solution may be restricted by some municipal sewer systems, but neutralization with sodium bisulfate will render it safe for disposal. Due to these hazards and limited applications, gluteraldehyde is not used frequently.

Steam

Sterilizing instruments or equipment with a steam sterilizer, or autoclave, is the most common method of sterilization that is used in veterinary clinics and hospitals. Most surgical instruments and equipment are designed to withstand autoclaving. Items that are electric, fiberoptic, plastic, rubber, or other similar material are not to be steam sterilized. Steam sterilization requires three parameters be met to consider items sterilized. Those three parameters are time, temperature, and pressure. If all three parameters are not met, it should be presumed that sterilization did not occur. There are two types of steam autoclaves – gravity displacement and vacuum assisted (Figure 3.137). With the gravity displacement autoclaves, as the steam enters

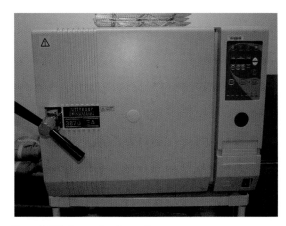

Figure 3.137 One style of autoclave.

the chamber, it pushes the air, or displaces it, out of the chamber, usually through the drain in the bottom of the chamber. The injection of superheated steam using pressure, then allows for the penetration of the steam into the items in the chamber. Sterilization, or killing of the microorganisms, then occurs. At the end of the sterilization cycle, the steam and pressure are removed from the chamber. The dry time portion of the cycle allows dry heat to dry the items in the autoclave but does not cool them. When the pressure reading reaches 0 psi, it is safe to open the autoclave. The operator should always stand behind the door of the machine because as it is opened, the residual steam in the chamber may burn the operator's face, arms, or hands if they are standing in front of the door. The door should be opened only 1–2″ to allow gradual cooling. The door should be left ajar for approximately 15 minutes before the packs are handled. When cooled sufficiently to allow safe handling, the packs are removed and placed on cooling racks to allow for full drying and cooling. When completely cool and dry, the packs can be placed into storage.

The vacuum-assisted autoclave has the same parameters that must be met. The main difference in machine operation is that with a vacuum sterilizer, the steam is forced into the chamber, which results in faster penetration of the packs. Similarly, at the end of the cycle, the vacuum evacuates the steam from the chamber resulting in faster removal of moisture-creating packs that are less wet. Cooling of items in the autoclave should be the same process as described for gravity displacement machines. Items sterilized by steam sterilization may be wrapped in cloth, paper, or peel pack pouches.

Recommended sterilization cycle times depend on the type of machine being used, whether or not the items to be sterilized are wrapped or not, and the type of item being sterilized. Table 3.9 shows recommended cycle parameters according to the Centers for Disease Control and Prevention Health Care Infection Control Practices Advisory Committee (HICPAC). It should be noted that pressure settings are not included. Presuming that temperature and time are met, the pressures should also be acceptable. Most pressure gauges on autoclaves merely report pressure readings with no option of altering the settings.

Loading the autoclave

Instrument packs to be sterilized in an autoclave must be placed flat on the tray. This position inhibits air pocket formation and/or condensation, both of which can prevent complete sterilization. Soft goods (cloth packs like gowns and drapes) wrapped for sterilization in an autoclave must be placed in the machine chamber vertically. This orientation allows better circulation of the steam and provides a greater possibility of adequate penetration of the steam. Wrapped packs should be placed with approximately 1″ between items. Additionally, items should not touch the chamber walls or ceiling. Peel pouches should not be stacked on top of one another, but rather placed in a rack for security and appropriate loading. If a rack is unavailable, the pouches can be placed in vertical orientation with the paper of one pouch against the plastic of the next pouch. This provides the opportunity for appropriate penetration by the steam. Items loaded plastic side to plastic side may not be sterilized as team penetration may be inhibited. After the autoclave is loaded, the door must be closed tightly and the cycle may be selected. Each time the autoclave is run, the reservoir should be checked for an acceptable water level. Autoclave manufacturers will indicate on the machine what determines an appropriate level of water. If water needs to be added only distilled water should be used. Water other than distilled can promote the build up of minerals in the pipes and tubing of the autoclave that will eventually cause a mechanical failure of the machine. Recordkeeping of sterilization loads is imperative in the event of an inadequate cycle. Maintaining a simple notebook for each sterilizer will allow the operator to list all the

Table 3.9 Sterilization guidelines.

Type of machine	Item being sterilized	Wrapped or unwrapped	Temperature	Time	Dry time
Gravity displacement	Instruments	Wrapped	250 F (121 C)	30 min	15–30 min
			270 F (132 C)	15 min	15–30 min
	Textiles	Wrapped	250 F (12 C)	30 min	15 min
			270 F (132 C)	25 min	15 min
	Nonporous items only (i.e., routine metal instruments, no lumens)	Unwrapped	270 F (132 C)	3 min	None
	Nonporous and porous items (e.g., rubber or plastic items, items with lumens) sterilized together	Unwrapped	270 F (132 C)	10 min	none
Pre-vacuum	Instruments	Wrapped	270 F (132 C)	4 min	20–30 min
	Nonporous items only (i.e., routine metal instruments, no lumens)	Unwrapped	270 F (132 C)	4 min	None
	Nonporous and porous items (e.g., rubber or plastic items, items with lumens) sterilized together	Unwrapped	270 F (132 C)	4 min	none
	Textiles	Wrapped	270 F (132 C)	4 min	5–20 min

items placed in the load. If an inappropriate cycle is determined at a later time, each item run will be able to be easily retrieved from the shelf for reprocessing.

Autoclave maintenance

Manufacturer's recommendations for autoclave maintenance should be strictly adhered to. In general a monthly cleaning of the chamber is advised. There are products available that are added to the reservoir and when a cycle is run, the chemical will move from the reservoir into the chamber and clean the surfaces while the cycle is running. Water left in the reservoir at the end of the week should be drained so that the chance of algae growing during non-use time is reduced. Lint residue buildup (a greater risk with paper wrappers/drapes than with cloth) can occur in the chamber, on the trays and in the piping of the machine and can also cause equipment failure. Annual inspection by a qualified repair technician will assist in the diagnosis of potential problems with the machine before it breaks down – usually at the most inopportune time.

Ethylene oxide sterilization (ETO, EtO, EO)

EtO is a toxic, flammable gas that uses low temperature and long periods of time to kill microorganisms on items by using alkylation to alter the DNA. Items that cannot survive steam sterilization should be sterilized with EtO (Figure 3.138). Fiberoptic cables, plastics,

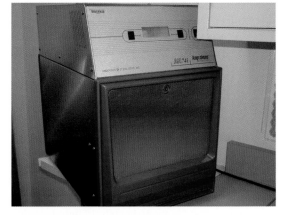

Figure 3.138 Ethylene oxide sterilizer.

electric equipment, cameras, rubber-based items are just a few examples of things that do well in an EtO cycle. The parameters that must be met for EtO are different than those for steam sterilization. EtO requires the four parameters of time, temperature, humidity, and EtO gas concentration be met in order for sterility to be achieved. Most items can be run for 12 hours, at a humidity of 20–40%, at a temperature of at least 68 °F and using one of the available premeasured EtO ampules. Tubing that is longer than 3' must be run for 24 hours using two ampules. Due to the dangerous nature of this chemical, it is imperative that personnel using the EtO sterilizers be well trained in proper loading, operation, and troubleshooting. Companies that sell this type of sterilizer may offer training sessions for personnel. Items sterilized with EtO may be wrapped in cloth, paper, peel pack pouches, or polyethylene peel packs. One of the more commonly seen EtO sterilizers requires that items be loaded into a company-designed plastic bag. The ampule containing the EtO liquid is placed in the bag on top of the items. Once the bag is purged of air, the ampule is broken and the bag is slid into the unit. The cycle (12 hours or 24 hours) is chosen and the cycle begins. Proper aeration following the cycle must be acknowledged and adhered to. Check with the manufacturer's recommendations regarding operation of the unit.

Plasma sterilization

Plasma sterilization is based on the theory of using ultra-violet photons and radicals to disrupt microorganisms. Hydrogen peroxide is the most common product used in vapor phase plasma sterilization and is becoming popular due to the safety of its use. Unlike EtO, hydrogen peroxide is neither toxic nor dangerous for operators or the environment. Current availability of machine size and expense, make this method of sterilization more common in academic facilities, but general practice use is uncommon. Items that have a lumen (tubing, instruments, cannulas, etc.) may need an H_2O_2 booster to insure proper sterilization is achieved. Currently theses boosters are not approved by the FDA for use in the United States. Special packaging must be used with products that are plasma sterilized as regular peel packs and linens are unacceptable. Currently there is one product available for use as a sterilization wrapper for all types of sterilizers (gravity and vacuum autoclaves, EtO, and Plasma). Items that are sterilized in a plasma sterilizer must have packaging specific to that system. Due to the nature of the sterilization process, no packaging products can be of organic nature.

Monitoring the sterilization process

Monitoring of the sterilization cycle is an important and often overlooked portion of the reprocessing procedure. Not only is assessment of the machine function important, but preventing the use of equipment that may not be truly sterile is critical to patient outcome. Monitoring

the efficacy of the sterilization process can be accomplished by combining any of the physical, chemical, or biological indicators that are available.

Physical monitors

Physical monitors are those methods available that verify the sterilization parameters are met by the equipment. Things like recording charts, digital readouts, gauges, or printouts on the machine will perform this assessment.

Chemical indicators

Chemical indicators are devices used to assess one or more parameters of the sterilization cycle. There are six classes of chemical indicators. Certain classes will be seen more commonly than other in veterinary use. Class 1 indicators are used externally. External indicators are used primarily to differentiate between processed and unprocessed equipment. This does not guarantee sterility, but rather merely that a pack was run through a sterilization cycle. Autoclave or EtO tape used to close packs is an example of a Class 1 indicator. Class 2 indicators are used to determine the sterilizer performance and are not used routinely with instrument packs. Bowie-Dick testing is an example of a Class 2 indicator and is used to detect air leaks, inadequate air removal, and so on from vacuum-assisted autoclaves. Class 3 indicators are internal indicators that are placed within a pack, generally at the most dense area of the pack. Indicators assess one of the parameters, such as whether or not the proper temperature was reached. Class 4 indicators assess multiple parameters, such as paper strips routinely place in the center of packs to be steam sterilized. Paper strips generally determine whether temperature and steam pressure were met (Figures 3.139, 3.140). Time, however is not evaluated. Class 5 indicators are designed to assess all parameters needed for a sterile cycle. The rigor of testing is equal to a biological indicator. Class 6 indicators are designed for specific cycle parameters. The response from these indicators does not correlate to a biological indicator. These indicators assess isolated information for each pack. Again, because it assesses only limited information, it does not guarantee sterility of the pack. For example, if the autoclave is not functioning properly, the steam may penetrate the pack but the proper time parameter will not have been met. Indicators are dependant on proper use by the operator, proper placement within

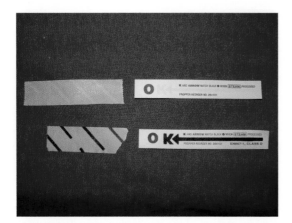

Figure 3.139 Before and after sterilization indicators for steam sterilization.

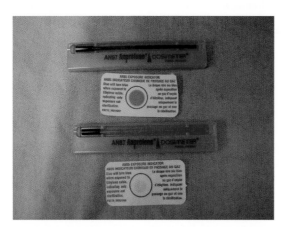

Figure 3.140 Before and after sterilization indicators for ethylene oxide sterilization.

the sterilizer, proper functioning of the sterilizer, and proper loading of the sterilizer by the operator. Steam sterilization indicators assess the three parameters of pressure, temperature, and time, whereas EtO indicators are sensitive to the four parameters of time, temperature, humidity, and EtO gas concentration.

Biological indicators

Biological indicators are considered the closest available option to the ideal monitor of sterilization cycles. Because of one of the most resistant microorganisms (Bacillus spores), the indicators measure the complete kill of a microorganism rather than merely assessing physical parameters of the sterilization cycle. The

premise of a biological indicator is that with a concentrated large number of bacteria that are more resistant than most contaminants that may be found on equipment, the result of killing those pathogens will strongly suggest that other pathogens that may be present will also be eradicated. The indicators are placed in the most challenging area of the sterilizer and run through the cycle. At the end of the cycle, the small vial is cracked with the provided device and incubated at 35 ˚F. The results of the vial should be checked every 12 hours for 48 hours before assuming a final result. A color change indicates a positive growth result and the items within the load should not be considered sterile. Steam biological indicators use *Geobacillus stearothermophils* and EtO biological indicators use *Bacillus atrophaeus*.

Shelf life

Date related shelf life is falling out of favor. Event-related shelf life is becoming the accepted method of storing sterilized items. Time does not determine whether an

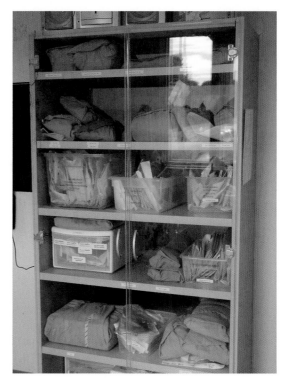

Figure 3.141 Closed cabinet for storage of sterilized items.

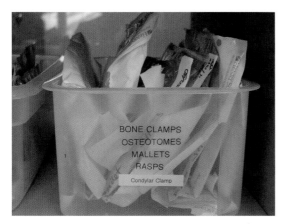

Figure 3.142 Avoid crushing peel packs and risking contamination.

item is contaminated, but rather handling and exposure to elements. More attention should be paid to storage conditions and frequency of handling rather than the calendar. Under ideal conditions, sterile items will remain sterile indefinitely. Storage should be in a closed cabinet to avoid dust contamination as well as exposure to air movement (Figure 3.141). Humidity should be less than 70% and a temperature of 75 °F should be maintained. The storage area should be 8–10″ above the floor surface, 18″ below the ceiling and 2″ from any outside wall. Items should be rotated so that the oldest item is the first one used. Excessive handling, rustling, and moving of the packs will add to compromising the integrity of the packaging. Especially with peel pack items, avoiding sliding, dropping, puncturing or compressing the packing should be practiced (Figure 3.142). Items should be inspected before each use. Any question as to the integrity should warrant repackaging and resterilization. Especially in the situation of large animal mobile veterinary services, extra care should be paid to sterilized packs. Storage in freezer Ziploc bags, plastic waterproof containers, or other such devices will greatly prolong the integrity of the packs.

References

Center for Disease Control (2008) Guideline for Disinfection and Sterilization in Healthcare Facilities

Darouiche, R.O.,Wall, M.J., Jr., Otterson, M.F., *et al.* (2010) Chlorhexidine – alcohol versus povidone-iodine for surgical-site antisepsis. The New England Journal of Medicine, 10.1056/NEJMoa0810988, Vol. 362, 18–26.

Fossum, T. (2007) *Small Animal Surgery*, 3rd edn. Mosby Elsevier, St.Louis, MO.

Healthcare Infection Control Practices Advisory Committee (1999) Recommendations from the CDC Guideline for Hand Hygiene in Healthcare Settings, Center for Disease Control and Prevention.

Hempel, Mike(1998) Research Animal Surgical Nursing, class handout, Madison Area Technical College.

Michalski, D.L. (2002) New Concepts of Sterilization and Disinfectants, AVMA Convention proceedings

Monnet, Eric (2011) Update on Laparoscopy, Proceedings from ACVS Symposium, Chicago, IL

Paulson, D.S. (2004) Hand Scrub products—performance requirements: versus clinical relevance. Association of Operating Room Nurses journal, 80 (**2**), 225–234.

Radlinsky, MaryAnn G. (2007) Minimally Invasive Instrumentation and Equipment, ACVS Symposium Proceedings, Chicago, IL.

Reuss-Lamky, Heidi Beating the "Bugs": sterilization is instrumental Veterinary Technician Journal, 2011 **32**, **11**.

Schultz, R. (2011) How to test & inspect scissors. In: *Inspecting Surgical Instruments; An Illustrated Guide*. Spectrum Surgical Instruments, Stow, OH.

Schultz, R. (2011) How to inspect needle holders. In: *Inspecting Surgical Instruments; An Illustrated Guide*. Spectrum Surgical Instruments, Stow, OH.

Sessum, J.D. (2003) Veterinary arthroscopy terminology and instrumentation. Veterinary Technician, 24 (**10**), 676–681.

Sigler, M., Sastyr, J., Stahl, J. *et al.* (2001) *Comparison of a Waterless, Scrubless CHG/Ethanol Surgical Scrub to Traditional CHG and Povidone-Iodine Surgical Scrubs*. 3M Health Care, St Paul, MN.

Tear, M. (2012) *Small Animal Surgical Nursing – Skills and Concepts*, 2nd edn. Elsevier, St. Louis, MO.

Wilson, D.G., Hartmann, F., Carter, V.R., *et al.* (2011) Comparison of three preoperative skin preparation techniques in ponies, Equine Veterinary Education 10.1111/j.2042-3292.2010.00203.x

Webliography

Chlorhexidine-alcohol tops povidone-iodine for surgical site antisepsis – www.thedoctorschannel.com/video/2820.html [accessed on 5 November 2014].

The Environmental Essentials to OR Cleaning – www.infectioncontroltoday.com [accessed on 5 November 2014]

This site discusses proper air handling in operating rooms – www.ehow.com/facts_7208379_ioeratubg-room-clean-air-stnadards.html [accessed on 5 November 2014].

Akridge, J Breathe Easy with the right air purification and filtration systems – www.hpnonline.com/inside/2004–10/Air Purification/Air Purification.html [accessed on October 2012].

Causes-of-corrosion-staining-pitting-marking.php. This is a surgical instrument company dedicated to instrumentcare– www.spectrumsurgical.com [accessed on 5 November 2014].

Ultrasonic cleaning. This is a surgical instrument company dedicated to instrument care – www.spectrum surgical.com [accessed on 5 November 2014].

Surgical instrument – lubrication. This is a surgical instrument company dedicated to instrument care – www. spectrumsusrgical.com [accessed on 5 November 2014].

This is another company dedication to the production and maintenance of surgical instruments – www.robox.com/ catalog%20pdfs/sterilizatoin_and_maintenance.pdf [accessed on July 2012].

This is a company that sells ultrasonic cleaners – www.unimax supply.com/equip/cleanequip/infoultrasonic.htm [accessed on 5 November 2014].

http://nasa.gov/policies/pdf/WFF_Autoclave_REcommenda tions.pdf. [accessed on 5 November 2014].

That's a Wrap. This company is a resource for sterilization and disinfection information – www.infectioncontroltoday .com/articles/2006/11/thats-a-wrap.apx. [accessed 25 July 2012]

http://medelcabalsa.blogspot.com/2009/06/surgical-scrub-technique.html [accessed on 5 November 2014]

http://cal.vet.upenn.edu/projects/saortho/chapter_09/09 mast.htm [accessed on 5 November 2014]

Kimberly – Clark Sterilization Wrap Receives FDA Clearance for ALL ASP STERRAD System Modalities – http:// www.infectioncontroltoday.com/news/2013/09/ kimberlyclark-sterilization-wrap-receives-fda-clearance-for-all-asp-sterrad-system-modalities.aspx [accessed on 5 November 2014]

http://www.cdc.gov/hicpac/Disinfection_Sterilization/4_0 efficacyDS.html#[accessed on 5 November 2014]

http://www.cdc.gov/hicpac/Disinfection_Sterilization/6_0 disinfection.html [accessed on 5 November 2014]

http://www.cfsph.iastate.edu/Disinfection/Assets/Dis infection101.pdf [accessed on 5 November 2014]

http://www.thecvc.com/cvc/data/html/cvc/352010/684325/ Hurley_Infectious_Disease_Control.pdf [accessed on 5 November 2014]

DiGangi, B.A (2009) Cleaning and Disinfection for the Spay-Neuter Clinic. www.sheltervet.org [accessed on 18 November 2014]

CHAPTER 4

Surgical Assistant and Circulating Nurse

One of the roles of the personnel working in a clinic or hospital that frequently goes unsupported by veterinary technicians is in the surgical suite – not an anesthetist or a circulating nurse, but rather a surgical assistant for the surgeon. Surgeons working without a surgical assistant are at the mercy of fate when it comes to speed and timely completion. Surgeons who work with a qualified and efficient assistant can attest to the benefit of the extra knowledgeable body. Working as a team, with the patient's best possible outcome as their goal, the surgeon and the assistant will set the tone and pace for the procedure.

A surgeon with a well-qualified proficient assistant can reduce the surgical procedure time significantly. Technicians that perform as assistants must be familiar with all instrumentation to be used and the process with which the surgeon will advance through the procedure. Assistants must master the skill of anticipation and ensure that the instrument/equipment is in the hand of the surgeon even before he/she even knows it is needed. Sometimes the surgeons' needs are made known nicely . . . . and other times, not so nicely (Beale, B.S. 2010).

Regardless of how the need is made known, it is the technician's job to make available at the right time what the surgeon is requesting.

Even before the patient is anesthetized, the surgical assistant is involved with the case. Making sure that the appropriate equipment and instrumentation is available is the most critical factor. Nothing can impede the progress of a surgery more than having to wait for equipment or instruments to be sterilized, or worse yet, not having the necessary item available at all. The assistant needs to be sure that the required instrument is functioning and ready for use. In addition to the assistant, the circulating technician in the operation room

can greatly influence the flow of the case. A circulating technician who knows what the surgeon needs, can find and open the item quickly and correctly, is a wonderful resource to have. Circulating technicians also grow to the point of being able to offer suggestions to the surgeon about equipment that may be useful to them. Sometimes when procedures do not go as planned, someone outside of the sterile field will have a different perspective of the situation, which allows them the ability to offer a suggestion that may not have otherwise been thought of.

Patient positioning

Once the patient is moved into the operating room, it is the responsibility of the surgical assistant to appropriately position the patient for the procedure to be done. Proper positioning of the patient is a critical step in the patient preparation process. Surgeons require the patient be positioned in a straight and anatomically correct fashion (Figure 4.1). One must consider first of all, the procedure being performed and the surgeons positioning preference. For example, for stifle surgery, sometimes the patient is positioned in dorsal recumbency with the instrument table over the chest of the patient (Figure 4.2). This positioning of the instrument table allows the surgeon to stand at the end of the surgery table and not have a non-sterile back of a gown facing the sterile instrument table. Although controversial in its safety, the author suggests that placement of the table be done judiciously. Other procedures where the patient is in dorsal recumbency, the instrument table will be placed behind the surgeon, exposing the instruments to the non-sterile back of the gown. Conversely, for forelimb surgery and most thoracic or abdominal procedures, the instrument table

Surgical Patient Care for Veterinary Technicians and Nurses, First Edition. Gerianne Holzman and Teri Raffel.
© 2015 John Wiley & Sons, Ltd. Published 2015 by John Wiley & Sons, Ltd.
Companion Website: wiley.com/go/holzman/surgical.

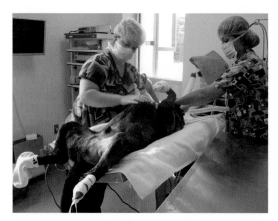

Figure 4.1 Positioning the patient on the surgery table.

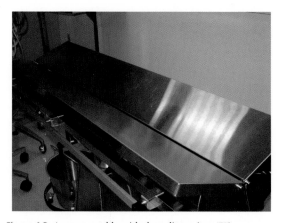

Figure 4.3 A surgery table with the split top in a "V".

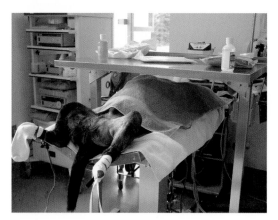

Figure 4.2 The instrument table over the chest of a patient having stifle surgery.

is placed over the caudal end of the patient. If it is a procedure to remove a mass from an unusual location, the technician must be certain that the positioning of the patient does not impede the surgeon's ability to perform the procedure. It is advised to have the surgeon verify the positioning of the patient on the surgery table before they scrub and before the final patient prep is performed. Patients in dorsal recumbency that are leaning to one side or another risk receiving an incision through the muscle layers of the abdominal wall instead of through the linea alba. Once a patient has been positioned to the surgeon's liking, the patient must not shift or move from that position until the end of the case.

The use of positioning aids will greatly assist in maintaining the animal in the desired position. Some surgery tables have a split top that allows either one or both sides of the table top to be adjusted (Figure 4.3). With this type of table, patients can be positioned in any manner from flat on the table to any degree of "V". For patients that need to be in dorsal recumbency, the use of the surgery table "V" may be all that is needed. For deep-chested dogs, long sandbags, as opposed to square sandbags, will be an effective method for supplementing the table top to maintain the patient in the proper position. Foam wedges may also be used but may slip and if contaminated by blood or other fluids, may be difficult to clean and disinfect. Additional positioning aids include Plexiglass/plastic positioners, vacuum bean bags, or similar devices and leg ties. All can be easily disinfected between patients by laundering or wiping down with a disinfecting solution. Vacuum positioning aids are extremely helpful in maintaining patients in unusual positions. These devices are especially helpful for ophthalmic procedures or thoracic cases that necessitate the patient be positioned in an oblique state, rather than a level lateral position. Because they can be conformed around the patient in any fashion, and then have the air vacuumed out to maintain the position, these devices are very unique. Leg ties are extremely common and in most cases, are the only positioning assistance that is needed. Soft ropes or commercially available leg ties are recommended. Roll gauze, IV tubing, or elastic bands are not recommended as they may apply too much pressure to the soft tissue and impede distal limb circulation. An adjustable loop on the leg tie should be placed just proximal to the carpus/tarsus; then a half hitch is placed just distal to those joints

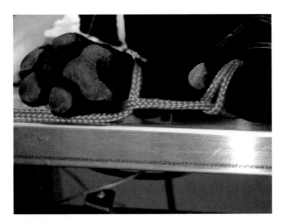

Figure 4.4 Leg with a half hitch.

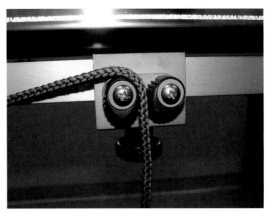

Figure 4.6 Leg tie through a roller style bracket on a surgery table.

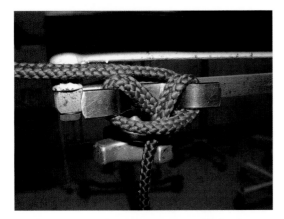

Figure 4.5 Leg tie in a figure 8 on a surgery table bracket.

(Figure 4.4). Double placement, as described, aids in the better distribution of pressure to reduce circulation issues. Most surgery tables have either brackets or side bar rollers on the side table rails, which are used to secure the leg ties. Brackets require a figure 8 method of securing the leg tie with a half hitch on the last loop to secure placement (Figure 4.5). Rollers are easier to use and simply require the leg tie be passed between the two rubber rollers to securely hold the rope (Figure 4.6). Care should be taken to avoid excessively extending the limbs to prevent unnecessary strain on joints or muscles. Limbs should be maintained in as normal a position as possible, depending on the position the patient is in. Some surgery-specific positioning aids are available such as an arthroscopy brace. It is used to position the limb of dogs having a stifle

arthroscopy performed. The brace holds the limb in a flexed position to assist the surgeon. The brace must be covered by a sterile drape before the limb can be placed on it.

The use of sand bags and/or vacuum aids is required in order to achieve and maintain proper positioning of the patient when a dorsal or ventral approach for a spinal surgery is indicated. Patients in this position must be monitored for adequate respiratory capability due to the potential respiratory complications from the compression on the chest wall required to keep the spine straight. The vacuum-positioning aids are quite stiff and hard following the evacuation of the air and are therefore not very forgiving at allowing the expansion of the chest wall if conformed too tightly to the patient. It is important to remember that whichever positioning aid is employed, it should not be wrapped around or laid over the chest of the patient, but rather gathered or formed along the sides of the chest. It is impossible to describe all the potential positions for surgical patients as it is dependent on the surgeon's preference. It is even difficult to make the statement that all patients for a certain procedure (i.e., stifle surgery) are always placed in the same position (i.e., dorsal recumbency). Factors such as procedure being done, size of the patient, and surgeon's familiarity all determine the positioning of the patient on a case–by-case basis. The most important thing to remember is that excellent communication must exist between the technician doing the positioning and the surgeon performing the procedure in order to avoid unnecessary delays.

Sterile patient prep

Following positioning of the patient, the sterile prep may begin. It is highly recommended that the patient has the clipping and initial skin prep (scrub) performed in an area outside of the surgery room. Once completed, the patient is moved to the surgical suite, positioned and a final sterile prep is done. A sterile surgical patient prep is done in a very similar fashion as the initial prep with the major difference being the use of sterile products. Prep sets can be made a couple of ways, depending on clinic choice. A small instrument pan (3″ × 8″) or a kidney (emesis) basin can be used as the pan. Two stacks of 10 4 × 4 gauze sponges are placed in the pan. An indicator strip should be placed in the middle of the sponges. A right hand glove (usually size 7 or 7 ½) can then be laid on top of the sponges (Figure 4.7). Some clinics prefer not to include the glove, which is an acceptable modification because it permits the flexibility of allowing any qualified person to perform the sterile prep, regardless of their glove size. The pan is double wrapped using the envelope style of wrapping and is sterilized in the autoclave.

In addition to the sterile prep set, squeeze bottles of the prep solutions also need to be available. The solutions and prep set should be set up in the surgery room when the rest of the packs and equipment are placed in the room. Once the patient is positioned, the prep set can be opened. Both wraps are aseptically opened to reveal the sterile contents. Before proceeding, the caps of the solution bottles should be opened. If a glove was not included in the sterile prep set, a pack of appropriate-sized gloves should now be aseptically opened and using the open gloving technique, a sterile glove is placed on the dominant hand. If a glove was included, it is now aseptically put on the dominant hand. Having one sterile hand and one non-sterile hand allows the technician the independence to perform the sterile prep without assistance. The non-sterile hand is also available to stabilize the suspended limb during the prep for orthopedic cases.

With the sterile, gloved hand, 1–2 sponges are picked up. The non-sterile hand picks up the surgical scrub bottle and aseptically applies some scrub solution to the sterile sponges. Care must be taken to ensure that the cap of the bottle does not touch the sponges. The prep now continues using the same pattern that the initial scrub used (Figure 4.8). New prep sponges should be retrieved as needed. The rinsing agent is aseptically applied to the sponges in the same manner as the scrub product. Be sure to save a few dry sponges to be used for the application of the final paint solution.

Once the final paint is applied, the draping may begin. Every effort should be made to allow the final solution

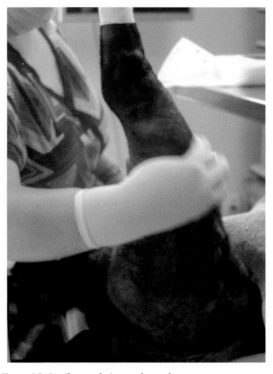

Figure 4.8 Sterile prep being performed.

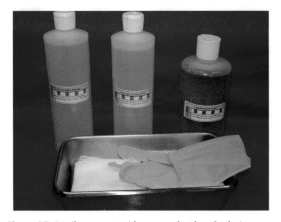

Figure 4.7 Sterile prep set with squeeze bottles of solutions.

to dry prior to draping the patient to encourage optimal efficacy of the product.

Patient draping

Once the patient has received the second, "sterile" prep, draping can begin. Assistants must be thoroughly knowledgeable about the procedure and the approach the surgeon will use in order to effectively drape the patient. Depending on the procedure to be done, draping may need to include extra wide margins away from the incision. For example, draping to allow access to the exit of a chest tube for a thoracic procedure or allowing access to a bone graft site for harvesting a graft for a fracture repair.

Especially during the draping sequence, but throughout the entire procedure, both the surgical assistant and the circulating technician must be acutely aware of strict asepsis in the surgical suite and sterile field. According to Dr. Brian Beale, "the surgical assistant should be cognizant of the need for strict asepsis and act as the asepsis police in the operating room" (Beale, B.S., 2010). Any question as to a break in aseptic technique must be treated as a valid break and corrective measures must be taken. Whether that means changing a pair of gloves, a gown, or an entire pack of instruments, it must be done. Although often times not very well liked by all members of the surgical team, the veterinary technician is acting as the patient's advocate and looking out for their well being. Breaks in asepsis are not to be argued or debated, but accepted and corrected.

Non-orthopedic draping (soft tissue, neuro, etc.)

Draping for non-orthopedic procedures is a fairly simple process. After the sterile drape pack has been opened aseptically by the circulating technician, and is available to the sterile team members, draping may begin using the four corner draping method. Usually ground/field drapes (also known as quarter drapes or huck towels) are placed first. It is important that before draping, all skin prep solutions (alcohol, paint solutions) have adequate time to dry/evaporate. Not only is this important for optimal efficacy of the prep products, it also decreases the complications from the use of electrocautery and/or lasers. Presuming the ground drapes are folded as described earlier, find the short

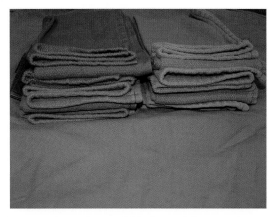

Figure 4.9 Short side, open folds of ground drape towels.

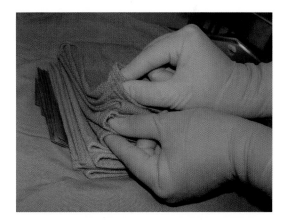

Figure 4.10 Fingers in the appropriate folds of the towel.

side of the drape that has the open folds (Figure 4.9). Place the index finger of each hand in the outermost opening and the thumb in the innermost opening (Figure 4.10). Using the thumb and middle finger of each hand, hold the drape and lift it up (Figure 4.11). The long side of the drape with the folds should be facing the ceiling. Holding the drape in front, move the hands away from each other to open the drape (Figure 4.12). Lift the thumb of each hand to allow the drape to unfold (Figure 4.13). Drapes should never be flipped, shaken, or fanned as that action may release dust and/or lint into the air and potentially onto the sterile field. Holding the towel with the index finger and the thumb of each hand, rotate the hands so all the fingers and palms are facing the operator (Figure 4.14). Rotate the hands again so the palms are down and the edges of the drape cover the gloved hands (Figure 4.15).

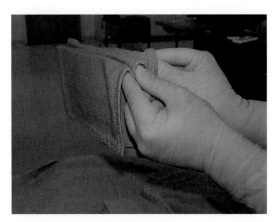

Figure 4.11 Picking up the towel.

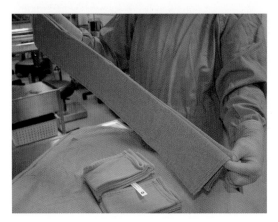

Figure 4.12 Opening the towel.

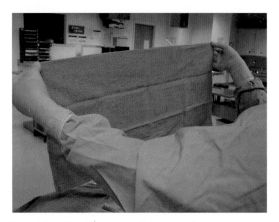

Figure 4.13 Lift each thumb and allow towel to open.

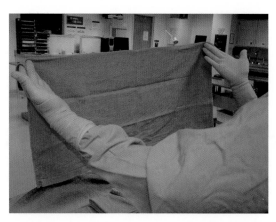

Figure 4.14 Rotate each hand so palms are facing the operator.

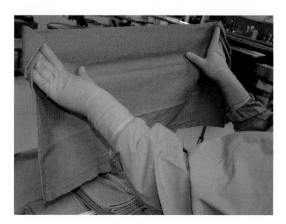

Figure 4.15 Pronate the hands so the fingers are protected by the towel.

This action protects the sterile hands from becoming contaminated as the drape is laid on the patient. This method of unfolding results in a crisp fold being closest to the incision, which helps the drape to lay as flat as possible. Communication with the surgeon prior to draping is strongly recommended in the event special draping requests may be made. Once a drape is placed on the patient, it cannot be moved or adjusted; therefore, proper initial placement is imperative. The side of the patient closest to the person draping should be draped first. As the drape is being placed, it is critical that no part of the sterile gown or sterile hands come in contact with a non-sterile surface. The folded edge of the drape should be placed 1/2″–1″ laterally to the proposed incision site. The second drape is placed opposite from the first. The person draping must *never* reach over the non-sterile area to place a drape. Walking around the table to place the drape is the only acceptable practice. The second drape should be placed at the same distance from the proposed incision site as the first drape. The third drape is placed on the cranial aspect of the proposed incision. As before, a 1/2″–1″ margin from the incision's cranial end should be followed. When placing the third drape, care must be taken to keep the front of the gown facing the surgery table. The person draping should turn just the arms and shoulders to place the drape. Especially with long haired patients, arms may need to be elevated to avoid sleeve contamination from the fur. After the third drape is placed, penetrating towel clamps should be placed at the intersecting corners of the towels to secure them to the patient. Penetrating towel clamps are used to pierce the skin and securely hold the drapes in place. Depending on the area of the body being draped, caution must be taken to avoid penetrating an important structure with the towel clamp (i.e., jugular vein, nerve, etc.).The caudal drape is the last to be placed using the same physical stance as with the cranial drape. The person draping the patient is not allowed to stand at the end of the surgery table to place the drape. In most cases, this would require reaching over the non-sterile table and that is a break in aseptic technique. Penetrating towel clamps can now be placed in the two remaining intersecting corners of the drapes. After all four ground drapes are placed and secured; the same draping process is repeated with larger drapes. The top drapes need to be large enough to completely cover the patient and table top to reduce the risk of contamination. Some surgeons will choose to use a large fenestrated drape instead of the four top drapes. Either option is acceptable. However, four corner draping (sometimes referred to as four quadrant draping) allows more flexibility, whereas the fenestrated drape is one fixed size and cannot be changed no matter the size of the patient. Fenestrations that are too large, risk over exposure of the patient's skin, thereby increasing infection risk. Fenestrations too small may hinder the surgeon's ability to visualize as needed due to a smaller incision. Top drapes can be secured with either penetrating or nonpenetrating towel clamps.

Orthopedic draping

When patients are having an orthopedic procedure and the limb has been suspended for the prep, the draping

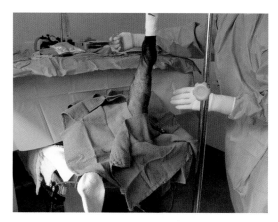

Figure 4.16 Securing ground drapes for an orthopedic case.

procedure is quite involved. After the drape pack has been aseptically opened for the sterile team, the first ground drape can be placed. In order to keep the limb freely moveable for the surgeon the ground drapes are placed approximately 1″ from the clipped margins at the proximal end of the limb. Ground drapes should be placed in the order which will allow the last drape placed to be the one by the IV pole that is suspending the limb (Figure 4.16). The risk of contamination is higher when placing that drape, and so it should be done last. After all ground drapes are placed and secured, the suspended limb will need to be cut down. To maintain the asepsis of the limb, the circulating tech should hold the foot of the suspended limb with one hand and use a scissors to cut the tape hanging the limb. The tape should be cut close to the foot to avoid any risk of a piece of tape from touching the prepped leg. The circulating technician can then move the IV pole away from the surgery table so the sterile team member can place the first large drape. This is done so a sterile area is provided on which to lay the limb, once the limb is ready to be laid down. The sterile team member can now take a sterile hand towel and take the foot from the circulating technician. It is imperative that the circulating tech not let go of the foot until it is known that the sterile member has control of the foot. Lack of observation of this detail can result in the limb being dropped, the sterile drapes, and potentially the sterile team members being contaminated and re-draping and re-gowning/gloving of the sterile team members will need to occur. The towel is wrapped around the foot of the patient to cover all the non-sterile tape and then

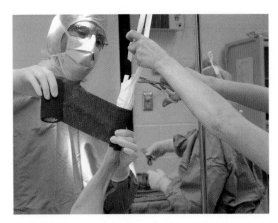

Figure 4.17 Surgeon grabbing the foot with sterile Vetwrap® while the circulating nurse cuts down the suspended limb.

secured with a towel clamp. Another option is to grab the foot with sterile Vetwrap® and cover all the tape (Figure 4.17). The limb can now be laid down on the sterile field. If a stockinette is used, it is now placed on the limb and unrolled proximally to cover all of the limb. As the stockinette reaches the proximal end of the limb, an operating scissors can be used to cut the remaining rolled portion of the stockinette so it can be completely unrolled. At this point, the remaining drapes can be placed in the following order: opposite the drape that is already on the table, cranial then caudal. It is important to remember that if the patient is in dorsal recumbency and the instrument table is over the chest of the animal, that table needs to be in place prior to beginning draping. In addition, if the table is over the patient, the caudal drape should be placed before the cranial drape. Some surgeons choose to use the povidone-iodine impregnated sticky drape for orthopedic cases. In most situations, the sticky drape is applied after all the drapes are in place. Making sure the limb is completely dry before application of the sticky drape will provide the greatest opportunity for good adhesion of the drape.

Other responsibilities

Other responsibilities of the surgical assistant include setting up the "back" or instrument table, passing surgical instruments, lavaging the tissue to insure tissue viability; providing hemostasis with either manual pressure with a gauze sponge or use of electrocautery; providing tissue retraction or limb manipulation as needed, and alerting the surgeon to any problem that may not have been noticed by the surgeon.

Setting up the instrument table

The surgical assistant is in charge of the "back" table or instrument table. The instruments should be laid out so the assistant can easily see the tips to quickly identify the instrument requested. For some surgical cases, the assistant will be standing opposite the surgeon on the other side of the surgery table. For other cases, they may be standing behind the instrument table at the caudal end of the surgery table. Some technicians like to assemble the instruments on the table so the "sharp" instruments (scalpel blades, scissors) are on one side and then progress across the table top to the "dull" instruments (hemostats). This order is logical and helps other sterile members find an instrument if need be.

Passing surgical instruments

Correctly and firmly passing an instrument to the surgeon or other sterile member is a critical skill. Communication or lack thereof, between the assistant and the surgeon can either enhance or negatively affect the flow of the case. Instruments handed with less than a firm "slap", may result in the instrument being dropped.

Scalpel handle and blade

Handing a scalpel handle loaded with a scalpel blade must be done safely because the risk of injury to the surgeon is great. Using an overhand grip the assistant should hold the handle with the blade facing them. The noncutting edge of the blade should be facing the palm. The handle and blade should be firmly placed in the waiting hand of the surgeon – noncutting edge first (Figure 4.18) (Tear, M. 2012).

Ring handled instruments

Ring-handled instruments should be held at the box lock or screw hinge in a vertical position, tips to the ceiling and ring handles to the floor (Figure 4.19). The instruments should be locked to the first ratchet or closed if no ratchet is present; so it is easier for the surgeon to grasp the ring handles. The instrument should be placed firmly in the palm of the waiting hand with the ring handles hitting the palm. Loading the needle holder with

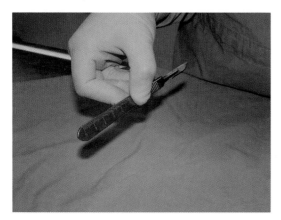

Figure 4.18 Proper method of passing a loaded scalpel blade and handle.

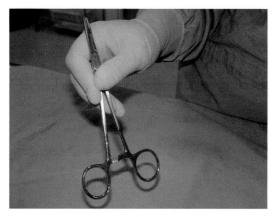

Figure 4.19   Proper method of passing a ring-handled instrument.

a suture needle should also be the assistant's responsibility. The needle holder should be placed about 3/4 of the way on the needle curve, closer to the suture attachment. The needle holder should never be clamped on the needle at the needle/suture junction. The needle should have the curve up so the surgeon is ready to place the first stitch.

Thumb tissue forceps

Thumb tissue forceps should also be held in a vertical fashion when being passed to the surgeon (Figure 4.20). The assistant should hold the thumb tissue forceps at the fused end with the tips facing the floor. Using this method will provide the surgeon with an instrument they can use right away instead of having to flip it

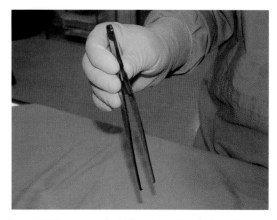

Figure 4.20 Proper method of passing a thumb tissue forceps.

around as well as keeping the assistant's hand out of the way of the surgeon accepting the instrument.

Lavaging

Maintaining the integrity of the tissue is a critical role of the surgical assistant. Sterile bowls should be filled, aseptically, with sterile saline and kept on the instrument table. The surgical assistant should hold the bowl off the sterile field to allow the circulating nurse to fill the bowl. The circulating nurse must be careful to not touch the bowl with the bottle of lavage fluid. Additionally, the bowl should not be overfilled, to avoid spillage once on the table (Figure 4.21). The bowl should be readily accessible, yet out of the way so as to avoid repeated bumping and spilling. Bulb syringes or gauze sponges are most commonly used to apply sterile

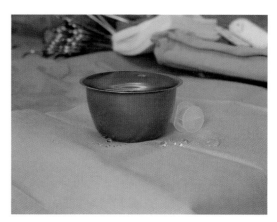

Figure 4.21 Fluid bowl too full.

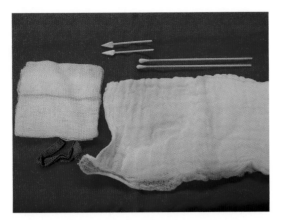

Figure 4.22 Options for hemostasis: radiopaque gauze sponge, radiopaque laparotomy pad, surgical spear, cotton-tipped applicator.

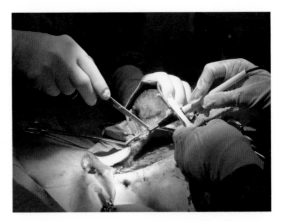

Figure 4.23 Assistant activating electrosurgery handpiece.

fluid to the exposed tissues. Tissue must be kept moistened at all times. Exposure to room air and heat from the surgical lights can lead to rapid dehydration and decreased viability. Tissues that may be exposed for long periods of time (exteriorized intestine, urinary bladder, etc.) should be covered with a saline-soaked radiopaque sponge or lap pad for increased moisture retention (Figure 4.22). Rehydrating the sponge, without removing it, can be done with a bulb syringe saturating the sponge as necessary. Surgeries that require using large amounts of lavage fluid (i.e., abdominal exploratory) should have warmed lavage fluids used. It is the responsibility of the circulating technician to warm the fluids. Continuous storage of the fluids in a warmer is ideal, but warm water bath warming is also an option. Warming fluids in a microwave is discouraged as hot spots within the bottle could result in fluids that are too warm damaging the patient.

Hemostasis

Electrosurgery, often called electrocautery, can be utilized by either touching the tissue/vessel directly with the electrocautery pencil, or by touching an instrument clamping a vessel or tissue (Figure 4.23). Technicians may be the one applying the electrosurgical pencil to the tissue or clamping the vessel with the hemostat. If electrosurgery is to be used, the cord from the hand piece must be secured on the sterile field to avoid having the hand piece slide off the field. Once the hand piece is on the sterile field, measure the cord to allow enough cord to reach all areas of the field. At the determined length,

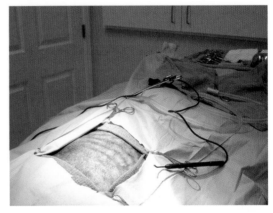

Figure 4.24 Electrosurgery pencil and suction tubing set up on the sterile field.

loop the cord in half and slip it through one ring handle of a towel clamp securing a drape. Then take the loop and place it around the other ring handle of the same instrument (Figure 4.24). This will secure the cord without inhibiting electric flow to the hand piece. Then the rest of the cord can be tossed off the sterile field so the circulating nurse can plug it in. Hemostasis can also be achieved by applying pressure with a gauze sponge. Small vessels or capillaries that are bleeding can often be controlled with pressure rather than using electrosurgery. A 16 ply 4″ × 4″ radiopaque sponge that is completely soaked will hold approximately 13 mls of blood. A 12″ × 12″ laparotomy sponge, soaking wet will hold ~65 mls. Radiopaque should ALWAYS be used on surgical fields. The radiopaque thread or strip in the sponge will allow for easy identification on a radiograph should a sponge be unaccounted for at the end of the procedure.

Hemostasis, as well as field vision, can also be controlled by the use of suction. Suction tubing can be secured in a similar fashion as the electrocautery. After determining the necessary length to remain on the sterile field, pass the tubing through one ring handle of a different towel clamp securing a drape, then pass it through the opposite ring handle of the same instrument. Make sure that the tubing is not kinked anywhere to compromise suction intensity. The rest of the tubing can be tossed off the table for the circulating nurse to connect to the suction unit.

Retraction

Excellent assistants will know exactly how much pressure can be placed on tissue with an instrument before damage occurs and will be able to recognize abnormalities in tissue appearance and will alert the surgeon. Ill colored tissue, a decrease in blood pressure (evidenced by decreased oozing), or malposition of tissue or an organ are all examples of what the surgeon may unintentionally miss. The surgeon is focusing on the problem of the patient that is to be corrected (as they should) and may not see "the whole picture" as the assistant does. In no way is it intended that the assistant insinuates the surgeon is not performing their duty, but rather the welfare of the patient is everyone's main concern.

Instrument maintenance

In addition to understanding all the instrumentation and equipment and how it works, the assistant is responsible for maintaining that equipment during the procedure. Blood and other gross material are very damaging to instruments if allowed to dry on the instrument. Not only does it instigate corrosion and pitting, but more importantly, it hinders the efficient function of the instrument. If a hemostatic forceps box lock and tip is covered in blood it will not open and close easily nor will it provide the 100% hemostasis and clamping pressure that it was designed to provide. That could prove catastrophic in an emergency situation. Surgical assistants must continually clean and wipe off instruments on the back table with sterile saline and gauze. It is important that the instruments are wiped clean and not allowed to soak in saline. Prolonged exposure to saline will cause pitting of the instrument

and is equally as damaging as allowing debris to dry on the instrument (Reuss-Lamky, H. 2011). Cleanliness of instrumentation is paramount in situations where the instrument will be repeatedly used such as drill bits and taps for screw placement, or rasps, or files in joint arthroplasty procedures. Each time the surgeon uses an instrument during a procedure, it needs to function as well as the first time it was used.

Loading the scalpel blade is the responsibility of the technician running the instrument table. Care should be taken to avoid injury while performing this seemingly easy yet dangerous task. First of all, using the correct instrument to seat the blade on the handle is paramount. The *only* instrument that should be used is a needle holder. Never use a hemostatic forceps as the grooves in the tip can be damaged by the metal of the scalpel blade and cause the forceps to perform inadequately when it needs to clamp a vessel. Another common method of loading the blade onto the handle is using one's thumb and index finger. This is extremely dangerous and should never be done; one slip and a career-altering injury can result. To correctly load the blade, use the needle holder and grasp the noncutting side of the blade (Figure 4.25). Hold the blade handle so the tip of the handle has the grooved edge facing up. Starting at the tip of the handle, place the opening of on the blade on the groove of the tip (Figure 4.26). Advance the blade until it seats securely on the blade handle (Figure 4.27).

There may be an audible "click" when the blade is firmly in place. Gently tug on the blade to insure its correct placement.

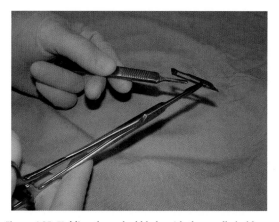

Figure 4.25 Holding the scalpel blade with the needle holder.

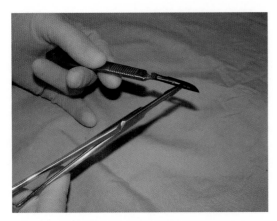

Figure 4.26 Begin placing the blade on the handle.

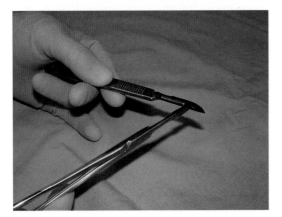

Figure 4.27 Fully seated blade.

Sponge/instrument count

Performing a sponge count and instrument count before the incision is made and before the incision is closed also falls to the surgical assistant. Knowing the status of all sponges and instruments is a critical role of the assistant. Sponges (and less frequently, instruments) have been left in small animal patients. This incident is unacceptable as it is completely avoidable, especially when a technician is the surgical assistant. To perform a sponge count, all sponges on the sterile field are counted before the incision is made and reported to the circulating nurse. A note should be made on the operating room report form. As sponges are added they should be counted, reported to the circulating nurse and added to the OR report form. As sponges are used, they should only be discarded in a designated place. Whether a specified sponge bowl on the sterile field or

a designated kick bucket on the floor, that is the only area dirty gauze from the surgical procedure should be found. Sponges open on a surgical field should be in one of three places: on the instrument table, in the hand of the surgeon and/or assistant or in the dirty sponge bucket located off the sterile field. *Never* leave a sponge just lying on the surgical field! Before the incision closure begins, the unused sponges on the instrument table should be counted by the assistant. The used sponges off the sterile field are counted by the circulating nurse. Both numbers are added and should equal the total number of sponges opened and reported on the OR report form. If there is a discrepancy the hunt must begin for the missing sponge(s). Sponges often hide under drape corners or are inadvertently thrown in the wrong kick bucket. Missing sponges must be accounted for before the wound is closed. Small 4″ × 4″ or 4″ × 8″ sponges should not be used to pack off organs in the abdomen or chest as they are too small and are easily forgotten or misplaced. Large radiopaque lap sponges (Figure 4.28) should be the only devices that can be packed into a body cavity. With a larger surface area and radiopaque indicator, they are more difficult to misplace or forget about.

Procedure-specific duties

Depending on the procedure, there may be additional expectations of the assistant. During an arthroscopy it is imperative that experienced hands are assisting the surgeon. Controlling the fluid flow in and out of the joint, manipulating the limb for maximum

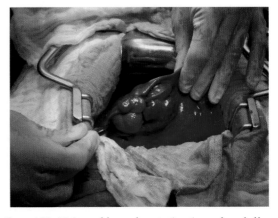

Figure 4.28 Moistened lap pad protecting tissues from balfour retractor.

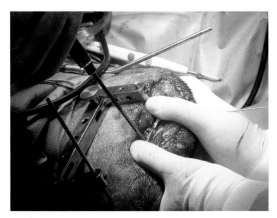

Figure 4.29 Assistant stabilizing limb for placement of a TPLO plate.

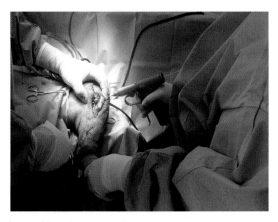

Figure 4.30 Assistant removing pins

visibility, monitoring the limb for fluid extravasation and assisting with instrument manipulation are all talents the surgeon expects of the assistant. Knowing the assistant will step up and perform, without being asked is invaluable to the surgeon. Other minimally invasive procedures have equally critical needs of the assistant. Making sure the circulating technician has the monitor positioned properly for a laparoscopy, knowing which trocar and cannula are needed before the laparoscope is placed can make a procedure run effortlessly. Stifle surgeries and fracture repairs can also benefit greatly from an efficient assistant being a member of the sterile team. Whether assisting with a Tibial Plateau Leveling Osteotomy (TPLO) (Figures 4.29 and 4.30) or a mid-humeral fracture repair with plates and screws, having an assistant that knows the order of the instruments needed for screw placement

(drill guide, drill bit, depth gauge, tap, tap sleeve, screw, and screwdriver) and hands them as the surgeon needs them, can save measurable time during a procedure.

Suture materials and suture patterns (MacPhail, C. 2007)

Another skill required of the surgical assistant is the knowledge of suture materials, suture patterns, and stapling devices that may be utilized during the procedure. In addition, the surgical assistant must be familiar with specific characteristics of each suture type, indications for use, patterns chosen by the surgeon and the stapling options available. If there were a perfect suture it would have the following characteristics:

- pliable for easy handling
- low tissue drag
- minimal tissue reactivity
- little memory
- consistent uniform diameter
- high tensile strength
- predictable performance

Many of these characteristics are achieved by the sutures currently available, but none is the ideal suture. Having said that, these characteristics as well as others will influence the decision regarding which suture is chosen. Often not only are the suture characteristics taken into consideration, but the surgeons personal preference as well. Availability of product, area of the body being sutured, the patient's overall health and the viability of the tissue being sutured also affect the decision (Table 4.1).

Characteristics

Pliability of the suture is an important factor to consider. The easier it is for the surgeon to handle and manipulate the suture, the faster the procedure will progress. Also, ease of handling generally equates to better knot security. Most frequently multifilament sutures will be easier to handle (Dunn, D.L. 2007).

Tissue drag means the suture moves easily through the tissues and therefore causes less irritation to the tissue. It is desirable for suture to have this characteristic to minimize tissue irritation and stress, which could compromise wound healing. Monofilament and coated sutures often provide minimal tissue drag.

Table 4.1 Suture characteristics.

Suture name	Generic name	Natural/ synthetic	Absorbable/ non-absorbable	Monofilament/ multifilament	Tensile strength	Absorption rate	Comments
Plain gut		Natural	Absorbable		Tensile strength loss affected by patient characteristics	Absorbed by enzymatic process	Available as yellowish tan and dyed blue
Chromic Catgut		Natural	Absorbable	Monofilament	Tensile strength loss affected by patient characteristics	Absorbed by enzymatic process	Available brown and dyed blue
PDS	Polidioxanone	Synthetic	Absorbable	Monofilament	70% remains at 2 wks 50% remains at 4 wks 25% remains at 6 wks	At 6 mo essentially complete	Available in clear, blue and violet
Biosyn®	Glycomer 631	Synthetic	Absorbable	Monofilament	75% at 2 wks; ~40% at 3 wks	Complete between 90–110 d	Excellent know security, minimal memory
Maxon		Synthetic	Absorbable	Monofilament	75% at 2 wks; 65% at 3 wks; 50% at 4 wks	Minimal for first 60 d; Complete within 6 mo	Excellent handling; minimal memory
Monocryl®	Poliglecaprone 25	Synthetic	Absorbable	Monofilament	50–60% remains at 1 wk 20–30% remains at 2 wks Lost by 3 wks	91–119 d shows completion	Available undyed and violet. Also available with antimicrobial coating
Caprosyn®	Polyglytone 6211	Synthetic	Absorbable	Monofilament	Lost by 21 d post implantation	Complete in 56 d	Excellent handling; excellent know security
Vicryl	Polyglactin 910	Synthetic	Absorbable	Multifilament	75% remains at 2 wks 50% remains at 3 wks 25% remains at 4 wks	56–70 d to completion	Available undyed and violet. Also available with antimicrobial coating
Dexon		Synthetic	Absorbable	Multifilament	65% at 2 wks; 35% at 3 wks	Complete between 60–90 d	Available dyed green or undyed
Ethilon	Nylon	Synthetic	Non-absorbable	Monofilament	Gradual loss over time due to hydrolysis	Gradual encapsulation over time	Available green, clear and violet
Prolene	Polypropylene	Synthetic	Non-absorbable	Monofilament	No degradation	Nonabsorbable	Available clear and blue
Silk		Natural	Non-absorbable	Multifilament	Gradual loss over time due to progressive degredation	Gradual encapsulation over time	Available in violet and white
Mersilene	Polyester	Synthetic	Non-absorbable	Multifilament	No change known to occur	Gradual encapsulation over time	Available in white and green

Memory is the act of the suture returning to its packaged coiled state, which provides challenges when working with it. Suture that coils tends to become knotted or tangled more easily. Multifilament sutures generally have less memory than other suture.

Tensile strength is the amount of force, in pounds, that the suture can withstand before breaking. This characteristic is important to consider when suturing tissues that are under a lot of physical stress. Frequently the tensile strength of a suture increases with the size (diameter) of the suture.

A uniform diameter size is critical for insuring quality knot security. If the suture is wider in section of the strand than in others, the knots will not be equally formed and therefore will not have good security. This characteristic is controlled by quality assurance practices of the suture manufacturer. Suture of lesser quality may not have the stringent quality control measures of higher grade materials.

Finally, predictable performance is important from the surgeon's perspective. Surgeon's preference often determines the suture chosen and if a surgeon has had a bad experience using a particular suture, it is safe to say it won't be chosen again.

Sizing

Suture material is sized according to USP (United States Pharmacopia) standards. The easiest way to remember suture sizing is to remember the following: The more zeros, the smaller the suture and the larger the whole number the larger the suture. Suture sizes can be written one of two ways – 000 is three zeros so it is called three ought. This could also be written 3–0. A suture that is 00000 is five zeros or five ought or 5–0 and is a smaller suture in diameter than the 3–0. Number 2 suture is a whole number and is therefore larger in diameter than 3–0. The size suture chosen by the surgeon has many factors influencing the decision including patient size and the tissue being worked with. Other things that are considered by the surgeon before selecting a size include intended purpose, tissue integrity, number of layers of closure to be used, and type of suture pattern placed. In general, surgeons will choose the smallest size possible to hold the tissue as it heals. This practice minimizes additional tissue trauma and results in the least amount of foreign material in the patient. Wounds over active joints (stifle, elbow) may need a larger size suture to bear the additional stress on the wound. Incisions on non-weight bearing areas (abdomen, medial limb) may be adequately closed with a smaller sized suture.

Classification

Sutures are classified by three areas: absorbable versus nonabsorbable; multifilament versus monofilament; and synthetic versus natural qualities.

Absorbable versus nonabsorbable (Figure 4.31)

The quality of absorbable versus nonabsorbable is fairly self explanatory. Absorbable sutures are broken down in the body by one of two different methods. Natural absorbable suture is broken down by enzymes that weaken the suture strand. Synthetic absorbable suture is hydrolyzed, which means water penetrates the strands and breaks down the polymers. This type of absorption causes much less tissue reaction than enzyme degradation. There is the rare instance of a nonabsorbable eventually breaking down (i.e., silk), but it is safe to say nonabsorbable suture will remain in the tissue for an indefinite time period following implantation. Absorbable suture is almost exclusively used on internal tissue. Absorbable sutures are most often used in general surgery except for cardiovascular, ophthalmic, and neurologic procedures. The experienced assistant will know what type of suture the surgeon is most likely to choose and the pattern of placement that will probably be employed. Although entirely the surgeon's decision/ preference and case dependence, the circulating technician can *anticipate* which material will be used, but will also be able to provide whatever the surgeon requests.

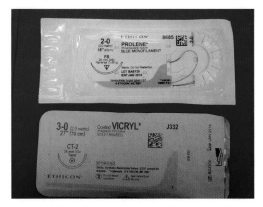

Figure 4.31 Absorbable (bottom) versus nonabsorbable.

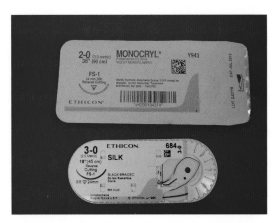

Figure 4.32 Monofilament (top) versus multifilament(braided).

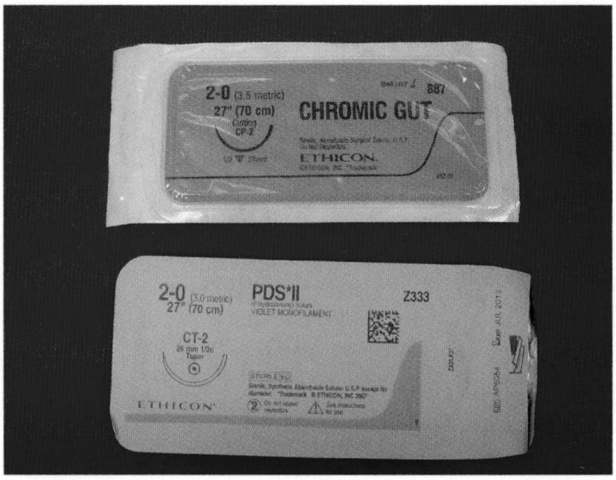

Figure 4.33 Natural (top) versus synthetic.

Monofilament versus multifilament (Figure 4.32)

Monofilament sutures are one solid strand of material. This type of suture is often chosen when the risk of infection is present as it does not harbor bacteria, which can cause an infection later. Another advantage of this type of suture is that it glides more easily through the tissues therefore causing less tissue resistance. Monofilament sutures usually ties easily, but care must be taken to avoid kinking the material while making knots. Kinking can weaken the suture and lead to premature breakdown of the strand. Multifilament sutures are multiple strands twisted or braided together. This type of suture has handles wonderfully, has little memory, and provides good knot security. The disadvantages include increased tissue resistance when passing through tissue, and increased risk of infection as it can "wick" or harbor harmful bacteria, which can cause infections.

Natural versus synthetic (Figure 4.33)

Natural sutures are made of materials found in nature, such as catgut and silk. Synthetic suture is that which is created as a product of man-made materials. Some examples of synthetic suture include those made of polypropylene or polymers.

Suture material

Absorbable sutures - monofilament

Catgut is one of the most commonly used absorbable sutures. It is made of sheep intestine submucosa or the serosal layer of beef intestinal. It is 97–98% pure collagen that is spun into strands and then polished into a monofilament product. Both plain gut and chromic gut are available. Plain gut has a very rapid absorption time (completed by 70 days) but tensile strength is maintained only for 5–7 days. Plain gut has very limited use in veterinary surgery and is therefore not seen very often. Chromic catgut is plain gut that has been treated with chromium salts, which resist enzymes and therefore extend the absorption time up to 90 days. With chromic gut tensile strength duration is doubled to 10–14 days. The treatment with chromium salts will turn the whitish/yellow plain gut into a brownish/tan-colored suture.

Other monofilament sutures that have been available for a while include polydioxanon (PDS®) and polyglyconate (Maxon®). Both are synthetic products that have varying absorption times from three months to six months, yet are known for maintaining their tensile strength for greater than 21 days. For gastrointestinal, respiratory, and urinary procedures, a monofilament absorbable suture will often be chosen. In a case where the tissues are more traumatized or diseased, this longer time frame may be desirable. Despite their inert property and ability to move easily through tissue, they do present some difficulties when working with them. These sutures are fairly stiff, have excessive memory, and require additional throws for good knot security. These properties illustrate that these sutures are not the best choices for subcutaneous or intradermal suture patterns.

Newer monofilament absorbable sutures include poliglecaprone25 (Monocryl®), glycomer 631 (Biosyn®), and polyglytone 6211(Caprosyn®). These products may be a better choice for uncompromised tissue that will regain strength rapidly. Urinary bladder cases as well as certain gastric procedures would be good indications for choosing these sutures. " ... suture should be chosen to match the healing rate of the tissue."[6] are words to live by in the operating room and assistants and circulating techs should feel comfortable suggesting alternatives to surgeons instead of using the same thing all the time. Other benefits of some of the newer monofilament absorbable products are increased ease of handling, significant tensile strength loss up to 14 days post-placement, minimal tissue reactions, and complete absorption as early as 56 days.

Absorbable – multifilament

Multifilament absorbable suture like polyglactin 910 (Vicryl®) and polyglycolic acid (Dexon®) are proven classics. These are also synthetic sutures that have absorption times from 42 to 70 days. As a multifilament, their use in visceral tissue is contraindicated; however, due to their ease of handling, they are often used as subcuticular sutures. Some multifilament sutures are available with a coating of lactide, glyclide, and calcium state, which allows the suture to pass through tissues with much less resistance. Some coated multifilaments are also available with the antibacterial agent Triclosan added to help inhibit colonizing of bacteria on the sutures. Many cases of tissue reaction at the incision when polyglactin 910 (Vicryl®) is used have created some hesitancy to use this suture. A new multifilament absorbable suture is Polysorb® and offers a new alternative to surgeons. Due to its tensile strength decreasing to 30% at 21 days and its complete absorption by 60 days post placement, the opportunity for tissue reaction is lessened, therefore resulting in fewer incisional issues.

Non-absorbable suture – monofilament

Monofilament nonabsorbable sutures are used primarily for skin closure, tube security or holding wound-covering devices in place. Occasionally, nonabsorbable suture material may be used internally, such as in stifle surgeries or in closure of the abdominal wall of a patient with adhesions or multiple surgery history where healing may be compromised. Cardiovascular procedures (graft placement, valve replacement, etc.) will use nonabsorbable suture to insure the integrity of the repair is not compromised by suture that can breakdown. Internal structures with limited blood supply (i.e., tendons, fascia) are often apposed with nonabsorbable suture due to the slow healing of the tissue. When using nonabsorbable suture for skin closure, the color of the suture should be taken into consideration based on the patient's hair coat color. For example, finding black nylon skin sutures on a black Laborador Retriever 14 days post implantation is quite a challenge. However, blue polypropylene sutures on the same patient would be much easier to see and accomplish the same end result. The most commonly seen monofilament nonabsorbable sutures are nylon (Ethilon®), and polyprolylene (Prolene®). Available in a variety of sizes, either suture is suitable for feline to equine patients. Nylon is available in both black monofilament and braided styles. Polyproylene (Prolene®) is another commonly used monofilament nonabsorbable suture. Colored a bright blue, it is easily distinguishable with almost every color hair coat. Stainless steel is another monofilament nonabsorbable choice. Although not used frequently in veterinary patients, it is sometimes chosen to help deter licking of the incision by anxious patients. Finally, polybutester (Novalfil™) and polyvinylidene glouride (Pronova™) are two other monofilament, nonabsorbable sutures. Polybutester is available as a clear or blue product. Due to the fact that seeing suture through the skin is not as important in veterinary patients, the blue may be a more common choice due to the ease of seeing the suture when suturing. Polyvinylidene is available in pigmented blue and is often used in cardiovascular and vascular surgeries.

Non-absorbable – multifilament

Braided nonabsorbable sutures include polyester (Mersilene®), silk and Vetafil®, or Fluorofil®. Polyester is a pliable braided suture indicated for internal use for all types of procedures including cardiovascular, ophthalmic, and neurologic cases. It is contraindicated as a skin suture due to its braided nature. Silk is another multifilament nonabsorbable suture that is frequently used for ligation or cardiovascular cases. Silk has long been regarded as the premier suture when it comes to ease of handling. The raw silk filament, which is produced by the silk worm is degummed and then braided into strands. The naturally occurring gum on the suture enables the cocoon to hold together but is of no benefit in surgery and needs to be removed by the degumming process. Although classified as a nonabsorbable suture, silk is relatively non-detectable in tissue 2 years after implantation. Vetafil is a synthetic nonabsorbable suture. It is basically a hollow suture that has multiple strands constructing the wall around a hollow middle. It is inexpensive compared to other nonabsorbable choices and therefore is often used as a skin closure material. As with the absorbable sutures, the final selection of a non-absorbable suture is the decision of the surgeon, however technicians can anticipate what will be requested. Circulating techs should refrain from opening any suture until either asked to do so or until they have checked with the surgeon.

Suture patterns

Some states allow credentialed technicians to suture skin incisions of surgical patients. Although it is a wonderful use of a surgical assistant, only a minority of states encourage this practice. Even if the technician will not be performing the suturing, it is important that they understand the placement process of the patterns. "Running" the suture during a continuous pattern or being ready to cut the sutures to the correct length during an interrupted pattern, are very important skills for the assistant. Suture patterns are either continuous or interrupted. Continuous patterns are placed by the surgeon without ever cutting the suture until at the end of the pattern. Interrupted patterns have the suture cut after each stitch is placed. Continuous patterns are faster to place but bear the risk of incisional dehiscence if even one stitch breaks down. Interrupted patterns take longer to place and use more suture, but the entire incision is not compromised if one stitch has issues.

Suture patterns are also classified by the way they appose tissue. Appositional patterns means the tissue edges just meet and healing occurs side to side. Everting patterns result in the skin edges turning out – away from the patient. These patterns usually result in more scarring as well as slower healing. Inverting patterns turn the tissue edges inward, toward the patient and are reserved for use on hollow organs such as intestines or the stomach.

Continuous patterns
Simple continuous
Probably the most commonly used continuous pattern is the simple continuous (Figure 4.34). It is used to close

muscle layers, body cavities, and even skin closures (Fossum, T. 2007). It is placed by taking a bite on one side of the tissue gap, passing the needle under the tissue gap and then the needle comes up on the other side, an equal distance from the gap as the initial bite. The suture is pulled tight to make the edges of the wound appositional. The next bite starts on the same side as the first bite, passes under the tissue, and comes up on the opposite side – following the same process as the first stitch. The suture is pulled to appose the edges and the pattern continues to the end of the wound. As the surgeon progresses through the wound closure, the assistant is responsible for holding the suture or "running" the suture (Figure 4.35). Holding

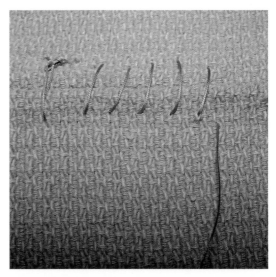

Figure 4.34 Simple continuous.

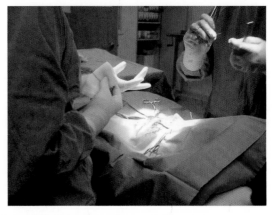

Figure 4.35 Assistant running suture for surgeon.

the suture out of the way for the surgeon will greatly assist in the speed with which the pattern can be placed. Maintaining enough tension, but not too much, on the suture also is the responsibility of the assistant. Ending the pattern can be accomplished by not pulling the suture tight with the last stitch. Leaving a loop provides a method of creating the knot to end the pattern. Depending on where the pattern is being placed, some people choose to bury the knot. This can be done only by cutting the loop strands of the knot. This leaves the long end of the suture still intact. The needle is passed under the tissue beyond the end of the suture line, and the needle re-surfaces approximately 1/2″ to 1″ beyond the end of the suture line and is pulled tight. This results in the knot being pulled under the tissue. The suture is cut close to the tissue so the suture end disappears once cut.

Ford interlocking

The Ford Interlocking continuous pattern is used less frequently in small animal surgery than in large animal surgery. This suture pattern resembles a "blanket stitch" for anyone familiar with sewing patterns (Figure 4.36). The benefit of a Ford Interlocking pattern is its strength and it is primarily used as a skin closure pattern. Having an assistant who can effectively run the suture with this pattern is especially helpful for the veterinary surgeon. When beginning the pattern the first bite is the needle starting approximately 1/2″ lateral to the incision, passing the needle under the tissue gap and then having the needle exit an equal distance from the incision on the opposite side. The suture strand is held parallel to

the incision and the needle passes over the long strand. The stitch is repeated in the same fashion, passing over the long strand each time to create the pattern.

Lembert, Cushing, Connell patterns

These three patterns are inverting continuous patterns used to close hollow organs. Surgical assistants are less frequently called upon to assist with organ closure, but may still need to run the suture for the surgeon placing one of these patterns.

Interrupted patterns
Simple interrupted

This is the most frequently used interrupted pattern (Figure 4.37). This pattern can be used internally, subcutaneously, or externally. To create this pattern, the needle is passed through the tissue approximately 1/2″ from the wound edge, under the incision or tissue gap and exiting on the opposite side, an equal distance from the wound. The suture is then tied with the knot off to one side so it isn't on the incision. If internal, this stitch should have the suture ends cut close to the knot, without cutting the knot. If placed externally, the suture strands should be cut approximately 1/2″–3/4″ in length so they can be found and held during suture removal.

Horizontal mattress

This suture pattern is often used in areas where there is a lot of tension. It is therefore, rarely seen as a skin suture, unless tension is present (Figure 4.38). To place this suture pattern, the needle is driven through the

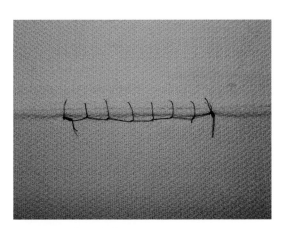

Figure 4.36 Ford interlocking.

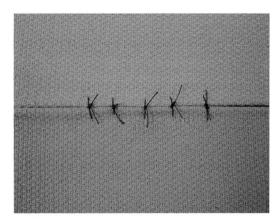

Figure 4.37 Simple Interrupted.

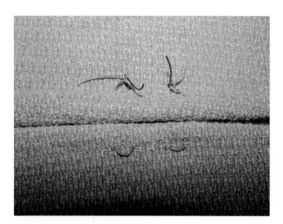

Figure 4.38 Horizontal Mattress.

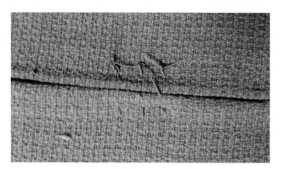

Figure 4.40 Vertical Mattress.

skin, approximately 1/2″ from the wound edge, on the far side and under the incision. The needle exits on the near side of the wound, approximately 1/2″ from the wound edge. The needle is then moved approximately 4 mm down the incision line and introduced from the near side. The needle passes under the wound and exits on the far side, approximately 1/2″ from the wound edge. The suture is then tied and the knot rests on the skin parallel to the wound. It is easy to evert this pattern, so if assistants are involved with the placement, care must be taken to avoid over pulling the suture and creating the eversion.

Cruciate pattern

This pattern is a variation of the horizontal mattress pattern and can be used internally as well as eternally

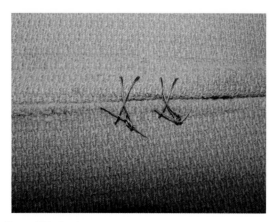

Figure 4.39 Cruciate.

(Figure 4.39). This pattern is started exactly the same way as the horizontal mattress. The needle is introduced through the tissue on the far side of the wound by placing the needle approximately 1/2″ from the wound edge. The needle is passed under the tissue gap and exits approximately 1/2″ from the edge of the wound on the opposite side. Now to make it different than the horizontal mattress, the needle is moved about 4 mm down the wound and passed through the tissue, starting on the far side. The suture is now tied and an "X" appears created from the suture over the wound. As with the simple interrupted, the knot is usually placed off the wound line.

Vertical mattress

The vertical mattress pattern may be placed where there is a lot of tension, as with the horizontal mattress (Figure 4.40). Known to be stronger than the horizontal mattress, it takes more time to place this pattern. The needle is introduced approximately 8 mm from the wound edge on the far side of the wound. The needle passes under the tissue gap and exits on the opposite side, again 8 mm from the wound edge. The needle is then reintroduced on the same side it just exited, half way between the exit site and the wound edge. The needle passes under the tissue gap and exits on the opposite side, again half way between the wound edge and the first puncture. The suture is then tied and the knot is on the side of the wound.

Knot tying

The knot between two pieces of suture material is the weakest point of the suture. A knot is described as two throws of suture on top of one another and then tightened. The method of placement of these throws can result in either a square knot or a granny knot. Granny knots, half hitches, or other misplaced throws can result in dehiscence of a wound due to poor knot security. Though many factors can influence the performance of a knot (i.e., the length of the cut ends, the material coefficient and the configuration of the knot) the configuration is the most reliable predictor of knot security. Superimposed square knots are the desirable configuration for the best knot security. It is possible to tie a suture knot using a couple of different methods. One way is to use the instruments to tie the knots. This method is generally more common in veterinary surgery due to the lack of waste of material. Another way to tie a knot is to do a hand tie. Whether doing an instrument tie or a hand tie, the rules for tying the knots are the same.

When typing knots it is important to pay attention to tension and hand position. When wrapping one suture end around another, the ends need to wind up facing the opposite direction. The suture ends should have equal and opposing tension as well as having the hands remain in the same plane (i.e., the hands remain level with one another). As the next throw is formed by wrapping the suture strands around one another, there is a very important step to remember. This time when the hands pull to tighten the suture, they need to move in an opposite motion from the first throw that was tightened. This action will result in the formation of a square knot. Failing to reverse the direction of the hands will result in a slip knot or half hitch.

Technicians allowed to suture in their state of employ, are referred to any veterinary surgical textbook for complete knot tying and suturing techniques.

Cutting suture

In addition to being knowledgeable about the pattern being placed and the characteristics of the suture, the surgical assistant must know how long or short to leave the suture ends when they are asked to cut the suture. The surgeon may give some indication of the length desired, but a great assistant will already know. Assistants must also know if they are cutting just one strand of the suture or both. Frequently, the surgeon will indicate "just one or both," but there is nothing

more frustrating than to have both strands cut when a continuous pattern was to be used.

Internal sutures

When cutting internally placed suture material, the assistant must know that the suture ends need to be short, but not so short that the knot is compromised or even cut. Internal sutures are generally cut short to decrease the amount of foreign material in the body that can potentially lead to inflammation and infection. To accomplish just the right consistent length, the blades of the operating scissors can be opened approximately 1/2″ and slid down the suture until the knot is reached. The scissor blades are then turned 45° and the suture is cut. This will provide for a short suture end without being too close to the knot (Figure 4.41).

External sutures

External sutures may vary in size depending on several factors. The surgeon must consider the number of layers of tissue already closed. When more layers are closed with suture, the dependency on the skin for strength with healing decreases. Also the surgeon must be considerate of the personality of the patient. This is where the technician can provide valuable information. If the patient has the type of personality that will lead to increased licking or chewing of the incision and sutures, then that information should be shared as it will affect what the surgeon chooses to use. Finally, the surgeon must think about the anatomic location of the wound. If it is a very tense skin closure (i.e., mastectomy) or an incision that will be exposed to a lot of motion due to

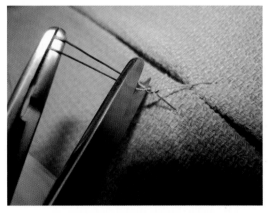

Figure 4.41 Scissor position for cutting internal sutures.

the fact that it is over a joint, the surgeon will have to adjust the suture type and pattern. Externally placed sutures, whether to secure drains, close an orifice (i.e., purse string suture) or skin incision sutures, must have suture "tails" or ends left long enough so they can easily be found when it is time to remove the sutures. Usually drain sutures or orifice sutures are removed shortly after they are placed (hours to days). Skin sutures are generally removed 7–14 days post placement. Patient healing status as well as other factors (medications such as corticosteroids, environment, patient tolerance), may affect that time frame. When cutting external sutures, generally a 1/2"–3/4" suture end is left. Often times, the surgeon may cross the two strands of suture and where the two meet is an indication of where to cut the suture (Figure 4.42).

Skin staples

External skin staples may be used to close the skin instead of conventional suture. The benefits of skin staples include shorter anesthesia time, faster wound closure, increased integrity due to the fact that staples can withstand more patient licking that suture, and relative ease of removal. Disadvantages include expense, poor performance in incisions with increased tension and tendency for rotation, which makes removal more challenging. Skin staples also easily evert the wound edges, which in turn makes the healing much less cosmetic. Skin staples are metal implants that are enclosed within a gun-like apparatus (Figure 4.43).

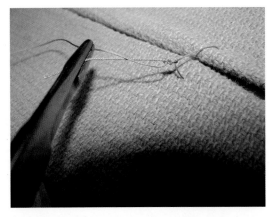

Figure 4.42 Suture strands crossed to indicate where to cut external sutures.

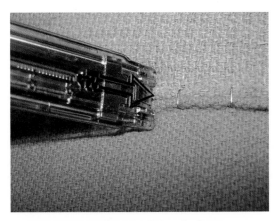

Figure 4.43 Proper approach for skin staple placement.

After the wound edges are apposed with a thumb tissue forceps, the stapler is fired and a staple is placed. Staples are not as secure as skin sutures and should be placed approximately 6 mm apart from one another. As with skin sutures, the number of staples placed should be recorded in the patient's medical record so that at the time of removal no staples or stitches are accidentally left in the animal.

Internal staples

Internal stapling devices are intended to be used instead of sutures. Although expensive, the benefit of shaving critical minutes off the procedure is overwhelmingly beneficial. Staples and the accompanying stapling devices are named for their function. The LDS™ *ligating dividing stapler* device discharges only one staple at a time. With a curved tip to slip under a vessel, this device will clamp (ligate), cut (divide), and occlude (staple) all in one smooth move with the pull of the trigger. This device proves very helpful when performing splenectomies or other highly vascularized tissue that needs to be excised (Figure 4.44). There are also individual clips that can be used to ligate vessels (Figure 4.45). The linear stapling devices available are the TA and GIA staplers (Figures 4.46 and 4.47). A TA™ *reusable stapler* is intended for thoraco-abdominal cases. TA staplers also have a number in the name, which indicates the length in millimeters of "B" shaped staples that will be placed. TA staplers are available in 30, 55, and 90 mm options. There is also a TA vascular device (TA30-V3), which places 3 staggered rows of B-shaped staples. This device was designed for use with

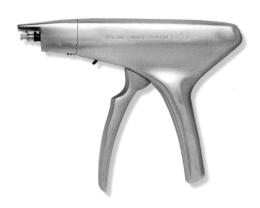

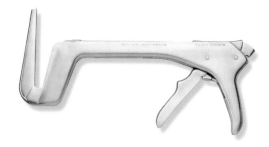

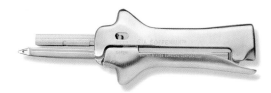

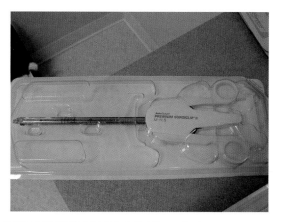

Figure 4.45 Single internal staple/clip applicator.

limited in veterinary surgery. Staples can be especially beneficial when performing an anastamosis due to the increased time that is consumed while suturing.

Almost all of the internal stapling devices discharge the entire cartridge when activated. Careful attention to loading and handling of the loaded device is critical to avoid a costly accidental discharge.

Circulating nurse

Another very important role of the technician within the surgical suite is that of the circulating nurse. The responsibilities of the circulator include setting up and preparing the operating room for the procedure, aseptically opening all needed equipment, anticipating the needs of the surgeon, retrieving any equipment or supply requested, and most importantly monitoring the asepsis of the procedure.

Setting up the room
Before any surgical case begins, the surgical suite needs to be prepared. All surfaces including tables, shelves, light fixtures, and so on must be wiped free of dust that may have settled. A cloth and 70% Isopropyl

large vessels. TA staples are used for lung lobectomies, tumor resections, partial splenectomies, partial gastrectomies, or intestinal anastomosis. The GIA™ *reusable stapler* is a linear device that has two interlocking rows of B-shaped staples and then cuts in between the two rows.

The GIA stapler is indicated for intestinal anastomosis or partial gastrectomies. When used with a TA stapler, a functional end-to-end anastamosis can be created. The EEA (end-to-end anastamosis) stapler is a device that places a circular double row of staples. The circular blade within the cartridge removes the excess inverted tissue, thus creating a new lumen. The cartridge size available and the challenging application process make the use of this device very alcohol are sufficient to accomplish this task. Next, the equipment necessary for the case must be placed in the room. Especially in a multi-doctor hospital, it may be helpful for the circulating nurse to have "case cards" for each surgeon/case. For instance, if Dr. Smith likes his patients positioned a certain way for a procedure, that information could be on the card as well as all the special equipment he wants for that procedure. Dr. Johnson, however, likes her patients positioned a different way for the same procedure and she uses different equipment. The case cards will help ensure that the room is ready with that surgeon's particular needs. Placing the packs and equipment in the proper location for ease of opening and flow of getting the procedure started is very important (Figure 4.48). Placing the electrosurgery ground plate on the table should also be the responsibility of the circulating nurse (Figure 4.49). Some electrosurgery ground pads are designed to adhere to the patient. Others are metal/vinyl plates and must be covered with a saline or water-soaked sponge to ensure proper grounding. Alcohol must *never* be used as it is flammable. Setting up the suction machine and ensuring anti fatigue mats are in place are additional steps in setting up the room. Determining that all needed equipment and suture is available is something that must be attended to by the circulating nurse prior to the procedure beginning.

Opening packs

Aseptically opening all the equipment and supplies used for a procedure is a very important task for the circulating nurse. Depending on the type of pack to be opened,

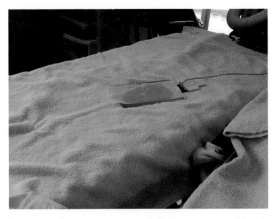

Figure 4.49 Electrosurgery ground plate on surgery table prior to the arrival of the patient.

the method of opening the pack can be different. For instance, if it is a gown pack, there is no sterile person to take the pack after the first wrapper is opened, so the circulating nurse must open both wrappers. To avoid dropping any of the contents of a gown pack as well as providing a sterile field for the person gowning, requires the pack to be sitting on a table as it is opened. When opening any pack, the first step is to determine that it is in fact the pack that is desired. Reading the tape label and performing a quick check to ensure the pack has been through a sterilizing cycle is very important. Remove the tape and the tab that is facing the opener should be pulled and unfolded *away* from the opener (Figure 4.50). Then either side is grasped at the corner of the wrapper and unfolded (Figure 4.51). Then the other side of the wrapper at the corner is grasped, and

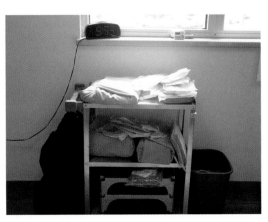

Figure 4.48 Equipment needed for procedure on cart in room.

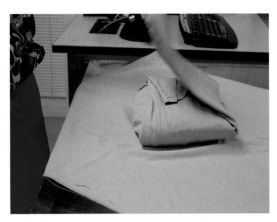

Figure 4.50 Opening first flap of wrapped pack.

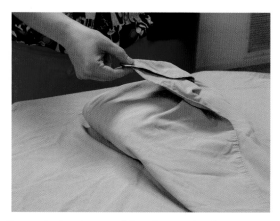

Figure 4.51 Opening second flap of wrapped pack.

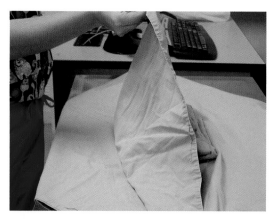

Figure 4.53 Opening final flap of wrapped pack.

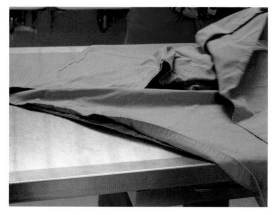

Figure 4.52 Opening third flap of wrapped pack.

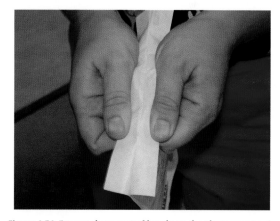

Figure 4.54 Proper placement of hands on the glove wrapper to open the pack.

unfolded. If at any time the wrapper is wrinkled or not lying flat, the circulating nurse is not allowed to touch the wrapper! Leave the wrinkle in the wrapper and the surgeon will work around it (Figure 4.52). The last tab should be grasped at the corner and unfolded toward the opener (Figure 4.53). The inner wrap is unfolded in exactly the same fashion. This method of opening encourages reduced opportunity for contamination of the pack contents. Once the gown is opened, the circulating nurse can open the gloves onto the sterile field created by the pack wrappers. Opening the glove wrapper should be done in a very controlled fashion in order to avoid contaminating the gloves within the pack. First of all, position the hands opposite one another grasping a flap of the wrapper in each hand (Figure 4.54). By slightly opening the sealed seam on either side of the wrapper first, the risk of the glove

wrapper tearing down the middle is reduced. With the hands holding the opening flaps, slowly pull the hands apart so the side seams of the wrapper unpeel. Continue opening the wrapper until the gloves are lying in a horizontal position in front of the opener (Figure 4.55). Now by simply rotating the wrists, the gloves will "fly" onto the sterile field (Figure 4.56). There is no need to throw the gloves. Now surgeon can gown and glove, while the circulating nurse is performing other duties. While the surgeon or assistant is gowning and gloving, the circulating nurse should be opening the instrument pack. With the pack sitting on the instrument table, the outer wrap, if an envelope style wrap, is opened using the same method as described for the gown pack. If it is a horizontal style wrap, the first side wrap is unfolded. Then the second side wrap is unfolded. The next flap

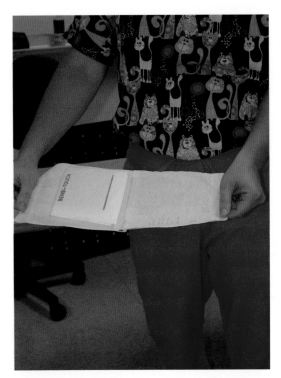

Figure 4.55   Opened glove wrapper in a horizontal fashion.

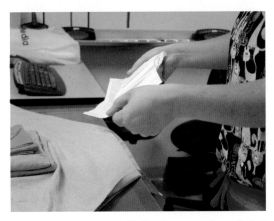

Figure 4.56   Turning wrists to flip the gloves onto the sterile field.

should be unfolded *away* from the circulating nurse. This is an important step because there should still be one flap covering the sterile inner pack protecting it from contamination. The final flap is unfolded toward the opener. The inner pack is sterile and should be left for the sterile person to unfold. Now that there is sterile person available to take other equipment from the

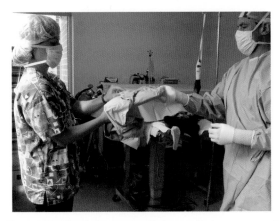

Figure 4.57   Circulating nurse offering sterile inner wrapped pack to surgeon.

circulating nurse, the remaining packs can be opened with a different method. Holding the pack in the hand with the fingers and thumb firmly holding the pack, the tape is removed after verification that it is the correct item to be opened. The tab of the outer wrap should be facing the opener. The tab is gently pulled toward the opener, and the flap is unfolded away from the opener. The next visible side flap should be opened with the corresponding hand to avoid crossing arms over the pack. The second side flap is then opened. If necessary, to avoid crossing arms over the pack, the hand holding the pack should be switched. The wrapper that is hanging below the pack should be gathered into one hand by the circulating nurse. The sterile inner pack can then be offered to the sterile member of the team (Figure 4.57). The circulating nurse may then continue to open items for the surgeon. Anything packed in a peel pack (suture, separate instruments, etc.) should be opened using the method described for opening gloves (Figure 4.58). Items opened for the surgical team may be handed to the team member or they may be flipped up onto the instrument table. Heavy instruments or delicate instruments are best handled by having the sterile member take the item from the circulating nurse. Lighter items such as suture, scalpel blades, and sponges may be deposited on the instrument table. Care *must* be taken to adhere to strict asepsis when opening items. At no time can the arms of the circulating nurse extend over the sterile field; this is a break in aseptic technique and could compromise the patient.

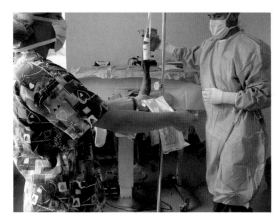

Figure 4.58   Circulating nurse opening peel pack item for surgeon.

Monitoring the aseptic technique

It is imperative that the surgical area be kept as microorganism free as possible. The risk to the patient from other uncontrollable factors is high enough, that every effort must be made to control those measures that pose a risk of infection for the patient. Not only do the patient's health status, immune system strength, age, and nutritional state affect healing; even factors outside of the patient too affect healing. The length of surgery, the surgical site (GI vs. bone), and the inadvertent introduction of pathogens to the surgical wound can also affect healing. It is a primary responsibility of the circulating nurse to act as the patient's advocate and monitor the surgical procedure and the people involved for breaks in aseptic technique. Often times sterile personnel do not realize they have inadvertently contaminated themselves and it is the responsibility of the circulating nurse to report such incidents. The patient's welfare and surgical healing are at stake, so the circulating nurses should not be shy about reporting observed breaks. Sterile members who have been informed that they have broken the technique must not argue or debate the report, but merely take measures to correct the situation. Often times, changing gloves is all that is needed, but changing gowns or entire instruments packs may also be necessary, depending on the severity of the break in technique. The rules of aseptic technique are found in Table 4.2.

Monitoring the room during the surgery

In addition to vigilant monitoring of the aseptic technique, there are other things that may occur during a

Table 4.2 Rules of aseptic technique.

Rule	Reason/example
Sterile personnel only touch sterile items; non-sterile members only touch non-sterile items.	Sterile members touching non-sterile items would result in cross contamination; non-sterile personnel touching sterile items would result in contamination
Talking is minimal	Aerosolized particles could contaminate instruments or the wound
Sterile member should pass each other back to back if passing one another is necessary	Any other orientation to each other would result in contamination of the sterile area of the gown/gloves
Air space over the surgical field is considered sterile and should not be invaded by non-sterile personnel	Shedding skin cells from arms of a non-sterile person, dust, lint or other particles may fall when reaching over a sterile field and contaminate the field
Anything below surgery table level is considered non-sterile.	Movement of items below the table cannot be controlled and are at risk of contamination
Sterile personnel may not cross their arms and place gloved hands in auxiliary regions.	Moisture from sweat in the auxiliary region may contaminate gloves
Sterile members should face the sterile filed at all times	The back of the gown is not considered sterile even if wearing a wrap around gown.
If the sterility of an item is in question, it should be considered non-sterile	Contamination of an item can occur and not be visible to the eye.
If a sterile member sits down during a procedure, they must remain seated for the entire procedure.	Items are considered sterile only if above the surgery table. Moving from sitting to standing would result in contamination of the field.

Adapted from Fossom (2007).

surgical case for which the circulating nurse is responsible. As items are opened, the cloth wrappers should be thrown in the laundry bag. The paper wrappers should be thrown in the trash. Ideally there would be a large trash bag in the surgery room for collecting the large volume of disposable items that will be generated, so as to not overflow the kick buckets in the room. Any trash from the sterile field that misses the kick bucket should be picked up right away and disposed of. Litter should not be allowed to accumulate on the floor of the operating room.

If the potential exists for fluid to fall from the sterile field, a kick buck should be positioned to catch as much of the run off as possible (Figure 4.59). Keeping the surgery room as clean and neat as possible during the procedure will permit a speedier clean up.

Connecting various pieces of equipment and accessories also falls to the circulating nurse. Plugging in the electrosurgery ground plate to the unit as well as plugging in the hand piece once that end is thrown off the sterile field should be done as soon as possible. Connecting the suction hose to the suction bottle is important to

do as soon as possible, especially if the procedure may have lots of fluid early in the procedure (i.e., evacuation of an abdomen before completing the approach). Other duties may include attaching a nitrogen-powered tool to the nitrogen tank, plugging in arthroscopic or laparoscopic cables, or even talking a surgeon through the set up or use of a piece of equipment they may not be familiar with. Another situation that arises too often in the operating room is troubleshooting equipment when it doesn't function as expected. Surgeons need to have the equipment ready for use, and if that is not the case, the circulating nurse needs to be able to figure out how to fix it.

Finally, but certainly equally important is the record-keeping responsibilities of the circulating nurse. Recording supplies used for accurate billing, making notes in the medical record (such a recording the number of skin sutures/staples placed) or completing discharge instructions as the surgeon is closing, are all examples of documentation that fall to the circulating nurse.

References

Beale, B.S. (2010) How to Make Yourself Indispensable as a Surgical Assistant. Proceedings from ACVS Symposium, Chicago, IL.

Association of Operating Room Nurses Board of Directors, (2005) Board of Directors Recommendations in AORN Journal.

Center for Disease Control (2008) Guideline for Disinfection and Sterilization in Healthcare Facilities

Dunn, D.L. (2007) *Wound Closure Manual*, 1st edn. Ethicon, Inc., Somerville, NJ.

Fossum, T. (2007) *Small Animal Surgery*, 3rd edn. Mosby Elsevier, St. Louis, MO.

MacPhail, C. (2007) *Suture and Staplers in Small Animal Surgery*. ACVS Proceedings, Chicago, IL.

Reuss-Lamky, H. (2011) Beating the "Bugs": sterilization is instrumental. Veterinary Technician Journal, 32 (**11**).

Tear, M. (2012) *Small Animal Surgical Nursing – Skills and Concepts*, 2nd edn. Elsevier, St. Louis, MO.

Webliography

http://www.aspjj.com/emea/sites/www.aspjj.com.emea/files/pdf/EN/STERRADFF_FamilyOfProducts.pdf [accessed on 6 November 2014]

Low –Temperature Oxidative Sterilization Methods for Sterilizing Medical Devices. "Joint Service Pollution Prevention Opportunity Handbook" revised 04/04 http://

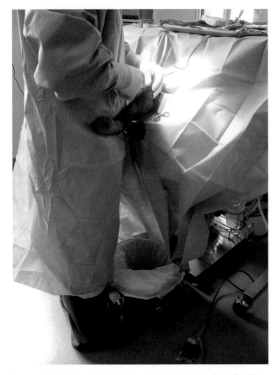

Figure 4.59 Kick bucket positioned to catch run off of fluid from a stifle surgery.

205.153.241.230/P2_Opportunity_Handbook/12_3.html. [accessed on 6 November 2014]

Guideline for Disinfection and Sterilization in Healthcare Facilities, 2008 http://www.cdc.gov/hicpac/disinfection_sterilization/7_0formaldehyde.html [accessed on 6 November 2014]

http://www.tuttnauerusa.com/sites/default/files/assets-usa/support/support_MAN_EZ.pdf [accessed on 6 November 2014]

http://www.covidien.com/imageServer.aspx?contentID=11850&contenttype=application/pdf [accessed on 6 November 2014]

http://veterinarynews.dvm360.com/dvm/Skin-staplers-offer-a-variety-of-surgical-closure-/ArticleStandard/Article/detail/73929 [accessed on 6 November 2014]

http://veterinarycalendar.dvm360.com/avhc/Medicine/Stapling-applications-in-abdominal-surgery-Proceed/ArticleStandard/Article/detail/571078 [accessed on 6 November 2014]

http://cal.vet.upenn.edu/projects/saortho/chapter_09/09mast.htm [accessed on 6 November 2014]

CHAPTER 5

Surgical Procedures

Veterinary technicians play major roles during surgical procedures as surgical assistants and circulating nurses. Important knowledge includes instrument identification, anatomical structures, and special needs of individual surgeries and surgeons. Surgeons' preferences will dictate specific information such as patient positioning and special instrumentation. This chapter outlines many *common and advanced surgical* procedures based on their anatomical location. It includes conditions, causes, clinical signs, corrective procedures, positioning, special instrumentation, the surgical assistant's role, and postoperative care. All patients require post-surgical monitoring, pain control, and perhaps some form of wound protection. *Advanced procedures, more commonly performed in referral practices, are indicated with a star (★).*

Orthopedic and neurosurgery (Piermattei *et al.* 2006a)

Elbow – elbow dysplasia (Schulz 2007a)
Fragmented medial coronoid process or fragmented coronoid process (FMCP or FCP)

a. Definition: portion of medial coronoid process of ulna separates from parent bone
b. Cause: unknown but breed disposition (large breeds), inherited and environmental factors contribute to the condition, found in young dogs
c. Clinical signs: forelimb lame, worse after exercise, stiff after rest, often bilateral, elbow pain, and effusion
d. Diagnosis: radiographs or CT of elbows
e. Surgery★: arthroscopy or open approach to remove fragment (Figure 5.1).
f. Positioning: Dorsal recumbency for both arthroscopic and open repair

g. Special instrumentation:
   i. Arthroscopic: Arthroscope 30° 1.9 or 2.4 mm scope, blunt(preferred)/sharp trocar, cannula, camera, arthroscopic hand instruments, ± motorized shaver, fluids, monitor, and tower
   ii. Open: Oschner (or other toothed) forceps, oscillating bone saw, battery or nitrogen tank to power saw, suction, bulb syringe, cautery
h. Assistant's role:
   i. Arthroscopic: Monitor fluid flow, manipulate limb for surgeon, set up arthroscope, set up motorized shaver if used.
   ii. Open: Assist with draping, set up suction/cautery, retract tissue with hand-held retractors, lavage field, suction field, set up bone saw, cut sutures.
i. Postoperative care: cryotherapy, restricted activity and physical rehabilitation

Osteochondritis dissecans (OCD) (distal humerus)

a. Definition: Incomplete endochondral ossification causes cartilage to remain, fissure in this cartilage creates a flap that may loosen causing a "joint mouse"(Figure 5.2).
b. Cause: Unknown but breed disposition (large breeds), genetic, and dietary (over nutrition = rapid growth) factors contribute to condition, found in young dogs
c. Clinical signs: Forelimb lame (unilateral or bilateral), worse after exercise, stiff after rest, pain, and elbow effusion if osteoarthritis is present
d. Diagnosis: Radiographs of elbows
e. Surgery★: Arthroscopy or open approach to remove cartilage flap (Figures 5.3 and 5.4).
f. Positioning: Dorsal recumbency regardless of technique of repair

Surgical Patient Care for Veterinary Technicians and Nurses, First Edition. Gerianne Holzman and Teri Raffel.
© 2015 John Wiley & Sons, Ltd. Published 2015 by John Wiley & Sons, Ltd.
Companion Website: wiley.com/go/holzman/surgical.

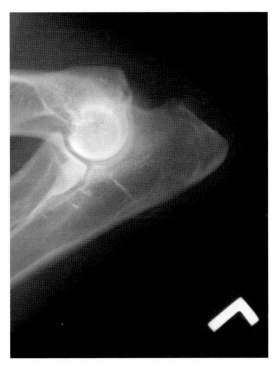

Figure 5.1   Radiograph of Left Fragmented Coronoid Process after removal. (Paul Manley, University of Wisconsin, Madison, WI. Reproduced with permission from Paul Manley.)

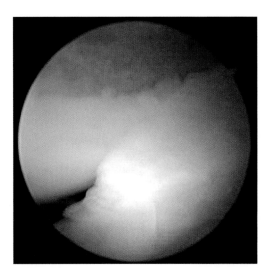

Figure 5.3 Arthroscopic view of distal humeral OCD flap. (Paul Manley, University of Wisconsin, Madison, WI. Reproduced with permission from Paul Manley.)

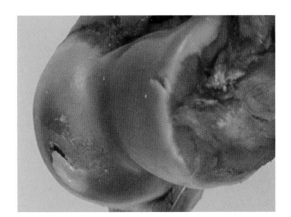

Figure 5.2   Distal Humeral Osteochondritis Dissecans (OCD) flap. (Paul Manley, University of Wisconsin, Madison, WI. Reproduced with permission from Paul Manley.)

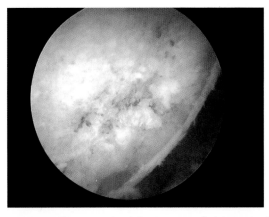

Figure 5.4 Arthroscopic view following removal of OCD. (Paul Manley, University of Wisconsin, Madison, WI. Reproduced with permission from Paul Manley.)

g. Special instrumentation:

i. Arthroscopic: Arthroscope 30° 1.9 or 2.4 mm scope, blunt(preferred)/sharp trocar, cannula, camera, arthroscopic hand instruments, ± motorized shaver, fluids, monitor and tower

ii. Open: Oschner (or other toothed) forceps, bone curette

h. Assistant's role:

i. Arthroscopic: Monitor fluid flow, manipulate limb for surgeon, set up arthroscope, set up motorized shaver if used

ii. Open: Assist with draping, set up suction/cautery, retract tissue with hand held retractors, lavage field, suction field, cut sutures

i. Postoperative care: No bandage or a soft-padded bandage for up to 1 week, cryotherapy, restricted activity, and physical rehabilitation

Ununited anconeal process

a. Definition: Anconeal process does not attach to proximal ulna

b. Cause: Center of ossification of the anconeous occurs separately from olecranon, disturbance of ossification of the juncture creates a fissure; large breed dogs, genetics, rapid growth, and trauma may contribute to condition

c. Clinical signs: Intermittent forelimb lame (unilateral), worse after exercise, stiff after rest, pain and elbow effusion, decreased elbow range of motion

d. Diagnosis: Radiographs (**after** five months of age) or CT scan of elbows (Figure 5.5).

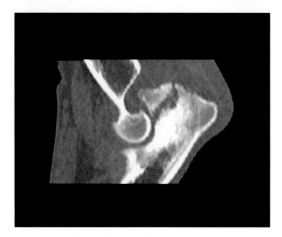

Figure 5.5 CT of united anconeal process (UAP).

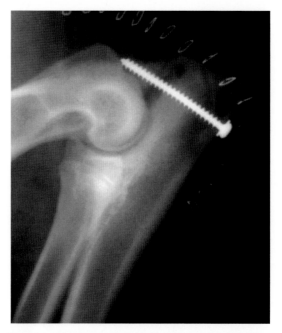

Figure 5.6 UAP repair with screw fixation (Paul Manley, University of Wisconsin, Madison, WI. Reproduced with permission from Paul Manley.)

e. Surgery★: Open approach to elbow to remove anconeal process or replacement with screw (Figure 5.6).

f. Positioning: Medial approach – dorsal recumbency; lateral approach – lateral recumbency with affected limb up

g. Special instrumentation: Gelpi self-retaining retractor, single action ronguer, oscillating saw if doing ulnar osteotomy, bone screws, screw placement instrumentation, power drill for lag screw placement

h. Assistant's role: Assist with draping, suction during drilling, hydrate field during osteotomy, cut sutures, retract tissue if necessary

i. Postoperative care: No bandage or a soft padded bandage for up to 1 week, cryotherapy, restricted activity and physical rehabilitation

Shoulder (Schulz 2007b)
Biceps tenosynovitis

a. Definition: Inflammation of the biceps brachii tendon and its synovial sheath

b. Cause: Trauma to the biceps brachii (bicipital) tendon including recurring injury or overuse, may become

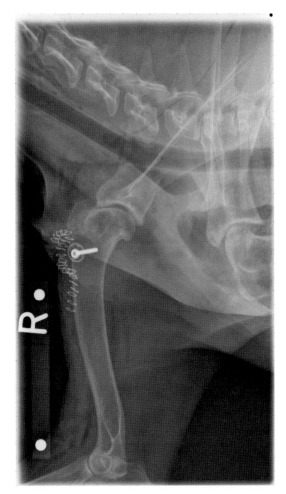

Figure 5.7 Radiograph post bicep tendon tenodesis with screw placement. (Paul Manley, University of Wisconsin, Madison, WI. Reproduced with permission from Paul Manley.)

mineralized or torn, often medium to large breeds and at least middle aged

c. Clinical signs: Unilateral forelimb lameness, may be progressive, pain on palpation of biceps tendon especially when shoulder is flexed and elbow is extended, patient is more lame if held in this position for two minutes.

d. Diagnosis: Radiographs of shoulders including skyline view ± arthrogram

e. Surgery: Arthroscopy★ or open approach to shoulder to transect the biceps tendon or tenodesis to change origin of tendon (Figure 5.7).

f. Positioning: Arthroscopic – lateral recumbency with affected limb up; Open repair – dorsal recumbency

g. Special instrumentation:
   i. Arthroscopy: Arthroscope, arthroscopy instrumentation, camera, monitor, and tower
   ii. Open repair: Gelpi self-retaining retractor, bone screws, bone screw placement instrumentation, power drill, suction, cautery

h. Assistant's role: Retraction of tissue, lavage of field, suction, cut sutures.

i. Postoperative care: Velpeau sling for 2–3 weeks (open approach), cryotherapy, restricted activity, and physical rehabilitation after sling removal or after arthroscopy

Osteochondritis dissecans (OCD) of proximal humerus

a. Definition: Incomplete endochondral ossification causes cartilage to remain, fissure in this cartilage creates a flap that may loosen causing a "joint mouse"

b. Cause: Unknown but breed disposition (large breeds), genetic, and dietary (over nutrition = rapid growth) factors contribute to condition, found in young dogs

c. Clinical signs: Forelimb lame (unilateral or bilateral), worse after exercise, improves with rest, pain on full shoulder extension

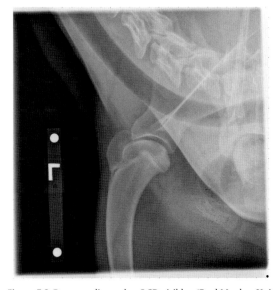

Figure 5.8 Pre-op radiograph – OCD visible. (Paul Manley, University of Wisconsin, Madison, WI. Reproduced with permission from Paul Manley.)

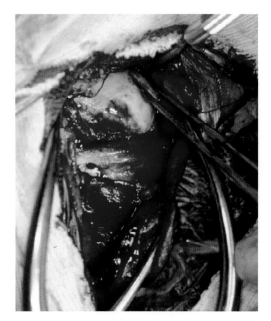

Figure 5.9 Arthrotomy to elevate proximal humeral OCD. (Paul Manley, University of Wisconsin, Madison, WI. Reproduced with permission from Paul Manley.)

d. Diagnosis: Radiographs of shoulders or CT scan (Figure 5.8).
e. Surgery: Arthroscopy★ or open approach to remove cartilage flap
f. Positioning: Dorsal recumbency for lateral approach
g. Special instrumentation:
   i. Arthroscopy – Arthroscope, arthroscopy instrumentation, camera, monitor, and tower
   ii. Open: Oschner forceps or other toothed forceps, bone curette suction, cautery, self-retaining retractor (Gelpi) (Figure 5.9).
h. Assistant's role:
   i. Arthroscopic: Monitor fluid flow, manipulate limb, set up arthroscope
   ii. Open: Retraction of tissue, suction, cut sutures
i. Postoperative care: Cryotherapy, restricted activity, and physical rehabilitation

Shoulder Instability

a. Definition: Increased range of motion of shoulder, most often medial-lateral
b. Cause: Tearing or stretching of ligaments and tendons of the shoulder, usually from long-standing trauma, medium to large breed active dogs

c. Clinical signs: Chronic unilateral forelimb lameness, increased angles of abduction, painful shoulder
d. Diagnosis: Not evident on imaging, physical exam findings
e. Surgery★: Conservative treatment first, if not successful: arthroscopic or open approach to shoulder to place bone anchors and suture to stabilize shoulder
f. Positioning: Lateral recumbency with affected limb up for arthroscopy; dorsal recumbency for medial approach for open repair
g. Special instrumentation:
   i. Arthroscopy: Arthroscope, arthroscopy instrumentation, camera, monitor and tower
   ii. Open: Gelpi self-retaining retractor, bone anchors, bone screws, bone screw placement instrumentation, large size monofilament nonabsorbable suture, suction, cautery
h. Assistant's role:
   i. Arthroscopic: Manipulation of limb, monitor fluid flow, set up arthroscope
   ii. Open: Suction field, hydrate tissues, stabilize limb for screw placement, hand screw placement instrumentation in correct order
i. Postoperative care: Velpeau sling or shoulder stabilization hobbles, restricted activity, physical rehabilitation (Figure 5.10).

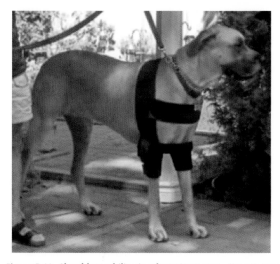

Figure 5.10 Shoulder stabilization from DogLeggs. (DoggLeggs Therapeutic and Rehabilitative Products, Reston, VA. Reproduced with permission from DogLeggs Therapeutic and Rehabilitative Products.)

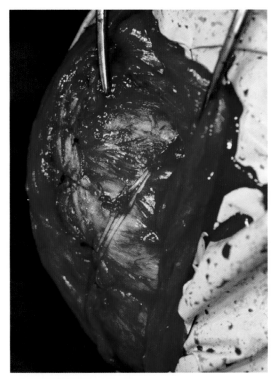

Figure 5.11 Leader line knotted for extra-capsular repair. (Paul Manley, University of Wisconsin, Madison, WI. Reproduced with permission from Paul Manley.)

Stifle
Cranial cruciate ligament (CCL) rupture

a. Definition: Partial or complete tearing of the cranial cruciate ligament
b. Cause: Thought to be related to chronic inflammation of the cranial cruciate ligament (CCL) causing long-term deterioration and eventual tearing, (Muir 2010) most common in large breed dogs, may have a genetic component (Wilke 2010)
c. Clinical signs: Acute to chronic grade 2–5/5 rear leg lameness, stifle effusion, painful during stifle manipulation, may sit to one side with affected leg in extension
d. Diagnosis: Positive cranial drawer test, positive tibial thrust test, radiographs to assess degree of inflammation, and degenerative joint disease
e. Surgery:
  i. Extracapsular repair, Lateral fabellar suture, "Fishing line" technique, (Schulz 2007c; Cook

2010) – stabilization of the stifle via suture outside the joint, suture material is monofilament nylon
  1 Surgery: Using heavy monofilament suture/leader line, a cruciate needle is passed around the fabella. Next, the suture is passed behind the patellar ligament. A hole is drilled through the tibial crest. With the stifle flexed the sutures is passed through the hole and tied or crimped. routine closure (Figure 5.11).
  2 Positioning: Lateral or dorsal recumbency
  3 Special instrumentation: Fishing or leader line, braided orthopedic suture, large monofilament nonabsorbable suture, suction, cautery, cruciate needle, metal crimper pieces, crimper tool
  4 Assistant's role: Stabilize the limb, suction field, provide hemostasis, cut sutures
  5 Postoperative care: Restricted activity for 8–10 weeks, physical rehabilitation to improve joint mobility and increase muscle strength
ii. Tibial plateau leveling osteotomy★ (TPLO) – mechanical stabilization of the stifle via a bone cutting procedure to change the tibial plateau angle, TPLO limits the shear force created by the compression of the stifle when weight-bearing and thus reducing tibial thrust (Milovancev and Schaefer 2010)
  1 Surgery: A medial approach to the joint provides visualization of the joint to allow for the bone saw to cut the tibia. As the osteotomy is completed the tibial plateau slope decreases, which allows for a more neutral or caudal cranial cruciate thrust. A TPLO bone plate is placed to stabilize the osteotomy site (Figures 5.12 and 5.13).
  2 Positioning: Dorsal recumbency or dorso-lateral oblique, tilted toward the affected limb, to allow the limb to lay flat on the surgery table top
  3 Special instrumentation: TPLO instrument set (including torque limiter, radial saw blades, jig), TPLO bone plate set, bone screw set (locking or non-locking), bone saw, bone drill, Gelpi self-retaining retractor (Figure 5.14).
  4 Assistant's role: Stabilize limb for sawing and/or drilling of screw holes, drill screw holes, place/remove k-wires/pins, retraction of patellar tendon during osteotomy, suction, hydrate field, cut sutures
  5 Postoperative care: Restricted activity for 8–10 weeks until radiographs show bony healing,

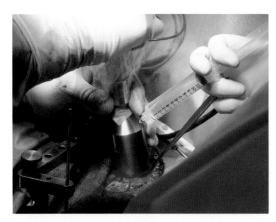

Figure 5.12 Using saw for Tibial Plateau Leveling Osteotomy (TPLO). Note: Assistant dripping fluid on bone to cool it while sawing.

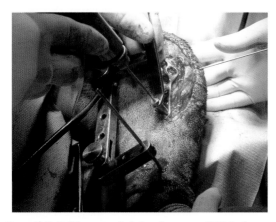

Figure 5.13 Drilling screw hole for placement of TPLO plate.

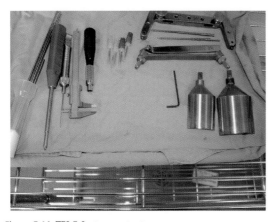

Figure 5.14 TPLO Instrument set.

physical rehabilitation to improve joint mobility and increase muscle strength (Figure 5.15).

iii. Tibial tuberosity advancement★ (TTA) - mechanical stabilization of the stifle via a bone cutting procedure to neutralize cranial tibiofemoral shear force (Boudrieau 2010)

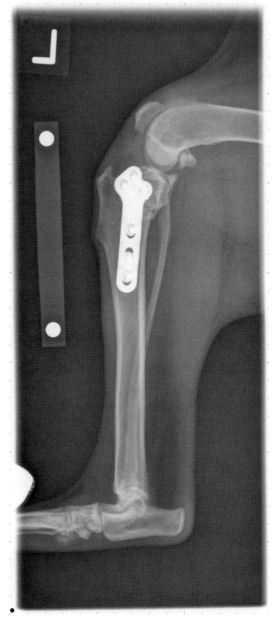

Figure 5.15 Post op radiograph of TPLO plate. (Paul Manley, University of Wisconsin, Madison, WI. Reproduced with permission from Paul Manley.)

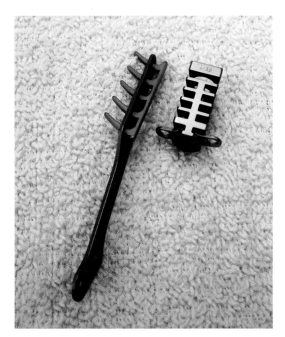

Figure 5.16 Tibial tuberosity advancement (TTA) cage, fork, and plate.

1 Surgery: Using an open approach to the stifle joint a partial tibial crest osteotomy is performed. A "cage" is secured with bone screws to keep the osteotomy site open. A TTA bone plate is used to stabilize the osteotomy site.

2 Positioning: Dorsal recumbency or dorso-lateral oblique, tilted toward the affected limb, to allow the limb to lay flat on the surgery table top

3 Special instrumentation: TTA implant set, power saw, periosteal elevator, TTA instrumentation set, Gelpi self-retaining retractor (Figure 5.16).

4 Assistant's role: Stabilize limb, suction, cut sutures, hold plate while first screw holes being drilled

5 Postoperative care: Restricted activity for 8–10 weeks, physical rehabilitation to improve joint mobility and increase muscle strength (Figure 5.17).

iv. Tightrope® – Stabilization of the stifle via suture technique outside the joint, suture material is braided fiber wire

1 Surgery: An ultra-high strength, braided synthetic ligament is passed through bone tunnels created in the distal femur and proximal tibia. The "ligament" is pulled tight and secured with

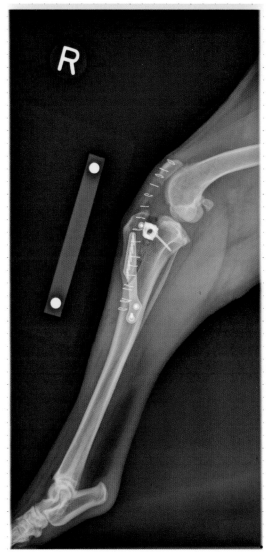

Figure 5.17 Post op radiograph of TTA surgery. (Paul Manley, University of Wisconsin, Madison, WI. Reproduced with permission from Paul Manley.)

a femoral button, simulating the normal cranial cruciate ligament.

2 Positioning: Dorsal recumbency

3 Special instrumentation: Power drill, drill bit, hand chuck, pin, ligament graft, femoral button, Gelpi retractor, suction cautery

4 Assistant's role: Stabilize limb while tunnels created, suction, cut suture, stabilization of leg as graft is tightened

5 Postoperative care: Restricted activity for 8–10 weeks, physical rehabilitation to improve joint mobility and increase muscle strength

Patella Luxation (Piermattei *et al.* 2006b)

a. Definition: Displacement of the patella, either medially or laterally

b. Cause: Congenital condition, medial luxation is most common, widespread in toy and miniature breeds but also occurs in large breeds and cats, bilateral complaint in 20–25% of patients

c. Clinical signs: Intermittent to continual non-weight bearing lame on affected leg, divided into the following grades:

   i. Patella easily luxates, is easily reduced, spends most of the time in correct position (surgery generally not indicated)

   ii. More frequent luxation than grade one, patella is easily reduced and most often in the correct position (may or may not require surgery)

   iii. Patella always luxated, reducible with effort (requires surgical correction)

   iv. Patella always luxated, not reducible (requires surgical correction)

d. Diagnosis: Stifle palpation, radiographs (Figure 5.19)

e. Surgery: A variety of surgeries correct this condition, they may be used singularly or in combination. The trochlear groove is deepened with a trochlear wedge, block recession or trochlear resection procedure. Additional procedures may be done to maintain placement of the patella in the newly created groove: Overlap of lateral or medial retinaculum, fascia lata overlap, patellar and tibial antirotational suture ligament, desmotomy and partial capsulectomy, quadriceps release, tibial tuberosity transposition (TTT) along with osteotomies if femoral deformities are present (Figure 5.18).

f. Positioning: Dorsal recumbency

g. Special instrumentation: Bone saw, number 20 blade, osteotome, mallet, ronguer, k-wires, power drill, self-retaining retractor, suction, cautery

h. Assistant's role: Stabilize limb, suction site if bone saw used, lavage field, cut sutures

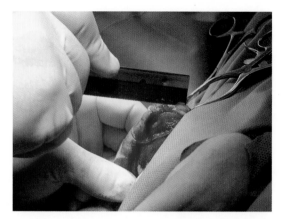

Figure 5.18 Cutting wedge for repair of MPL (medial patellar luxation).

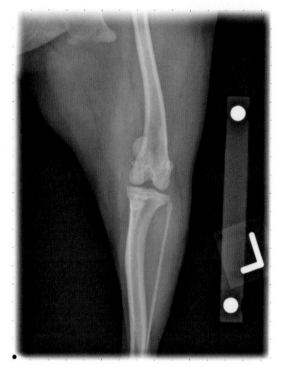

Figure 5.19 Cranial-caudal radiographic view of medial patellar luxation – pre op. (Paul Manley, University of Wisconsin, Madison, WI. Reproduced with permission from Paul Manley.)

i. Postoperative care: Restricted activity for 4 weeks, physical rehabilitation to improve joint mobility and increase muscle strength, encourage weight bearing, sling support under abdomen to assist walking if bilateral procedure (Figure 5.20).

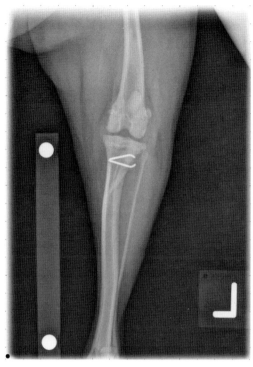

Figure 5.20 Cranial-caudal radiographic view of corrected medial patellar luxation – post op. (Paul Manley, University of Wisconsin, Madison, WI. Reproduced with permission from Paul Manley.)

Pelvis
Hip dysplasia

a. Definition: Malformation of the femoral head and acetabulum causing joint laxity leading to degenerative joint disease, often bilateral
b. Cause: Genetic and environmental
c. Clinical signs: Reduced activity, difficulty rising, "bunny hopping" gait, muscle atrophy of rear limb(s)
d. Diagnosis: Radiographs, positive Ortolani sign (young, sedated patient), painful hip range of motion, crepitus in older patients (Figure 5.21).
e. Surgery: Conservative therapy consisting of exercise modification, medical, and dietary management may be indicated pending the severity of the patient's clinical symptoms. The type of surgical procedure is dependent upon the age of the patient, clinical severity, and the client's expectations. For example, a performance or working dog may have a better outcome and greater return to function with a

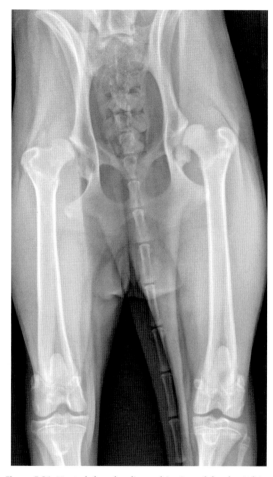

Figure 5.21 Ventral-dorsal radiographic view of dysplastic hips. (Paul Manley, University of Wisconsin, Madison, WI. Reproduced with permission from Paul Manley.)

total hip replacement than with a femoral head ostectomy.

i. Femoral head ostectomy (FHO) or Femoral head and neck excision (FHNE) (Piermattei *et al.* 2006c) – removal of the head and neck of the femur to create a fibrous false joint to relieve pain from bone on bone contact, surgery is a salvage procedure for end-stage degenerative joint disease (may also be performed following femoral head/neck fractures or acetabular fractures).

1 Surgery: A craniolateral approach to the hip is made to allow intentional luxation of the hip. The round ligament is incised (if still intact) and the femoral head is subluxated. The head and neck is then be excised.

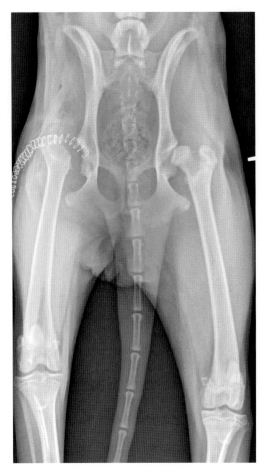

Figure 5.22 Post op ventral-dorsal radiographic view of hips post femoral head osteotomy (FHO). (Paul Manley, University of Wisconsin, Madison, WI. Reproduced with permission from Paul Manley.)

2 Positioning: Lateral recumbency with affected limb up

3 Special instrumentation: Power saw, osteotome, mallet, ronguer, rasp, suction, cautery, Gelpi self-retaining retractor, lavage fluid

4 Assistant's role: Lavage field, drip saline on bone as osteotomy is performed, cut sutures, rotate/stabilize limb, load saw blade on power saw

5 Postoperative care: Restricted activity for two weeks, then encourage limb use, physical rehabilitation to improve joint mobility and increase muscle strength (Figure 5.22).

ii. Juvenile pubic symphysiodesis (JPS) (Piermattei *et al.* 2006d) – pubic bone physis closure via stapling

or electrocautery causing improvement in the acetabular angle and thus more coverage of the femoral head by the acetabulum, degenerative joint disease (DJD) prevention, performed at 12–16 weeks of age. PennHIP® radiographs determine a distraction index (DI) – if DI is greater than or equal to 0.70, surgery is not effective in preventing DJD (Dueland *et al.* 2010).

1 Surgery: A ventral midline incision over the pubis allows dissection/retraction of muscle to expose pubic symphysis. Cautery is set at 40 watts and ablation is performed every 2–3 mm along pubic symphysis

2 Positioning: Dorsal recumbency

3 Special instrumentation: Small malleable retractor, suction, cautery

4 Assistant's role: Retraction of muscle, suction, cut sutures

5 Postoperative care: Moderate exercise for 2–3 months

iii. Total hip replacement/Arthroplasty★ (THR/THA) (Piermattei *et al.* 2006e) – removal of the femoral head/neck and replacement with a stainless steel or titanium head/stem as well as reaming of the acetabulum and replacing it with a high-density polyethylene cup, surgery is a salvage procedure for end-stage degenerative joint disease (also may be performed for femoral head/neck fractures) (Figure 5.23).

1 Surgery: A craniolateral approach is made to the hip. The hip is luxated and the round ligament is incised. The femoral head and neck are excised. The femoral canal is broached and prepped for implant placement. The acetabulum is reamed and prepped for acetabular placement. After implant placement the hip is repositioned, range of motion is evaluated prior to closure.

2 Positioning: Lateral recumbency with surgical hip up, use THA positioner may be used to insure pelvic alignment (Figure 5.24).

3 Special instrumentation: Cemented/cementless femoral prosthesis, femoral head implant, acetabular implant, power saw/drill, total hip instrumentation set, Gelpi self-retaining retractor, deep muscle retractor (Myerding), cement (if needed), evacuation bowl, Hohmann retractors, suction, cautery, lavage fluid (Figures 5.25 and 5.26).

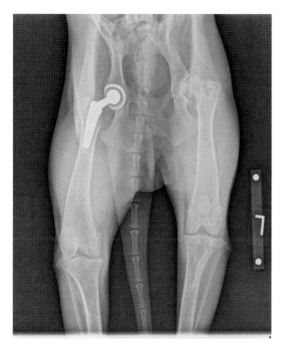

Figure 5.23 Post op VD view of total hip arthroplasty (THA) implants. (Paul Manley, University of Wisconsin, Madison, WI. Reproduced with permission from Paul Manley.)

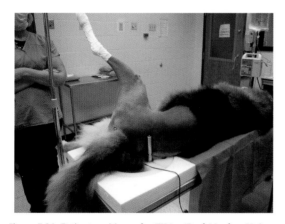

Figure 5.24 Patient positioner for THA. (Paul Manley, University of Wisconsin, Madison, WI. Reproduced with permission from Paul Manley.)

4 Assistant's role: Strict enforcement of asepsis, mix cement, muscle retraction, stabilize limb, hand instruments during joint prep in correct order, keep instruments clean between use, cut sutures

5 Postoperative care: *Very restricted* activity for four weeks, use of sling for walking at all times

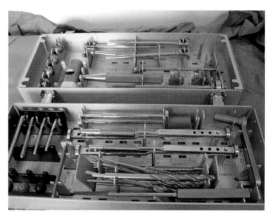

Figure 5.25 THA instruments and implant template set. (Paul Manley, University of Wisconsin, Madison, WI. Reproduced with permission from Paul Manley.)

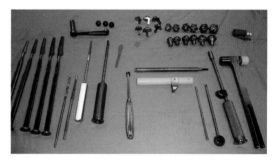

Figure 5.26 THA instruments from different company laid out on instrument table. (Paul Manley, University of Wisconsin, Madison, WI. Reproduced with permission from Paul Manley.)

to avoid slipping and luxation of implants, rehabilitation starting 2–4 weeks postoperative, slow increase in activity after 4–8 weeks

iv. Triple/double pelvic osteotomy★ (TPO/DPO) (Piermattei *et al.* 2006f) – cuts made in the ilium and pubis (DPO) as well as ischium (TPO) to allow rotation of the acetabulum and provide more coverage of the femoral head, performed only in skeletally immature dogs (4–12 months) without degenerative changes, reduces degenerative joint disease from hip dysplasia (Figure 5.27).

1 Surgery: An incision is made over the pectinius muscle to allow dissection and access to pubis. An osteotomy is performed on the medial wall of the acetabulum. The incision is closed. An ischial

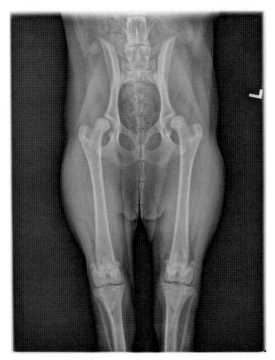

Figure 5.27 Pre op VD radiograph of patient needing a TPO (Triple pelvic osteotomy). (Paul Manley, University of Wisconsin, Madison, WI. Reproduced with permission from Paul Manley.)

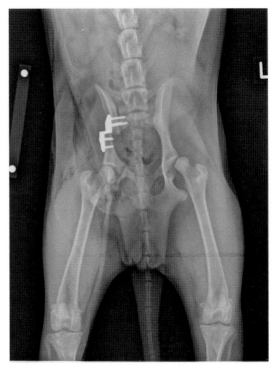

Figure 5.28 Post op VD radiograph of patient having had a TPO performed (Paul Manley, University of Wisconsin, Madison, WI. Reproduced with permission from Paul Manley.)

approach is made and the ischial osteotomy is performed. The ischial osteotomy is centered over the obturator foramen. Finally the ilial approach and osteotomy is performed. The pelvis is realigned to permit the application of a bone plate to stabilize the pelvis.

2 Positioning: Dorsal recumbency/lateral recumbency with affected hip up *Note: Re-positioning of patient may be necessary to allow access to pelvic osteotomy sites*

3 Special instrumentation: Power bone saw, bone plates, bone screws, bone screw placement instrumentation, osteotome, mallet, bone holding forceps, Gelpi self-retaining retractors, Hohmann retractors, periosteal elevator, second set of drapes, instruments (if repositioning of patient is necessary to access pelvic osteotomy sites)

4 Assistant's role: Suction during osteotomies, lavage field as osteotomy performed, muscle retraction, handing of screw placement instruments in proper order when screws are being placed, cut sutures

5 Postoperative care: Exercise restriction for 4–6 weeks, physical rehabilitation, sling walk when on slippery surfaces (Figure 5.28).

Avascular necrosis (Legg-Calvé-Perthes disease)

a. Definition: Femoral head necrosis and distortion, may be bilateral

b. Cause: Unknown etiology but results in lack of blood flow to the head of the femur

c. Clinical signs: Reduced activity, difficulty rising, "bunny hopping" gait, muscle atrophy, most common in young small breed dogs

d. Diagnosis: Radiographs, pain on hip palpation and or range of motion, crepitus

e. Surgery: Femoral head/neck excision or total hip replacement – see above for procedure and nursing care

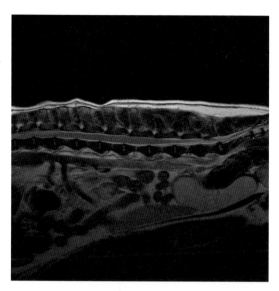

Figure 5.29 MRI performed on patient needing a hemilaminectomy.

Spine (Shores 1985)
Intervertebral disc disease (IVDD) – not cervical

a. Definition: Degeneration and protrusion of intervertebral disc material into the spinal canal, may cause compression of the spinal canal

b. Cause: Genetics: most common in chondrodystrophic (abnormal cartilage) breeds such as dachshund, Pekinese, beagle, basset hound, and American cocker spaniel; trauma may also cause a sudden protrusion of a intervertebral disc

c. Clinical signs: Paresis or paralysis of the rear limbs, knuckling or dragging of the feet, inability to urinate, back pain, weakness, reluctance to rise, collapse, trembling

d. Diagnosis: Neurological exam checking proprioception, reflexes, pain response; radiographs, myelogram, CT, MRI ± contrast (Figure 5.29).

e. Surgery: Hemilaminectomy★ – decompression of the spinal cord via removal of a portion of a vertebral body to relieve pressure; provides access for removal of extruded intervertebral disc material. Following a dorsal midline incision, dissection continues until vertebral bodies are reached. Ronguers and a drill are used to remove the dorsal lamina until an appropriate "window" is created to allow decompression.

A fat graft is harvested and placed over the defect prior to closure

f. Positioning: Sternal recumbency with spine perfectly straight, positioning aids are often required

g. Special instrumentation: Hall air drill, neuro instruments (dural hooks, dental spatula, delicate thumb tissue forceps), Frazier suction tip, single action ronguers, double-action ronguers, Kerrison ronguer, laminectomy retractor, Gelpi Self-retaining retractor, periosteal elevator, Gelfoam®, bone wax

h. Assistant's role: Hold stay sutures to elevate dura, drip saline as burring of vertebral roof is occurring, suction, cut sutures, lavage field, elevate dorsal spinous processes with towel clamp

i. Postoperative care: Intensive care, bladder expression, maintain spine in an even plane, rehabilitation, sling walking to encourage walking, cart if never regains function of rear limbs

Intervertebral disc disease (IVDD) – cervical and cervical vertebral instability (wobbler syndrome)

a. Definition: Degeneration and protrusion of intervertebral disc material into the spinal canal, may cause compression of the spinal canal

b. Cause: Genetics: most common in chondrodystrophic (abnormal cartilage) breeds such as Dachshund, Pekinese, Beagle, Basset Hound, and American Cocker Spaniel; Wobbler Syndrome most common in larger breed dogs particularly Doberman Pinschers and Great Danes. Trauma may also cause a sudden protrusion of a intervertebral disc

c. Clinical signs: Painful neck, paresis or paralysis of all four limbs

d. Diagnosis: Neurological exam checking proprioception, reflexes, pain response; radiographs, myelogram, CT, MRI ± contrast

e. Surgery: Ventral Slot★ – decompression of the cervical spinal cord via removal of a portion of a vertebral body to relieve pressure, provides access for removal of extruded intervertebral disc material. A ventral midline incision is made. Dissection and muscle retraction proceeds until the affected vertebral body/bodies are reached. Ronguers remove ventral spinous processes. An air drill is used to create a window and allow removal of herniated disc material. No graft is used to fill the deficit. Routine closure follows the procedure.

f. Positioning: Dorsal recumbency with forelimbs extend caudally toward chest; head in hyperextension with a rolled up towel under the neck; mandible taped to table.

g. Special instrumentation: Pneumatic drill and burrs, cautery, suction, Gelfoam®,#11 blade, ronguers, periosteal elevator, bone wax, dental spatula, dural hooks, 3–0/4–0 bone curettes.

h. Assistant's role: Irrigate wound following drilling, suction, lavage field, muscle retraction, hand instruments, cut sutures

i. Postoperative care: Intensive care, bladder expression if needed, maintain spine in an even plane, rehabilitation, sling walking (front and rear) to encourage walking, quadriplegic cart if never regains function of limbs

Fractures

a. Definition: Fractures may occur in any bone. They are classified as: Transverse (defect from cortex to cortex), Oblique (defect runs diagonally to the long axis of the bone), Spiral (defect wraps around the long axis of the long bone), Comminuted reducible (no more than two large fragments), Comminuted nonreducible (multiple small fragments) and Compound (any break in the skin whether from the bone moving outward or foreign object moving inward) Grade I, II or III. Physeal fractures: Salter Harris I (runs through the physis), Salter Harris II (through physis and portion of metaphysis), Salter Harris III (runs through physis, epiphysis and generally are articular). Salter Harris IV (articular fractures that run through the epiphysis, physis and metaphysis), Salter Harris V (crushing injuries of the physis)

b. Cause: trauma, neoplasia, osteoporosis, osteomyelitis

c. Clinical signs: Lameness, pain, swelling, redness, bone protruding through skin

d. Diagnosis: Known trauma, palpation, radiographs

e. Surgery★: Internal fixation (plate, pin, interlocking nail, wires, screws) or external fixation (external skeletal fixator – bars, ring fixators) – approach and dissection to reveal fractured bone. Reduction of fracture and stabilization with bone holding forceps, implants of choice are placed, bone graft may/may

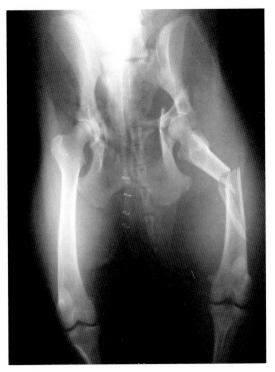

Figure 5.30 Pre op radiographs of fractured pelvis and femur. (Paul Manley, University of Wisconsin, Madison, WI. Reproduced with permission from Paul Manley.)

not be harvested and implanted. Closure follows (Figures 5.30–5.34).

f. Positioning: Depends entirely on the bone that is fractured and the approach being used; however often the repair will be done with the animal in lateral recumbency with the affected limb up

g. Special instrumentation: Power drill, battery, or nitrogen tank for drill, self-retaining retractors, bone holding forceps, suction, cautery, periosteal elevators, curette (if bone graft harvested), implant of choice, plate benders (Figures 5.35–5.40).

h. Assistant's role: Hand instruments for screw placement in proper order (drill bit, drill guide, depth gauge, tap, tap sleeve (if tapping needed), screw, screwdriver), keep drill bit/tap clean between uses, moisten tissues, guard harvested bone graft to avoid accidental disposal

i. Postoperative care: Dependent upon fracture and fixation – generally exercise restrictions, physical rehabilitation, wound care ± external coaptation

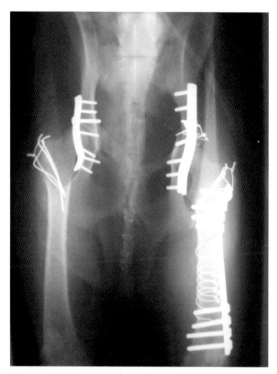

Figure 5.31 Post op radiographs of repaired fractured pelvis and femur using plates and screws (Paul Manley, University of Wisconsin, Madison, WI. Reproduced with permission from Paul Manley.)

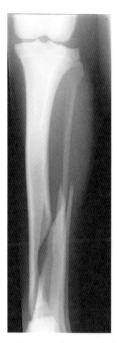

Figure 5.32 Pre op radiograph of fractured tibia. (Paul Manley, University of Wisconsin, Madison, WI. Reproduced with permission from Paul Manley.)

Joints – arthroscopy★

a. Definition: Internal visualization of a joint through a camera and employing instruments through ports to perform intra-articular surgery or for diagnosis, less invasive than an arthrotomy

b. Cause: Joints may be explored for a variety of conditions including inspection of the internal structures (cruciate ligaments, menisci) during stabilization of a CCL injury. Other reasons include septic joints for flushing and as outlined above for elbow dysplasia and shoulder conditions.

c. Clinical signs: Varies with reason for surgery; lameness, joint effusion, drainage from open wound

d. Diagnosis: Varies with condition; may include imaging, arthrocentesis, physical exam

e. Surgery: The cannula and arthroscope are placed along with a fluid inflow line. A fluid outflow portal is placed as well as a portal for hand instruments. Evaluation and repair of the joint occurs if possible.

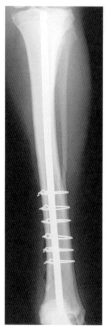

Figure 5.33 Post op radiograph of repaired fractured tibia using pin and wire. (Paul Manley, University of Wisconsin, Madison, WI. Reproduced with permission from Paul Manley.)

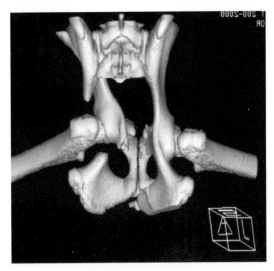

Figure 5.34 VD view of three dimensional CT fractured pelvis. (Paul Manley, University of Wisconsin, Madison, WI. Reproduced with permission from Paul Manley.)

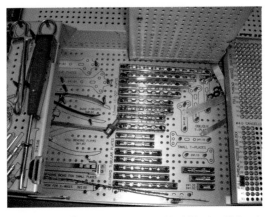

Figure 5.35 Small Fragment DCP set. (Paul Manley, University of Wisconsin, Madison, WI. Reproduced with permission from Paul Manley.)

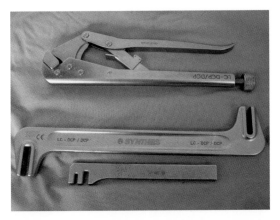

Figure 5.36 Plate benders used to manipulate bone plate to better conform to recipient bone. (Paul Manley, University of Wisconsin, Madison, WI. Reproduced with permission from Paul Manley.)

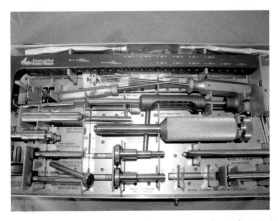

Figure 5.37 Interlocking nail implant set. (Paul Manley, University of Wisconsin, Madison, WI. Reproduced with permission from Paul Manley.)

Upper respiratory system (Hedlund 2007a)

Stenotic nares

Evaluation of the joint may also result in performing an arthrotomy (Figure 5.41).

f. Positioning: Depends entirely on procedure and joint having arthroscopic evaluation. Refer to surgeon preference.

g. Special instrumentation: Arthroscope, camera, arthroscopic instrumentation, monitor tower, extra fluids (Figures 5.42–5.45).

h. Assistant's role: Monitor fluid flow during procedure to avoid extravasation

i. Postoperative care: Varies with disease, generally exercise restrictions for 2–4 weeks, rehabilitation

a. Definition: Nostrils with very narrow openings (Figure 5.46).

b. Cause: Congenital condition in brachycephalic breeds

c. Clinical signs: Dyspnea, exercise intolerance, collapse

d. Diagnosis: Physical exam: medial deviation of nares ± respiratory distress, radiographs to determine if any other underlying cardiac, or thoracic abnormalities

e. Surgery: This procedure may or may not be performed in a surgical suite. Resection of some dorsolateral cartilage or horizontal or lateral tissue

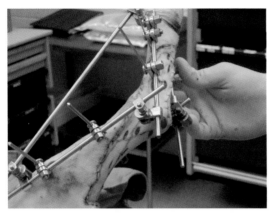

Figure 5.38 External fixator. (Paul Manley, University of Wisconsin, Madison, WI. Reproduced with permission from Paul Manley.)

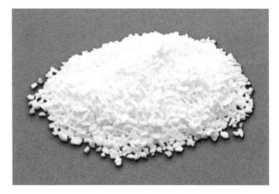

Figure 5.40 Bone graft granules. (Paul Manley, University of Wisconsin, Madison, WI. Reproduced with permission from Paul Manley.)

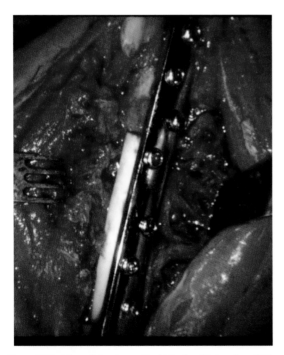

Figure 5.39 Allograft in place. (Paul Manley, University of Wisconsin, Madison, WI. Reproduced with permission from Paul Manley.)

wedge resections of the nares will result in widened nares.

f. Positioning: Sternal recumbency, head taped to table for stability
g. Special instrumentation: Number 11 blade, cautery
h. Assistant's role: Not usually present

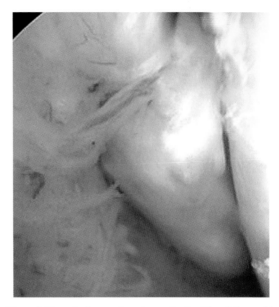

Figure 5.41 Arthroscopic view of shoulder joint with osteoarthritis. Osteophyte visible through scope. (Paul Manley, University of Wisconsin, Madison, WI. Reproduced with permission from Paul Manley.)

i. Postoperative care: Close monitoring for respiratory distress, prolonged intubation in immediate postop period, Elizabethan collar to protect surgery site, weight reduction if indicated

Elongated soft palate

a. Definition: Soft palate extends 1–3 mm caudal to the epiglottis (Figure 5.47).

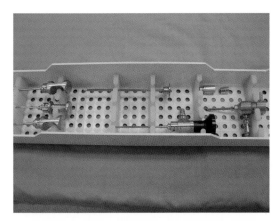

Figure 5.42   Arthroscope and tray.   (Paul Manley, University of Wisconsin, Madison, WI. Reproduced with permission from Paul Manley.)

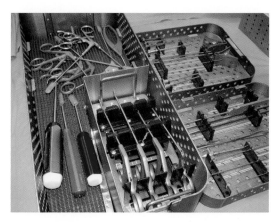

Figure 5.44   Arthroscopy instruments.   (Paul Manley, University of Wisconsin, Madison, WI. Reproduced with permission from Paul Manley.)

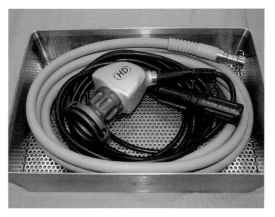

Figure 5.43   Arthroscope camera and cable.   (Paul Manley, University of Wisconsin, Madison, WI. Reproduced with permission from Paul Manley.)

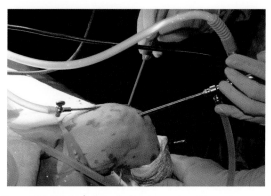

Figure 5.45   Triangulation of arthroscope, hand instrument, and outflow portal.   (Paul Manley, University of Wisconsin, Madison, WI. Reproduced with permission from Paul Manley.)

b. Cause: Congenital condition in brachycephalic breeds
c. Clinical signs: Noisy breathing, exercise intolerance, increased respiratory effort
d. Diagnosis: Pharyngeal exam, radiographs to determine if any other underlying cardiac or thoracic abnormalities
e. Surgery: Following evaluation of the soft palate, the surgeon places stay sutures along the intended line of resection. Minimal handling of the soft palate is encouraged. Metzenbaum scissors are used to transect small amounts of excessive tissue. Closure of the

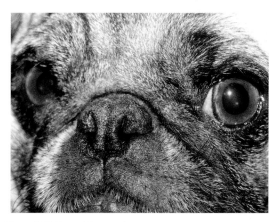

Figure 5.46   Pug with stenotic nares.

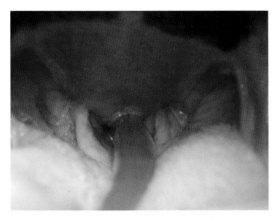

Figure 5.47 Pre-operative view of an elongated soft palate in an English Bulldog. (Robert Hardie, University of Wisconsin. Madison, WI. Reproduced with permission from Robert Hardie.)

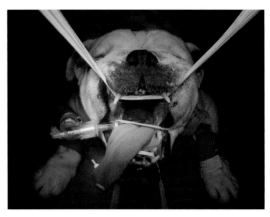

Figure 5.49 Positioning for elongated soft palate reduction. (Robert Hardie, University of Wisconsin Veterinary Care. Madison, WI. Reproduced with permission from Robert Hardie.)

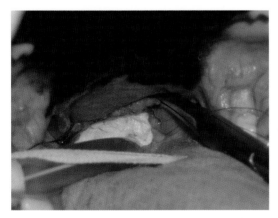

Figure 5.48 Right angle clamp on transected palatal tissue. (Robert Hardie, University of Wisconsin Veterinary Care. Madison, WI. Reproduced with permission from Robert Hardie.)

wound with a simple continuous pattern of monofilament absorbable suture follows each small resection. This alternating pattern of cut/suture continues until all tissue is removed (Figure 5.48).

f. Positioning: Sternal recumbency with a piece of roll gauze through mouth, just caudal to canine teeth, used to suspend maxilla from IV pole. Roll gauze is passed just caudal to the mandibular canines and taped to the table to keep the mouth open (Figure 5.49).

g. Special instrumentation: Long instruments if available, light source, cautery

h. Assistant's role: Provide lateral retraction of tissue by holding hemostats attached to stay sutures.

i. Postoperative care: Close monitoring for respiratory distress, prolonged intubation in immediate postop period ± oxygen therapy, provide small amounts of water when fully awake, delay feeding for 18–24 hours postop, slowly feed soft food formed into meatballs for 5–7 days to slow ingestion, use harness instead of neck collar for 2–4 weeks to avoid trauma to the surgery site

Laryngeal paralysis

a. Definition: Failure of the arytenoid cartilages to open through inspiration and close during swallowing, they remain stationary

b. Cause: Muscles and nerves that cause abduction of the arytenoid cartilage cease to function, may be idiopathic or congenital, more common in older large breed, male dogs

c. Clinical signs: Hoarse barking, exercise intolerance, inspiratory stridor

d. Diagnosis: Laryngoscopy, radiographs to determine if any other underlying cardiac or thoracic abnormalities and to assess aspiration pneumonia and esophageal function

e. Surgery:

   i. Arytenoid lateralization – approach to larynx is through a lateral incision, transection of the interarytenoid ligament, monofilament suture is used to abduct the arytenoid cartilage moderately lateral.

ii. Partial Laryngectomy – oral approach – a long handled scalpel or Metzenbaum scissors is used to resection the corniculate process and the proximal half and base of the cuneiform process. Hemostasis is provided with gauze sponges or cautery.

iii. Partial laryngectomy – ventral approach – a ventral approach is made to expose the larynx. Excision of the corniculate, cuneiforma, and vocal processes over the arytenoid cartilage is performed. Vocal folds are also excised. Defect is closed with small monofilament absorbable suture, routine muscle, and skin closure.

f. Positioning:

i. Arytenoid cartilage lateralization – lateral or dorsal recumbency, rolled towel placed under neck to elevate ipsilateral mandible. Tape head to table.

ii. Partial laryngectomy – oral approach – sternal recumbency with the maxilla elevated via roll gauze placed caudal to the maxillary canines. Mandible can be held open by assistant, taped to table or place roll gauze just caudal to the mandibular canines and tape gauze to table.

iii. Partial laryngectomy – ventral approach – dorsal recumbency with head extended and taped to table.

g. Special instrumentation:

i. Arytenoid cartilage lateralization – cautery, suction

ii. Partial laryngectomy – oral approach -long instruments

iii. Partial laryngectomy – ventral approach – Gelpi, small (4-0 – 6-0) monofilament suture

h. Assistant's role: Visualize larynx through mouth at surgeons request for the ventral approach, suction, cut sutures, tissue retraction

i. Postoperative care: Close monitoring for respiratory distress, provide small amounts of water when fully awake, delay feeding for 18–24 hours postop, slowly feed soft food formed into meatballs for 5–7 days to slow ingestion, use harness instead of neck collar for 2–4 weeks to avoid trauma to the surgery site, restrict exercise for 6–8 weeks, minimize barking, monitor closely for aspiration, may need elevated feedings.

Cardiovascular (heart and lungs)

Patent ductus arteriosus (PDA), persistent right aortic arch (PRAA), Thoracic tumor/abscess, etc.

a. Definition: Congenital conditions effecting the flow of blood through the heart and lungs (PDA/PRAA), tumors of various types, infection (Figures 5.50–5.52).

b. Cause: PDA and PRAA are congenital conditions; other reasons for thoracic surgery include trauma, neoplasia, lung torsion, infection, and so on.

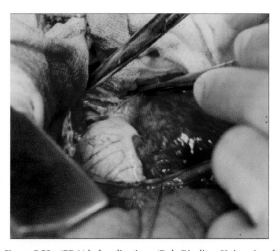

Figure 5.50 (PDA) before ligation. (Dale Bjorling, University of Wisconsin, Madison, WI. Reproduced with permission of Dale Bjorling.)

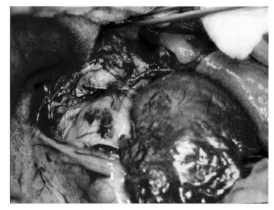

Figure 5.51 PDA after ligation. (Dale Bjorling, University of Wisconsin, Madison, WI. Reproduced with permission of Dale Bjorling.)

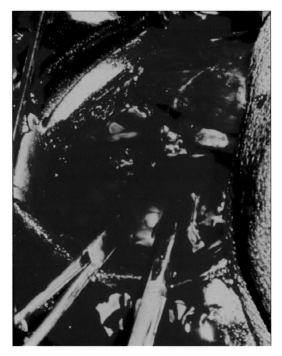

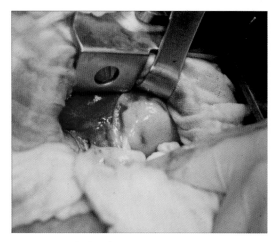

Figure 5.53 Caudal lung lobe abscess. (Dale Bjorling, University of Wisconsin, Madison, WI. Reproduced with permission of Dale Bjorling.)

Figure 5.52 PDA hemorrhaging. (Dale Bjorling, University of Wisconsin, Madison, WI. Reproduced with permission of Dale Bjorling.)

c. Clinical signs: dependent upon cardiac disease but generally decreased respiratory ability, increased lung sounds, low exercise tolerance, and heart murmur.

d. Diagnosis: Thoracic radiographs, chest auscultation, known trauma

e. Surgery: Thoracotomy★ (Fossum 2007a) – surgical incision into the chest wall between two ribs or through the sternum. Surgical approach to the thoracic cavity can be accomplished with a ventral midline sternotomy or a lateral intercostal incision. Depending on the procedure, there may be vessel ligation, tissue resection, or organ resection. Closure depends on approach used (Figures 5.53–5.55).

f. Positioning: Dorsal recumbency or lateral recumbency, left or right lateral will be determined by procedure being performed

g. Special instrumentation: Finiochetto retractor, lap pads, lavage fluid, chest tube, Heimlich valve, cardiovascular instruments, internal staplers, suction, cautery, long instruments. If *sternotomy* performed – bone saw, orthopedic wire, wire twister, wire cutter (Figures 5.56 and 5.57).

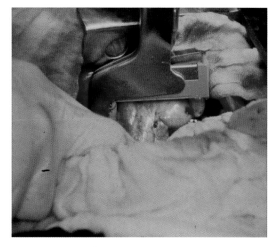

Figure 5.54 Internal stapler in position for lung lobectomy. (Dale Bjorling, University of Wisconsin, Madison, WI. Reproduced with permission of Dale Bjorling.)

h. Assistant's role: Keep tissues moist, retract lungs, load internal staplers if used, suction, run suture, cut wires if sternotomy performed

i. Postoperative care: Close monitoring of respirations – if insufficient, radiograph for pneumothorax, evaluate blood gas for adequate ventilation, nasal oxygen or oxygen cage may be required, possible chest tube placement, provide pain control, critical care monitoring (Figures 5.58 and 5.59).

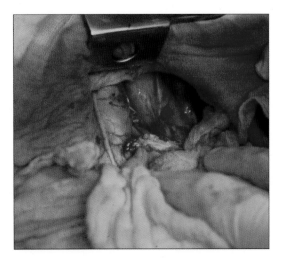

Figure 5.55 Post lung lobectomy with internal stapler. (Dale Bjorling, University of Wisconsin, Madison, WI. Reproduced with permission of Dale Bjorling.)

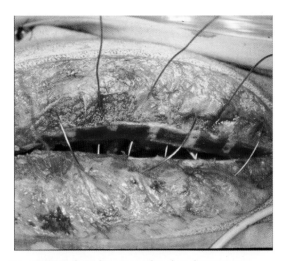

Figure 5.57 Orthopedic wire used to close the sternum.

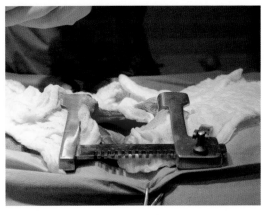

Figure 5.56 Finiochetto retractor in chest.

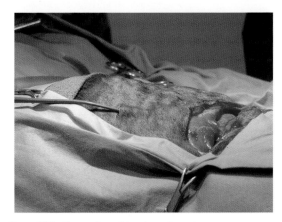

Figure 5.58 Chest tube exiting thoracic cavity.

Arrhythmia

a. Definition: Irregular heartbeat may be related to bradycardia or heart block
b. Cause: Disruption of the heart's electrical activity
c. Clinical signs: Bradycardia, tachycardia, irregular cardiac rhythm
d. Diagnosis: Cardiac auscultation, electrocardiogram, echocardiogram, thoracic radiographs
e. Surgery: Pacemaker Placement★ (Fossum 2007b) – insertion of a pericardial device to control abnormal heart rhythms *Epicardial* placement requires a celiotomy and diaphragmatic incision. The cardiac

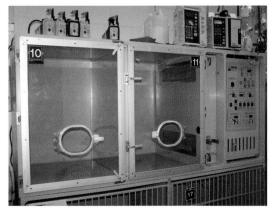

Figure 5.59 Oxygen cages benefit patients following thoracic surgery and other conditions with respiratory distress.

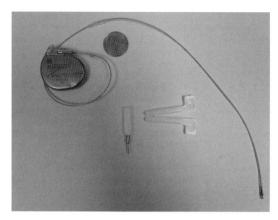

apex is visualized through the diaphragm and the pericardium is incised. Electrode lead is passed through the diaphragmatic incision and screwed into the apex of the heart. The other end is attached to the generator. The generator is placed in a muscle pocket created in the abdominal wall. Routine closure follows. *Endocardial* placement in the right ventricle is achieved via the jugular vein. This approach requires cardiac catheterization capabilities.

f. Positioning: Dorsal recumbency
g. Special instrumentation: Pacemaker implant, pacemaker wires, suction, cautery (Figure 5.60).
h. Assistant's role: Retract pericardium, suction, provide hemostasis, appropriate handling of pacemaker generator and electrode wires
i. Postoperative care: Close monitoring of pacemaker for first 48 hours via electrocardiogram, then follow-up every 3–6 months, monitor for exercise intolerance

Abdominal

Liver – portosystemic shunt (PSS) (Fossum 2007c)

a. Definition: Blood vessels bypass the liver and drain from the stomach, intestines, spleen, and pancreas directly into the circulatory system thus partially eliminating the liver's filtering properties – may be intrahepatic or extrahepatic[1]
b. Cause: *Congenital* (intrahepatic) when ductus venosus does not close at birth, *congenital* (extrahepatic) when an anomalous vessel allows blood to flow directly from the portal vein to the general circulatory system, *acquired* (extrahepatic) from portal hypertension in patients with liver disease, most common in young, pure bred dogs and shorthair cats, hereditary in Yorkshire Terriers
c. Clinical signs: Small size for breed, vomiting, seizures, behavioral changes
d. Diagnosis: Radiographs, positive contrast portography, ultrasound, laboratory tests including liver function and pre/post prandial bile acids
e. Surgery★:
   i. Extrahepatic: A ventral midline incision is made. Dissection occurs to identify the shunt. Placement of a constrictor or cellophane band occurs. Occasionally ligation is performed. Routine closure (Figure 5.61).
   ii. Intrahepatic: Caudal sternebrae/cranial abdominal ventral midline incision, the shunt is identified and ligated.
f. Positioning: Dorsal recumbency

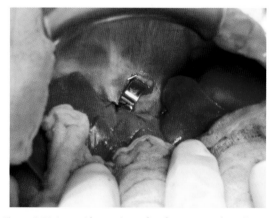

---

[1] http://en.wikipedia.org/wiki/Portosystemic_shunt

g. Special instrumentation:

i. Extrahepatic: Ameroid constrictor, Balfour retractor, lap pads, suction, cautery, cellophane band if ameroid constrictor not used, right angle forceps.

ii. Intrahepatic: umbilical tape, $3\frac{1}{2}$ or 5 fr. Polypropylene catheter, right angle forceps, silk ligature, or suture requested by surgeon

h. Assistant's role: Lavage, tissue retraction, cut sutures

i. Postoperative care: Critical care monitoring for portal hypertension, painful abdomen and seizures, low protein diet for 2–3 months until recheck liver values show return to normal function

Spleen

a. Definition: A variety of conditions may affect the spleen

b. Cause: Trauma, tumor, or torsion

c. Clinical signs: Enlarged spleen, possibly anemia

d. Diagnosis: Palpation, radiographs, laboratory tests

e. Surgery: Splenectomy★(Fossum 2007d) – partial or total removal of the spleen, ventral midline approach to the abdomen with visualization of spleen, careful exteriorization of the spleen, double ligation, or stapling of all splenic vessels, routine closure (Figures 5.62 and 5.63).

f. Positioning: Dorsal recumbency

g. Special instrumentation: Lap pads, ± Balfour retractor, internal stapler (usually LDS), lavage fluid, ligature suture if stapler not used, suction, cautery, specimen container, comparative measure device (ruler), camera

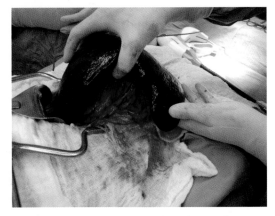

Figure 5.62 Spleen being exteriorized. (Robert Hardie, University of Wisconsin Veterinary Care. Madison, WI. Reproduced with permission from Robert Hardie.)

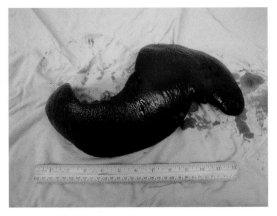

Figure 5.63 Spleen following excision from abdominal cavity. (Robert Hardie, University of Wisconsin Veterinary Care. Madison, WI. Reproduced with permission from Robert Hardie.)

h. Assistant's role: Load stapler if used, run suture, cut suture if ligatures used, moisten tissues

i. Postoperative care: Monitor closely for postoperative hemorrhage and disseminated intravascular coagulation (DIC), blood transfusions if indicated for anemic patients

Digestive (stomach and intestines)

Abdomen

a. Definition: A variety of conditions may require surgical exploration of the abdomen

b. Cause: Varies based on diagnosis – neoplasia, chronic disease (i.e., porto-systemic shunt)or emergency conditions (i.e., gastric torsion, foreign body, trauma)

c. Clinical signs: Dependent upon condition being treated

d. Diagnosis: Abdominal palpation, laboratory tests, radiographs, dependent upon assumed disease, or injury

e. Surgery: Abdominal Exploratory (Celiotomy) (Fossum 2007e) – surgical incision into the abdominal cavity, ventral midline approach to the abdomen, exploration of entire abdomen, biopsy, or excision of affected organ (Figures 5.64 and 5.65).

f. Positioning: Dorsal recumbency

g. Special instrumentation: Balfour retractor, lap pads, biopsy instruments if indicated, internal staplers if indicated, suction, cautery, formalin jars for samples, lavage fluid (Figure 5.66).

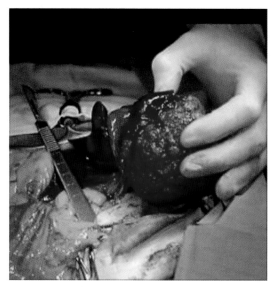

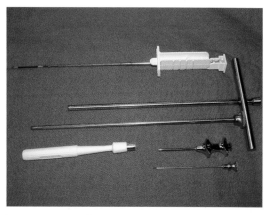

Figure 5.66 Various biopsy instruments (soft tissue and orthopedics).

Figure 5.64 Liver tumor. (Dale Bjorling, University of Wisconsin, Madison, WI. Reproduced with permission of Dale Bjorling.)

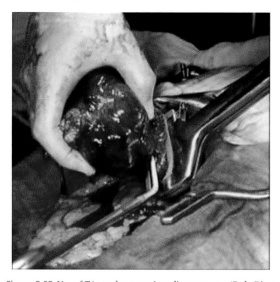

Figure 5.65 Use of TA stapler to excise a liver tumor. (Dale Bjorling, University of Wisconsin, Madison, WI. Reproduced with permission of Dale Bjorling.)

h. Assistant's role: Lavage tissue, suction, provide hemostasis, hand biopsy instruments, cut sutures

i. Postoperative care: Monitor incision for redness, swelling, drainage, dehiscence, Elizabethan collar, or body stocking to protect the surgical site, exercise restrictions until sutures removed

Gastric dilatation volvulus (GDV or bloat) (Hedlund and Fossum 2007)

a. Definition: Stomach is twisted causing enlargement (may have simple dilation without volvulus (twisting) (Figure 5.67).

b. Cause: Gastric outflow is blocked causing gas and fluid to accumulate in stomach, etiology unknown although may be related to overeating and anatomic conditions, most common in large, deep-chested dogs

c. Diagnosis: Obvious distended abdomen on palpation and radiographs

d. Surgery: Ventral midline approach to the cranial abdomen, reduction of dilation, and/or volvulus of stomach, resection of necrotic gastric tissue if necessary, possible gastropexy, routine closure (Figure 5.68).

e. Positioning: Dorsal recumbency

f. Special instrumentation: Lap pads, suction, cautery, lavage, nonabsorbable, monofilament suture if performing gastropexy, internal stapling device if partial gastrectomy performed

g. Assistant's role: Moisten tissue, suction, tissue retraction, cut sutures

h. Postoperative care: Monitor electrolytes and acid-base balance especially potassium as patients tend to become hypokalemic, feed small amounts of water and soft low fat diet during first few days postop, incisional care as with celiotomy

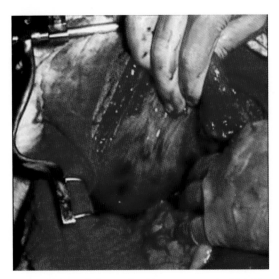

Figure 5.67 Distended stomach with spotty necrosis. (Dale Bjorling, University of Wisconsin, Madison, WI. Reproduced with permission of Dale Bjorling.)

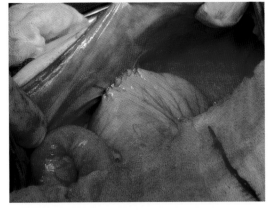

Figure 5.68 Gastropexy. (Dale Bjorling, University of Wisconsin, Madison, WI. Reproduced with permission of Dale Bjorling.)

Gastric foreign body

a. Definition: Ingestion of anything that cannot be digested such as plastic, clothing, string, yarn, ribbon, and may include bones and rawhide chews
b. Cause: Dogs will eat anything; cats enjoy playing with yarn, and so on.
c. Clinical signs: Vomiting, known ingestion of foreign material

d. Diagnosis: Possible abdominal pain, may see string attached to tongue, endoscopy, radiographs, ultrasound
e. Surgery: None if retrievable by endoscopy, ventral midline approach to the abdomen, placement of stay sutures to elevate stomach, incise stomach and remove foreign body. Inspect stomach for compromised tissue, lavage abdomen after closure of stomach. Change to second set of instruments, gloves, and drapes for closure to avoid contamination from stomach contents.
f. Positioning: Dorsal recumbency
g. Special instrumentation: Lap pads, lavage, second set of drapes, and instruments
h. Assistant's role: Hold stay sutures to elevate stomach, suction, cut sutures, hydrate tissues on field
i. Postoperative care: Monitor for vomiting, food and water as tolerated, feeding tube may be indicated, incisional care as with celiotomy

Intestinal foreign body

a. Definition: Ingestion of anything that cannot be digested such as plastic, clothing, string, yarn, ribbon, and may include bones and rawhide chews, may be partial or complete obstruction, can lead to intestinal necrosis and perforation
b. Cause: Items may be small enough to pass through the esophagus and stomach but become trapped in the smaller diameter of the intestine
c. Clinical signs: Anorexia, constipation and vomiting, abdominal pain, possible known foreign body ingestion, cats are more prone to linear foreign bodies
d. Diagnosis: Physical exam findings of abdominal pain, bunched intestines may be evident with linear objects, radiographs, contrast imaging, ultrasound, known ingestion of foreign object
e. Surgery: Ventral midline approach to the abdomen, evaluation of entire intestinal tract, enterotomy for simple foreign body, resection and anastomosis for linear foreign body (Figures 5.69–5.72).
f. Positioning: Dorsal recumbency
g. Special instrumentation: Balfour retractor, intestinal clamps, internal staplers, second set of drapes, gowns, gloves, instruments, lavage, suction, cautery, camera
h. Assistant's role: Occlude intestine with index finger and third finger of each hand if resection and anastomosis performed, load internal stapler if used,

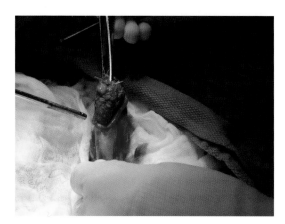

Figure 5.69 Intestinal foreign body. (Robert Hardie, University of Wisconsin Veterinary Care. Madison, WI. Reproduced with permission from Robert Hardie.)

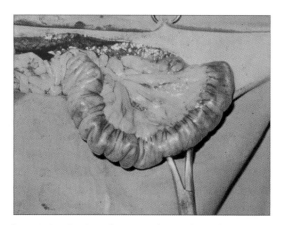

Figure 5.72 Plication of intestine from a linear foreign body. (Dale Bjorling, University of Wisconsin, Madison, WI. Reproduced with permission of Dale Bjorling.)

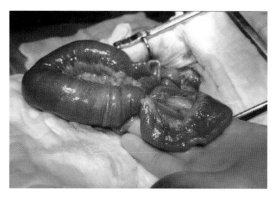

Figure 5.70 Intestinal intussusception before reduction. (Dale Bjorling, University of Wisconsin, Madison, WI. Reproduced with permission of Dale Bjorling.)

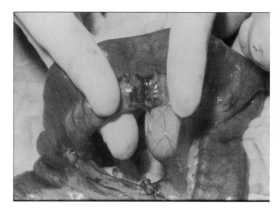

Figure 5.73 Assistant occluding intestine prior to resection.

moisten tissue, suction, cut sutures (Figures 5.73 and 5.74).

i. Postoperative care: Monitor for vomiting and peritonitis, correct fluid and electrolyte imbalances if present, food and water as tolerated, incisional care as with celiotomy

Urogenital (Hedlund 2007b)

Obstetrics

a. Definition: Removal of fetuses, may be performed with an ovariohysterectomy
b. Cause: Fetuses are not able to be delivered without intervention; may be performed for dystocia or elective procedures for specific breeds or patients with a

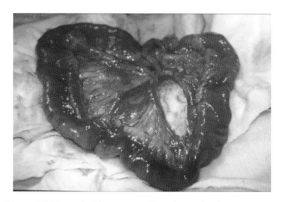

Figure 5.71 Intestinal intussusception after reduction – not compromised vascularity. (Dale Bjorling, University of Wisconsin, Madison, WI. Reproduced with permission of Dale Bjorling.)

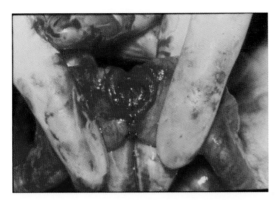

Figure 5.74 Assistant occluding intestine for anastamosis.

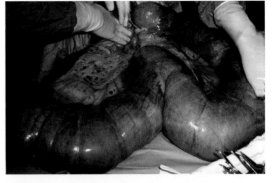

Figure 5.75 Gravid uterus exteriorized from abdomen. (Jonathan McAnulty, University of Wisconsin-Madison, Madison, WI. Reproduced with permission from Jonathan McAnulty.)

decreased pelvic canal opening e.g., following pelvic fracture

c. Clinical signs: Difficulty giving birth (dystocia), end term pregnancy (elective)

d. Diagnosis: Palpation ± radiographs

e. Surgery: Cesarean Section (C-Section) – incision into the uterus (hysterotomy) to remove fetuses, may be performed with an ovariohysterectomy, ventral midline approach to the abdomen, exteriorize gravid uterus. Incise uterus for removal of fetuses. Clamp and transect umbilical cord of each fetus prior to handing them off the sterile field to an assistant, close uterus, lavage abdomen, redrape, change gloves, and open new instruments for closure to avoid contamination (Figures 5.75–5.78).

f. Positioning: Dorsal recumbency *Note: Much of the prep of the patient is performed prior to anesthesia to decrease anesthetic effects on the fetuses.*

g. Special instrumentation:
  i. Bitch/Queen: Lap pads, suction, cautery, Oxytocin in room, lavage fluids, extra hemostats
  ii. Newborns: Warm environment, suture to ligate umbilicus, bulb syringe for suctioning nares, dry towels, intubation supplies (small endotracheal tubes (ET) – 18 gauge × 2″ IV catheters may be used for ET tube), oxygen source

h. Assistant's role: Assist with elevation of gravid uterus out of abdomen, suction, hand instruments quickly as newborns are removed, hand off newborns to waiting circulating tech or other non-sterile assistant

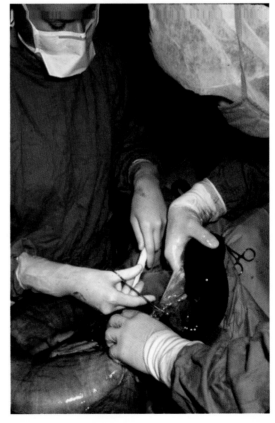

Figure 5.76 Removal of a puppy and clamping of umbilicus of puppy. (Jonathan McAnulty, University of Wisconsin-Madison, Madison, WI. Reproduced with permission from Jonathan McAnulty.)

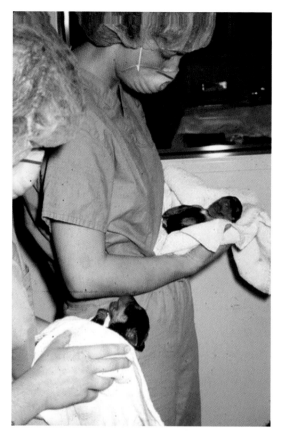

Figure 5.77 Resuscitation of newborn. (Jonathan McAnulty, University of Wisconsin-Madison, Madison, WI. Reproduced with permission from Jonathan McAnulty.)

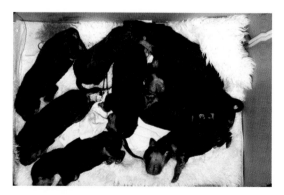

Figure 5.78 Happy ending!. (Jonathan McAnulty, University of Wisconsin-Madison, Madison, WI. Reproduced with permission from Jonathan McAnulty.)

i. Postoperative care:

   i. Newborn care includes suctioning nares, briskly rubbing, and drying to stimulate respiration, keep warm.

   ii. Bitch or queen: Monitor incision for redness, swelling, drainage, dehiscence, Elizabethan collar or body stocking to protect the surgical site as needed, exercise restrictions until sutures removed, encourage lactation

Intact male – orchiectomy (neuter/castration)

a. Definition: Sterilizing a male dog/cat to prevent breeding, decrease aggressive behavior and prevent hormone-related diseases such as prostate conditions and perineal hernias

b. Cause: Intact male animal, testicular condition such as tumor

c. Clinical signs: Generally normal physical exam, intact male animal

d. Diagnosis: Determine if both testes are descended, evaluate prostate

e. Surgery:

   i. Canine: A prescrotal incision is made and testicles are squeezed out of incision one at a time. Ligation and transaction of testicular structures, closure of scrotum may or may not include skin sutures

   ii. Feline: A scrotal incision is made over each testicle. The testicle is removed and ligated or self-tied, no scrotal closure (Figures 5.79 and 5.80).

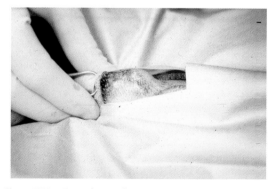

Figure 5.79 Draped area for canine castration. (Jonathan McAnulty, University of Wisconsin-Madison, Madison, WI. Reproduced with permission from Jonathan McAnulty.)

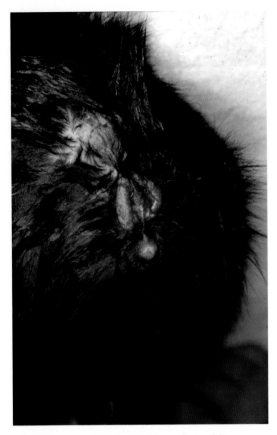

Figure 5.80   Postoperative incisions from feline neuter. (Jonathan McAnulty, University of Wisconsin-Madison, Madison, WI. Reproduced with permission from Jonathan McAnulty.)

f. Positioning: Dorsal recumbency; lateral recumbency may be used for felines

g. Special instrumentation: None needed

h. Assistant's role: Not usually present

i. Postoperative care: Monitor incision for redness, swelling, drainage, dehiscence, Elizabethan collar to protect the surgical site as needed, exercise restrictions until sutures removed

Intact female – ovariohysterectomy (OHE/neuter/spay)

a. Definition: Sterilizing a female dog/cat to prevent breeding and prevent hormone-related diseases such as mammary tumors and pyometra

b. Cause: Intact female, uterine condition such as pyometra

c. Clinical signs: Generally normal but may have enlarged uterus, purulent, or bloody vaginal discharge indicating estrus or infection

d. Diagnosis: Check for vaginal discharge, enlarged vulva

e. Surgery:

  i. Routine: Ventral midline abdominal approach, identification of ovaries, uterine horn and uterus, ligation and removal of ovaries, uterine horns and uterus, routine closure

  ii. Laparoscopic: Minimally invasive procedure for the removal of ovaries, uterine horns and uterus, ligation or electrosurgical sealing of transected tissue (Figure 5.81).

f. Positioning:

  i. Routine: Dorsal recumbency

  ii. Laparoscopic: Dorsal or lateral recumbency

g. Special instrumentation:

  i. Routine: None needed

  ii. Laparoscopic: Laparoscope, laparoscopic instrument set, CO_2 insufflator (Figure 5.82).

h. Assistant's role:

  i. Routine: Usually not present

  ii. Laparoscopic: Monitor insufflation pressure, manipulate scope as needed, cut sutures

i. Postoperative care: Monitor incision for redness, swelling, drainage, dehiscence, Elizabethan collar to protect the surgical site as needed, exercise restrictions until sutures removed

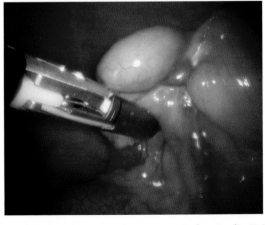

Figure 5.81 Ovariectomy via laparoscope. (Robert Hardie, University of Wisconsin Veterinary Care. Madison, WI. Reproduced with permission from Robert Hardie.)

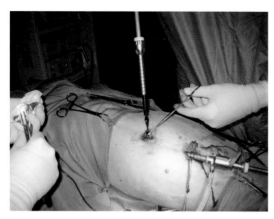

Figure 5.82 Set up for laparoscopic OHE. (Robert Hardie, University of Wisconsin Veterinary Care. Madison, WI. Reproduced with permission from Robert Hardie.)

Urethral blockage – male cats

a. Definition: Inability to urinate
b. Cause: Feline lower urinary tract disease (FLUTD), urethral calculi, tumor, trauma, more common in overweight, middle-aged, indoor cats, less commonly found in dogs,
c. Clinical signs: Inappropriate urination, hematuria, anuria, anxious, anorexia, vomiting
d. Diagnosis: Palpable large bladder that cannot be expressed, radiographs
e. Surgery: Perineal urethostomy (PU) (Fossum 2007f) (penile amputation to alleviate chronic urethral obstruction not relievable by other means), dissection and release of caudal urethra, extension of urethra allows suturing of pelvic urethra to the skin to allow a wider path for the passage of urine, increased urethral width decreases risk of reobstruction, caudal urethra, and penis are removed/amputated
f. Positioning: Ventral recumbency with hind limbs hanging over the end of the surgery table, rolled up towel underneath hips to prevent pressure/nerve damage, tail taped up to allow access to perineal area, purse string suture placed in anus
g. Special instrumentation: Head loops, tom cat catheter, ophthalmic instruments (baby Metzenbaum scissors, delicate thumb tissue forceps), surgical spears for hemostasis, small needle holder (Derf, Short Mayo/Olsen Hagar)

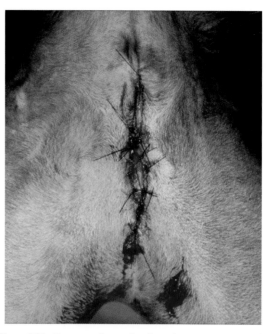

Figure 5.83 Postoperative perineal urethrostomy site. (Dale Bjorling, University of Wisconsin, Madison, WI. Reproduced with permission of Dale Bjorling.)

h. Assistant's role: Hemostasis, manipulation of urinary catheter, cut sutures
i. Postoperative care: Shredded paper or commercially available paper source litter, Elizabethan collar to prevent licking until sutures removed, gentle cleaning of surgical site with damp cotton swab, Vaseline® around urethral opening if needed for urine scald, sedation required for suture removal, intermittent monitoring for urinary tract infection (Figure 5.83).

Chronic renal failure

a. Definition: Progressive loss of kidney function that eventually becomes insufficient to support life
b. Cause: Variety of reasons: obstruction, infection, toxins, age
c. Clinical signs: Anorexia, vomiting, polydipsia, polyuria
d. Diagnosis: Increased creatinine and blood urea nitrogen levels, ultrasound, radiographs
e. Surgery: Renal transplant★(implantation of kidney from a compatible donor) After the donor kidney is harvested it is placed in solution to maintain its viability. A ventral midline abdominal approach

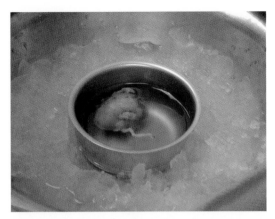

Figure 5.84 Maintaining kidney viability. (Jonathan McAnulty, University of Wisconsin-Madison, Madison, WI. Reproduced with permission from Jonathan McAnulty.)

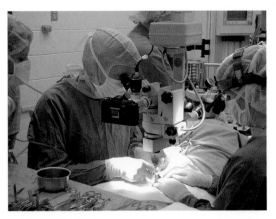

Figure 5.86 Delicate instrumentation. (Jonathan McAnulty, University of Wisconsin-Madison, Madison, WI. Reproduced with permission from Jonathan McAnulty.)

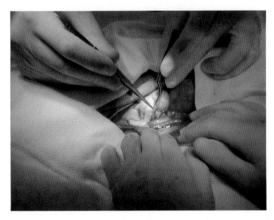

Figure 5.85 Viewing surgical site via microscope for anastamosis of vessels during a renal transplant. (Jonathan McAnulty, University of Wisconsin-Madison, Madison, WI. Reproduced with permission from Jonathan McAnulty.)

is made and the diseased kidney is dissected and excised. A surgical microscope is positioned to allow anastomosis of the renal artery, vein, ureter, and so on to implant the new kidney (Figures 5.84 and 5.85).

f. Positioning: Dorsal recumbency, at the end of the table

g. Special instrumentation: Surgical microscope, Balfour, lap pad, ultra small (10–0) suture, delicate/ophthalmic instrumentation aneurysm clips (Figure 5.86).

h. Assistant's role: Lavage field, pass kidney, cut sutures, hand instruments

i. Postoperative care: Monitor incision for redness, swelling, drainage, dehiscence, Elizabethan collar to protect the surgical site as needed, exercise restrictions until sutures removed, patients are maintained on lifelong immunosuppressive therapy to avoid graft rejection

Other surgery

Onychectomy (Declaw) (Hedlund 2007c) – routine

a. Definition: Removal of the third phalanx of each digit, usually only performed on the front feet

b. Cause: To prevent cats from scratching

c. Clinical signs: Normal kitten, fastest recovery when performed at early age

d. Diagnosis: Usually normal kitten, confirm number of toes as some cats may be polydactyl

e. Surgery: Third phalanx is flexed to facilitate dissection with a number 12 or number 15 scalpel blade. All structures around third phalanx are transected including all tendons and ligaments (Figure 5.87).

f. Positioning: Lateral recumbency with surgical paw up

g. Special instrumentation: Tourniquet placed distal to elbow, number12/number15 scalpel blade, bandage material, tissue adhesive

h. Assistant's role: Apply tourniquet, stabilize/elevate limb

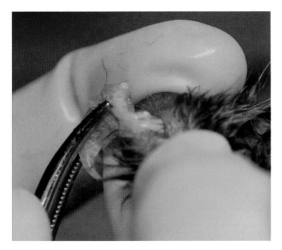

Figure 5.87   Dissection of claw and all surrounding ten-dons and ligaments.   (Jonathan McAnulty, University of Wisconsin-Madison, Madison, WI. Reproduced with permission from Jonathan McAnulty.)

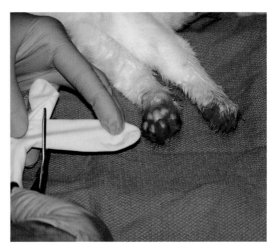

Figure 5.89   Declaw bandage step 2: Cut off middle finger of glove.

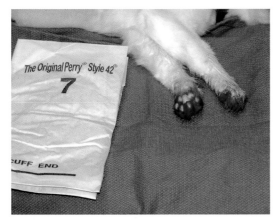

Figure 5.88   Declaw bandage step 1: After declaw procedure; open a package of size 7 sterile gloves.

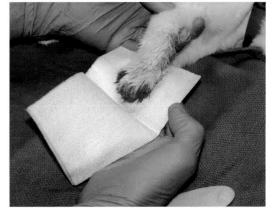

Figure 5.90   Declaw bandage step 3: Unfold two 3 × 3 gauze sponges, cover paw with gauze, creating a tube shape.

i. Postoperative care: Bandage feet for 12–24 hours, shredded paper litter or commercially available paper source litter for two weeks, monitor for hemorrhage as well as persistent lameness and pain (Figures 5.88–5.93).

Onychectomy (declaw) – laser

a. Definition: Removal of the third phalanx of each digit, usually only performed on the front feet
b. Cause: To prevent cats from scratching

c. Clinical signs: Normal kitten, fastest recovery when performed at early age
d. Diagnosis: Usually normal kitten, confirm number of toes as some cats may be polydactyl
e. Surgery: Third phalanx is flexed to facilitate dissec-tion with the laser. Entire third phalanx is removed.
f. Positioning: Lateral recumbency with surgical paw up
g. Special instrumentation: *Note: No alcohol can be used in surgical prep of patient*, protective eyewear specific to laser wavelength (Figure 5.94).

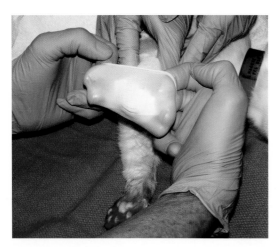

Figure 5.91 Declaw bandage step 4: Stretch glove finger over gauze to secure gauze in place.

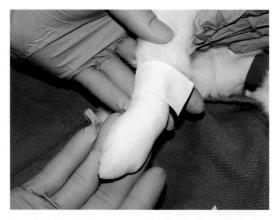

Figure 5.93 Declaw bandage step 6: Create "tab" on end of tape to ease removal. On the day after surgery, remove the bandages by gently detaching the tape strip and cutting the glove finger. Monitor the patient closely for bleeding.

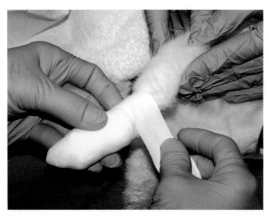

Figure 5.92 Declaw bandage step 5: Apply adhesive tape (1″) strip to edge of glove finger so one half of the width of the tape is on the glove and the other half of the width is on the hair.

h. Assistant's role: Suction smoke plume, monitor safety

i. Postoperative care: Bandage feet for 12–24 hours, shredded paper litter or commercially available paper source litter for 2 weeks, monitor for hemorrhage as well as persistent lameness and pain

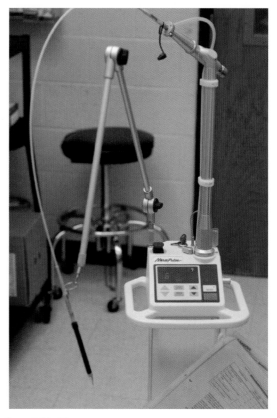

Figure 5.94 CO_2 Laser.

References

Boudrieau, R.J. (2010) Tibial tuberosity advancement. In: Muir, P. (ed), *Advances in the Canine Cranial Cruciate Ligament*. American College of Veterinary Surgeons and Wiley-Blackwell, Ames, IA, pp. 177–187.

Cook, J.L. (2010) Extracapsular stabilization. In: Muir, P. (ed), *Advances in the Canine Cranial Cruciate Ligament*. American College of Veterinary Surgeons and Wiley-Blackwell, Ames, IA, pp. 163–168.

Dueland, R.T., Patricelli, A.J., Adams, W.M. *et al.* (2010) Canine hip dysplasia treated by juvenile pubic symphysiodesis. Part I.: two year results of computed tomography and distraction index. Veterinary and Comparative Orthopaedics and Traumatology, 23 (**6**), 472.

Fossum, T.W. (2007a) *Small Animal Surgery*, 3rd edn. Mosby Elsevier, St. Louis, MO, pp. 867–879.

Fossum, T.W. (2007b) *Small Animal Surgery*, 3rd edn. Mosby Elsevier, St. Louis, MO, pp. 810–816.

Fossum, T.W. (2007c) *Small Animal Surgery*, 3rd edn. Mosby Elsevier, St. Louis, MO, pp. 539–553.

Fossum, T.W. (2007d) *Small Animal Surgery*, 3rd edn. Mosby Elsevier, St. Louis, MO, pp. 624–629.

Fossum, T.W. (2007e) *Small Animal Surgery*, 3rd edn. Mosby Elsevier, St. Louis, MO, pp. 317–322.

Fossum, T.W. (2007f) *Small Animal Surgery*, 3rd edn. Mosby Elsevier, St. Louis, MO, pp. 698–701.

Hedlund, C.S. (2007a) Surgery of the upper respiratory system. In: Fossum, T.W. (ed), *Small Animal Surgery*, 3rd edn. Mosby Elsevier, St. Louis, MO, pp. 817–838 842–846.

Hedlund, C.S. (2007b) Surgery of the reproductive and genital systems. In: Fossum, T.W. (ed), *Small Animal Surgery*, 3rd edn. Mosby Elsevier, St. Louis, MO, pp. 702–720.

Hedlund, C.S. (2007c) Surgery of the integumentary systems. In: Fossum, T.W. (ed), *Small Animal Surgery*, 3rd edn. Mosby Elsevier, St. Louis, MO, pp. 251–253.

Hedlund, C.S. & Fossum, T.W. (2007) Surgery of the digestive system. In: Fossum, T.W. (ed), *Small Animal Surgery*, 3rd edn. Mosby Elsevier, St. Louis, MO, pp. 425–433 and 462–467.

Milovancev, M. & Schaefer, S.L. (2010) Tibial plateau leveling osteotomy. In: Muir, P. (ed), *Advances in the Canine Cranial Cruciate Ligament*. American College of Veterinary Surgeons and Wiley-Blackwell, Ames, IA, pp. 169–175.

Muir, P. (2010) Role of synovial immune responses in stifle synovitis. In: Muir, P. (ed), *Advances in the Canine Cranial Cruciate Ligament*. American College of Veterinary Surgeons and Wiley-Blackwell, Ames, IA, pp. 87–91.

Piermattei, D.L., Flo, G. & DeCamp, C.E. (2006a) *Handbook of Small Animal Orthopedics and Fracture Repair*, 4th edn. WB Saunders Co, Philadelphia, PA, pp. 49–68.

Piermattei, D.L., Flo, G. & DeCamp, C.E. (2006b) *Handbook of Small Animal Orthopedics and Fracture Repair*, 4th edn. WB Saunders Co., Philadelphia, PA, pp. 562–582.

Piermattei, D.L., Flo, G. & DeCamp, C.E. (2006c) *Handbook of Small Animal Orthopedics and Fracture Repair*, 4th edn. WB Saunders Co, Philadelphia, PA, pp. 501–506.

Piermattei, D.L., Flo, G. & DeCamp, C.E. (2006d) *Handbook of Small Animal Orthopedics and Fracture Repair*, 4th edn. WB Saunders Co, Philadelphia, PA, pp. 491.

Piermattei, D.L., Flo, G. & DeCamp, C.E. (2006e) *Handbook of Small Animal Orthopedics and Fracture Repair*, 4th edn. WB Saunders Co, Philadelphia, PA, pp. 495–501.

Piermattei, D.L., Flo, G. & DeCamp, C.E. (2006f) *Handbook of Small Animal Orthopedics and Fracture Repair*, 4th edn. WB Saunders Co, Philadelphia, PA, pp. 483–489.

Schulz, K.S. (2007a) Diseases of the Joints. In: Fossum, T.W. (ed), *Small Animal Surgery*, 3rd edn. Mosby Elsevier, St. Louis, MO, pp. 1197–1213.

Schulz, K.S. (2007b) Diseases of the joints. In: Fossum, T.W. (ed), *Small Animal Surgery*, 3rd edn. Mosby Elsevier, St. Louis, MO, pp. 1176–1197.

Schulz, K.S. (2007c) Diseases of the joints. In: Fossum, T.W. (ed), *Small Animal Surgery*, 3rd edn. Mosby Elsevier, St. Louis, MO, pp. 1255–1276.

Shores, A. (1985) Intervertebral disk disease. In: Newton, C.D. & Nunamaker, D.M. (eds), *Textbook of Small Animal Orthopaedics*. Lippincott, Williams & Wilkins, Philadelphia, PA.

Wilke, V. (2010) Genetics of cranial cruciate ligament rupture. In: Muir, P. (ed), *Advances in the Canine Cranial Cruciate Ligament*. American College of Veterinary Surgeons and Wiley-Blackwell, Ames, IA, pp. 53–58.

CHAPTER 6

Wound management

Patients come to the veterinary hospital with a huge variety of wounds. They range from simple scrapes to burns and huge gaping contaminated injuries. While basic wound management starts the same for any injury, the extent of care varies greatly. A Labrador Retriever with a pad laceration from stepping on a piece of glass needs far different care than a Chihuahua attacked by a Mastiff causing bite wounds and internal abdominal damage or a cat caught in a house fire. Postoperatively and sometime preoperatively, patients require wound and surgical incision care that may include drains, bandages, and external coaptation. The veterinary technician is an integral part of the team in daily (or more frequent) assessment of patients' wounds. A wound is damage to the skin and underlying structures (Hosgood 2012). There are many types of injuries.

Types of wounds

- **Abrasion:** Although painful, abrasions are less than full skin thickness deep, have a minimal amount of bleeding, and heal quickly with little intervention
- **Puncture:** Full penetrating injury, punctures go deep into the tissues through a small opening resulting in contamination and destruction – examples include stick penetration, bite, and gunshot wounds
- **Laceration:** Sharp skin edges characterize lacerations although the edges may be ragged, they may be deep or superficial, and include surgical incisions
- **Degloving:** Much skin and underlying tissue is lost or torn away thus severing the blood supply, most often found on distal limbs

- **Burn:** Resulting from a heat source near or directly on the skin, burns vary in severity: superficial partial (epithelial), deep partial (epithelial and partial dermal), and full thickness, burns may worsen in severity over time due to delayed microvascular damage
- **Decubital ulcer:** A compression injury, decubital ulcers form when skin and soft tissues are compacted between a bony prominence (e.g., elbow, hock, and hip) and a hard surface (e.g., deficiently padded bed), tissue damage can be extensive and is most common in recumbent patients

Phases of wound healing (Cornell 2012)

Wounds follow a specific pattern of healing. (Table 6.1)

1 Inflammation: When a wound occurs, inflammation begins. Endothelin protein is produced along with other mediators; it initially causes vasoconstriction. The coagulation cascade begins to create hemostasis. Thrombin and growth factors attract cells to the site to begin wound healing. Neutrophils and macrophages travel to the wound within 24–48 hours to remove bacteria. These cells die as they ingest material and produce fluid. This is the purulent material seen in wounds. (Figure 6.1) Soon after, prostaglandins, histamine, and other factors initiate vasodilation and increased blood flow to the area. This creates the characteristic inflammatory signs of redness, heat, and swelling.
2 Proliferation: This constructive phase begins after wound debridement and from about day four through day twelve following injury. It is delayed when foreign material, infection, necrotic debris, or

Surgical Patient Care for Veterinary Technicians and Nurses, First Edition. Gerianne Holzman and Teri Raffel.
© 2015 John Wiley & Sons, Ltd. Published 2015 by John Wiley & Sons, Ltd.
Companion Website: wiley.com/go/holzman/surgical.

Table 6.1 Wound healing chronology.

Time	Wound
1–3 d	Cellular debridement, inflammation in minimally traumatized (ideal) wound
3–5 d	Granulation bed forming and visible
7 d	Collagen deposition increases, minimal increase in wound strength
7–14 d	Rapid increase in wound strength
14 d	Wound begins to strengthen
6 wk	Full contracture of properly managed wound
Months to years	Scar maturation; gradual strengthening

Jonathan McAnulty, University of Wisconsin-Madison, Madison, WI. Reproduced with permission from Jonathon McAnulty.

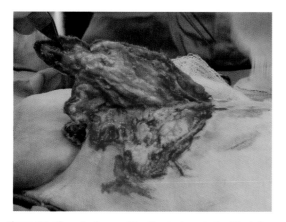

Figure 6.1 Phase 1 of wound healing is characterized by *inflammation*, redness and purulent material accumulating within the wound from cell death. (Robert Hardie, University of Wisconsin Veterinary Care. Madison, WI. Reproduced with permission from Robert Hardie.)

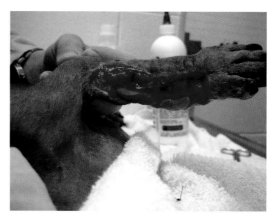

Figure 6.2 Phase 2 of wound healing includes *proliferation* of tissue and granulation bed formation. (Robert Hardie, University of Wisconsin Veterinary Care. Madison, WI. Reproduced with permission from Robert Hardie.)

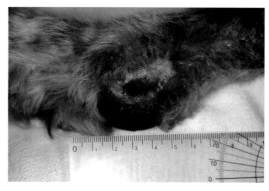

Figure 6.3 Phase 3 of wound healing is the *maturation* of the cells as collagen forms and strengthens while the wound continues to shrink in size. (Robert Hardie, University of Wisconsin Veterinary Care. Madison, WI. Reproduced with permission from Robert Hardie.)

a hematoma is present. The scope of the wound, its location, and patient condition influences the duration of this period. Capillaries grow into the wound from surrounding vasculature, collagen is produced and the wound contracts and eventually closes. A network of small blood vessels within the wound provides oxygen and nutrients and eventually develops into granulation tissue, which is very resistant to infection (Figure 6.2).

3 Maturation: The remodeling and strengthening phase is the longest; primarily it begins in 5–9 days and lasts 4–5 weeks but can extend to eighteen months. During this time, the initial type of collagen changes and becomes stiffer, stronger, and thicker collagen. If continual bending occurs at the wound site, such as over a joint, this phase of healing is prolonged. The initial collagen continues production and abnormal healing may occur by contracture causing decreased function of the joint (Figure 6.3).

Delays in wound healing

In addition to contamination with foreign material, infection, and necrotic tissue, other factors can affect wound healing. Patients' general conditions can delay injury healing. Systemic disorders such as diabetes,

Cushing's disease, chronic steroid use, renal and liver disease, cancer, starvation, chemotherapy, and so on all affect a patient's ability to heal. Wounds must be well perfused to provide oxygen critical to healing. Systemic antibiotics cannot reach the injury without sufficient blood flow. Shock and hypotension as well as arterial and venous impairment limit hemoglobin (oxygen) delivery to the wound. Hematomas and seromas impair healing by physical disruption, increased pressure on the wound bed, increasing dead space and providing an ideal environment for bacterial growth. Large wounds heal slower due to the greater affected surface area than smaller wounds. Partial wound closure, where appropriate, reduces this factor.

Good surgical techniques can *decrease* delays in healing. These include minimizing tissue trauma, minimizing debris, maintaining moist tissues, minimizing surgical time, avoiding tension on the wound (incision), and providing drainage as needed. Factors that can *increase surgical wound infection* are many.

1 Bacterial contamination: Surgeries are classified according to their likelihood of infection, (Mangram *et al* 1999) higher classifications have a much-increased chance of postoperative complications. Wounds are classified as:

I. Clean: no trauma, infection or inflammation and respiratory, gastrointestinal, genitourinary, and oropharyngeal cavities are *not* entered – infection rate: 2–4.8%

II. Clean-Contaminated: respiratory, gastrointestinal, genitourinary, and oropharyngeal cavities are entered under controlled conditions – infection rate: 3.5–5%

III. Contaminated: open, fresh, accidental wounds, operations with major breaks in sterile technique or gross spillage from gastrointestinal tract – infection rate: 4.6–12%

IV. Dirty-Infected: old traumatic wounds with devitalized tissue, existing clinical infection, foreign bodies, perforated colon, infective organism present prior to surgical procedure – infection rate: 6.7–18.1% (National Research Council Wound Classification System 2012).

2 Propofol use (Brown 2012a): Lipid-based emulsions may support microbial growth. Prompt use of prepared syringes of propofol and avoiding the use of the same syringe on multiple patients decreases this source of infection.

3 Operating room personnel: Inadequate aseptic technique and increased number of personnel in the surgical suite increases the source of contamination.

4 Patient's sex: Intact males produce androgenic hormones leading to immunomodulation (Brown 2012b).

Despite best surgical practices, surgical wound infection remains a concern in small animal hospitals. The United States Centers for Disease Control created guidelines defining surgical site infection (SSI) (Table 6.2).

Table 6.2 Centers for Disease Control criteria for defining a surgical site infection (SSI).

Type of infection	Timing	Infected tissue	Signs – at least one present
Superficial incisional SSI	Within 30 d of surgery	Skin or subcutaneous	1 Superficial purulent discharge 2 Positive culture 3 Pain, tenderness, swelling, redness or heat
Deep incisional SSI	Within 30 d of surgery or 1 year if implant in place and infection related to procedure	Deep soft tissue of incision: fascia or muscle	1 Deep purulent discharge 2 Incision spontaneously dehisces 3 Abscess present in deep tissue
Organ/space SSI	Within 30 d of surgery or 1 year if implant in place and infection related to procedure	Any part of anatomy opened or manipulated during surgery excluding incision	1 Purulent drainage from drain placed into organ or space 2 Positive culture 3 Abscess present in organ/space

Data from Mangram *et al.* (1999).

General wound care

Upon admittance, along with evaluating the entire patient, an assessment is made of the patients' wounds for degree and duration of injury. Patient's life-threatening injuries are always addressed first including the ABCs – Airway, Breathing and Circulation. Despite the initial reaction to want to manage huge gaping wounds, even these do not generally require immediate attention unless the patient is hemorrhaging.

The facilitation of healing without infection is the goal of wound management. Contamination is the presence of bacteria on the surface of a wound. If unattended, this leads to colonization where the microbes are increasing. If still not addressed, colonization becomes infections where the bacteria and other organisms invade the tissues. Class 1 wounds are less than 6 hours old with minimum contamination and trauma. These first 6 hours are the *golden period* where there are an insufficient number of microbes to cause infection. Class 2 wounds, 6–12 hours old, show organism replication but they may not have reached the critical level (10^5 colony forming units(CFU) per gram of tissue) to create infection. Class 3 wounds of greater than 12 hours show great bacterial and other organism growth and develop infection.

First intention healing occurs when the surgeon *primarily closes* a wound within hours of occurrence. Most class 1 injuries and surgical incisions are secured by this method. Class 2 wounds may be amendable to primary closure if there is minimal wound contamination and trauma. Surgical debridement occurs prior to closure and includes the removal of devitalized tissue, bacteria, and foreign matter. In the face of mild contamination and trauma, Class 2 wounds benefit from *delayed primary closure* happening within 3–5 days of injury.

Second intention healing occurs when a wound is left to heal without primary closure. This occurs, over time, by *granulation and contraction*. While many wounds can heal this way, it is a long, often inefficient process and may create an unfavorable result. Excessive granulation tissue may form keeping the skin edges from completely constricting. Likewise, abnormal wound contracture may cause scarring and decreased function of the injured area. Wounds most suited for open wound management (second intention healing) are dirty and contaminated. They often require extensive and

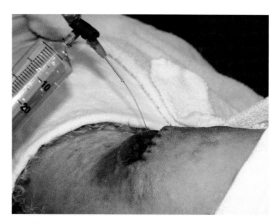

Figure 6.4 Irrigating a wound with saline removes debris, contaminants, and purulent material.

prolonged cleaning and debridement. With time, these wounds may progress enough for secondary closure.

Third intention healing occurs when a wound is repaired by *secondary closure*—more than 3–5 days after injury. These wound have undergone extensive cleansing to remove severe contamination. The tissue is healthier and granulation tissue is present protecting the wound from infection. The surgeon closes the wound over the granulation bed.

Open wound management allows for lavage and debridement to remove debris and microbial contamination (Figure 6.4).

Isotonic saline in large volumes or under high pressure, aids in cleaning wounds. The use of an administration set attached to a fluid bag produces copious amounts of irrigation at low pressure. An 18-gauge needle attached to a 35 ml saline filled syringe creates high pressure of 7–8 psi. Commercial jet pressure (70 psi) units quickly remove contaminants but may force more bacteria into underlying tissues and cause edema. The addition of antiseptics to the irrigation solution is unnecessary and can have cytotoxic effects (McAnulty, 2014). The goal of open wound management is to convert a contaminated, traumatized wound into one that is clean and healthy. This creates an injury that can be closed with great confidence of healing successfully with minimal complications.

Debridement of a wound removes any remaining foreign material and necrotic tissue. The clinician may surgically remove damaged skin and fascia to clean up the wound. Assorted topical treatments also provide wound debridement (Table 6.3).

Table 6.3 Topical treatments.

Material	Indication	Example
Hypertonic saline dressing	20% saline, antimicrobial	Commercially available hypertonic saline gauze
Honey	Antibacterial, reduces inflammation and edema, augments granulation and epithelialization	Medical grade honey
Sugar	Hyperosmotic effect	Sugar from store shelf
Gauze – wet to dry	Debridement*	Sterile gauze moistened with sterile saline
Enzymatic agents	Debridement	Trypsin, collagenase
Maggots	Digestive enzymes dissolve necrotic tissue	Medicinal maggots
Topical antibiotic ointment	Lessens surface bacteria	Triple antibiotic
Silver	Infected wounds	Silver sulfadiazine, silver impregnated dressing
Hydrogel	Minimal exudate, keeps wounds moist	Hydrogel dressings
Hydrocolloid	Absorbs moderate exudate, promotes granulation while keeping wound moist	Hydrocolloid dressings
Alginate	Absorbs excessive exudate, promotes granulation while keeping wound moist	Calcium alginate dressings

Adapted from Hosgood (2012).

*The use of wet-dry gauze bandage is controversial. Based on the author's consultation with veterinary surgeons, this continues to be a viable wound management technique.

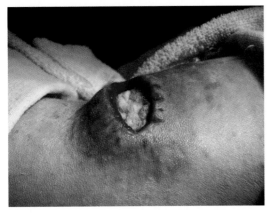

Figure 6.5 Wet gauze applied to a wound is a traditional method of removing accumulating discharge.

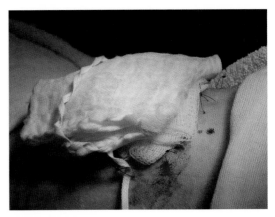

Figure 6.6 The dry part of a wet-dry bandage absorbs drainage while maintaining moisture within the "wet" layer. A tie-over bandage is secured in place with loose sutures acting as loops for lacing umbilical tape.

Based on the extent of the injury, debridement may be a one-time occurrence or continue for several days or even be performed more than once per day. Infected sites benefit from extended treatment to minimize microorganism growth prior to wound closure. (Figures 6.5–6.7) This may include a combination of lavage and debridement to remove purulent and necrotic tissue.

Topical broad-spectrum antimicrobial ointments, gels, and creams applied to a wound aid in controlling contamination and decreasing microbe population.

Collection of a wound culture and sensitivity prior to applying antimicrobials provides important information for choosing a systemic antibiotic. Narrowing the spectrum of coverage of a systemic antibiotic, based on culture sensitivity results, reduces the incidence of the development of resistant microorganisms (Hosgood 2012). Topical antimicrobials are of little use after a healthy granulation bed has formed. The topical

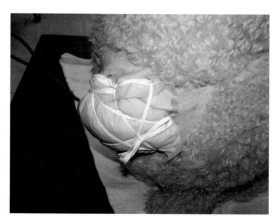

Figure 6.7 A tie-over bandage in place on an open wound over the hip of a Labradoodle. This difficult location to bandage is served well with this type of wrap. Chux padding covers the underlying gauze to protect the gauze from contamination.

Oil impregnated gauze

- Stainless steel container with cover (e.g., cold sterilization tray)
- 4 X 4 or 4 X 8 gauze sponges
- Petrolatum (Vaseline®)

Put gauze in container and cover with petrolatum. Autoclave until petrolatum melts. This does not sterilize the gauze but the process melts the petrolatum to permeate the gauze sponges. Sponges are removed individually with a sterile forceps. The entire tray is reautoclaved weekly to prevent bacteria growth.

Figure 6.8 Oil emulsion gauze is easily made in a clinic following the recipe. (University of Wisconsin Veterinary Care Surgical Suite Technicians. Reproduced with permission.)

treatment may impede healing and a sound granulation bed is resistant to infection.

Application of a dressing following lavage, debridement, and topical treatment shields the wound from further contamination. The bandage also absorbs exudate and protects newly forming granulation tissue from trauma. The first layer of a protective bandage is a nonadherent dressing, which comes in many types, sizes, and shapes. Telfa® pads, while nonadherent, do not allow exudate to migrate away from the wound. Sterile oil-emulsion gauze sponges do not stick to the skin and allow fluid to move away from the wound into surrounding padding. This type of bandage is commercially available or readily created in the clinic (Figure 6.8).

Layered gauzed is unfolded to open up the thread space allowing more drainage. All areas of the wound bed are covered to provide protection and to maintain moisture. (Petrolatum applied to the normal skin surrounding the wound protects it from irritation and scald from any exudate.) The next bandage layer is absorbent to soak up wound fluid and pull it away from the wound surface. Roll cotton and cast padding are great products for this purpose. The thickness of the layer depends on the amount of exudate expected and the amount of additional support needed e.g., wounds on limbs may also need support for bone or tendon injuries. Following the padding layer, stretch gauze is applied to hold the cotton in place. Depending upon the amount of padding applied as well as the

area to be bandaged and the needs of the bandage, the stretch gauze may be applied tightly to provide compression. (Never apply a bandage tight enough to restrict breathing or inhibit blood flow – unless needed to stop hemorrhage.) The final bandage layer is impermeable. Its primary purpose is to keep the underlying layers clean and avoid environmental contaminants. This layer is made of self-adhering flexible bandage tape (e.g., Vetrap™ – 3M™), adhesive elastic bandage tape (e.g., Elastikon™ – Johnson & Johnson) or white adhesive tape. Care is taken to avoid over tightening the bandage when using tapes with elastic properties.

Negative pressure wound therapy

Negative pressure wound therapy (NPWT) or vacuum wound therapy is a treatment in human medicine for patients requiring skin grafts as well as those suffering from infected wounds and burns among other conditions. Although anecdotal reports are available, limited publications have been written on the subject in veterinary medicine. A study performed at Michigan State University in 2010 experimentally compared healing by traditional open wound management methods and with NPWT (Demaria *et al.* 2011). Identical wounds were created on both forelimbs of ten dogs to resemble a minor shear injury. One side was treated as a control using traditional open wound care of absorbent dressing and padding until a granulation bed formed. Upon granulation, a non-adherent dressing and padding covered the wound until the close of the study – 21 days post injury. The bandages were changed at appropriate intervals following standard wound care. The dogs' opposite limbs received NPWT. Foam or gauze covered the wounds followed by an impermeable adhesive drape incised with an evacuation tube leading to the vacuum apparatus. The NPWT was continued throughout the study and the bandages changed at the same intervals as the control limb. Wound measurements, granulation tissue assessment, biopsies, and cultures were obtained throughout the study. The study found advantages and disadvantages of NPWT over traditional open wound therapy. If initialized, NPWT should continue for no more than 10 days to lessen its effects on contraction and epithelialization.

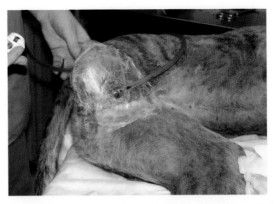

Figure 6.9 Negative pressure wound therapy (NPWT) is applied to a non-healing wound, post amputation, in a Greyhound dog.

- NPWT Advantages
  - earlier granulation tissue
  - superior smoother granulation tissue
  - less-exuberant granulation tissue
  - earlier acute inflammatory stage
  - potential for longer time intervals between dressing changes
  - decreased need for patient sedation for traditional bandage changes
- NPWT Disadvantages
  - initially more retraction of wound edges
  - decreased wound contraction and epithelialization
  - higher bacterial load but no clinical infection noted in study
  - tissue surrounding wound erythema
  - vacuum system requires monitoring to maintain negative pressure
  - commercial system to deliver constant vacuum required

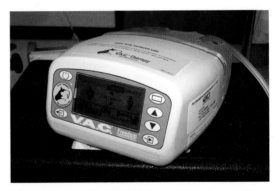

Figure 6.10 Vacuum Assisted Closure (VAC) units provide constant negative pressure to NPWT.

Figures 6.9 shows a Greyhound who had undergone a right rear leg amputation. The surgical wound dehisced. Due to the location of the wound and the thinness of the patient's pelvis, traditional bandaging, and wound care was unsuccessful. The patient underwent NPWT. The suction tubing attached to the wound is connected to a Vacuum Assisted Closure unit (Figure 6.10). The unit contains a cassette that collects the wound exudate (Figure 6.11). This cassette is changed as it fills with material.

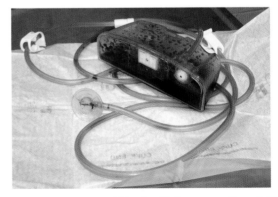

Figure 6.11 Cassette within the VAC system collects fluid removed via NPWT.

Burns

Severe burns are one of the most difficult injuries to treat in human and veterinary medicine. They range greatly in severity-burns that are more extensive carry a graver prognosis. Burns are classified according to the source of injury, depth of wound, and percentage of patient that is injured. The source of the burn divides into three mains types of injury. Burns are *thermal* from either extreme heat or extreme cold (frostbite). Most often, however, thermal burns are considered coming from a heat source. This may be fire, liquids (scalds), hot objects, superheated air in a house fire, or radiation. *Chemical* burns occur when a chemical interacts with the skin and/or produces a hyperthermic or hypothermic reaction. Animals chewing on electric cords can suffer from *electric* burns.

Thermal burns (Bohling 2012)

Thermal burns are graded according to the degree of injury based on the depth of tissue affected (Figure 6.12 and Table 6.4).

This section concentrates on thermal injuries due to hyperthermia. (Hypothermic burns (frostbite) are described in a separate section.) Burn injuries occur rapidly. A skin temperature of 104 °F–111 °F can begin cell death. Partial thickness burns can happen in one second if the skin temperature reaches 140 °F and full thickness in less than a second if temperature exceeds 158 °F. Depending on the source of the flame, house fires can exceed 1000 °F.

Another, perhaps more accurate, classification for assessing burn injury is based on percentage of body surface area affected. The "Resuscitation Burn Card" is based on the size (8.5 × 5.3 cm or 45 cm^2) of an ordinary credit card (Figure 6.13). The burn is compared to the size of the card (or multiple cards) to determine the square centimeters of body surface injured compared to the patient's entire body surface area. The patient's body surface area is taken from a standard body weight to surface area chart. The number of cards is multiplied by 0.45 and divided by the body surface area in square meters to reach a percentage of total body surface area (TBSA) affected.

Burned tissue is divided into three areas:

1 Zone of coagulation (or necrosis or destruction): Center of the wound, area of greatest injury, and no viable tissue

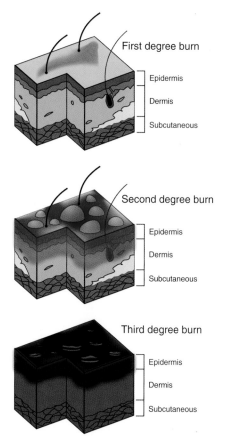

Figure 6.12 Burn diagram demonstrating the depth of injury in the three degrees of thermal burns. (By K. Aainsqatsi at en.wikipedia (Original text: K. Aainsqatsi) [GFDL (www.gnu.org/copyleft/fdl.html) or CC-BY-SA-3.0 (http://creativecommons.org/licenses/by-sa/3.0/)], from Wikimedia Commons).

2 Zone of stasis: Next farthest out from zone of coagulation, less blood perfuses this area, tissue may remain viable if no further damage occurs
3 Zone of hyperemia: Furthest away from the center of the wound, tissue is viable and inflammation occurs to aid in healing

Burn wounds heal slower than other wounds due to lack of normal wound healing cytokines and other growth factors.

Thermal burn treatment

Patients caught in building fires commonly suffer smoke inhalation in addition to thermal injuries. Home materials produce toxic substances and carbon monoxide from the smoke inhibits the lungs and other systems from

Table 6.4 Degree classification of thermal burns.

Degree	Symptoms	Depth	Treatment
First	Erythema, premature skin sloughing, mild discomfort	Partial skin thickness – epidermis	First aid
Second – superficial	Fluid exudate, blistering, sensitive to light touch	Partial skin thickness – epidermis and superficial dermis	First aid and pain control
Second – deep	Skin white and poorly vascularized, less sensitive	Partial thickness – epidermis and most of dermis	May require wound excision ± grafting
Third	Skin dry and leathery without blisters	Full thickness – epidermis, dermis, and into subcutaneous	Wound excision and grafting
Fourth	Skin leathery or missing	Full thickness – extends to muscle and/or bone	Extreme measures to preserve area of injury

Data from http://www.medstudentlc.com/page.php?id=84

absorbing and producing oxygen. As with all emergencies, airway, breathing and circulation is addressed prior to treating other injuries. Many body systems are affected by burns. After establishing a patent airway and providing ventilation support, other metabolic areas are treated in addition to the burn itself. Among the many systems affected by burns are:

1 Cardiovascular: The vascular systems leakage of plasma and evaporation cause hypovolemia, the heart has decreased contractility in very severe burns, carbon monoxide causes decreased cardiac output

2 Gastrointestinal: Gastrointestinal barrier is compromised allowing translocation of bacteria, endotoxins, and cytokines leading to septic shock, decreased gut motility

3 Renal: High burn percentages of TBSA are linked to acute renal failure; decreased cardiac output provides less blood flow to the kidneys

4 Neurologic: Severe pain is present in all burns both initially and as tissue heals and is managed

Burn patients are treated with strong aseptic techniques to minimize contamination. Initially first aid is applied to wounds, and then aggressive fluid therapy is initiated as well as treating inhalation damage, pain, and providing nutritional support. Finally, the burn wound itself is addressed.

Initial care of a burn is application of cold running water (35–60 °F). This provides analgesia and improves healing as it stops the burning. Treatment with ice *is not indicated* and it does not provide a benefit to the patient. Many ointments, creams, herbs, and plants have been used as burn remedies. None of these is scientifically proven superior to plain cold running water. After initial cooling, the wound is covered with a sterile nonadherent dressing. Small partial thickness wounds often heal well from second intention with minimal scarring. Patients are provided with analgesia and the injury is protected from further damage including infection. A topical antibiotic is applied to the wound followed by a moist layer. Padding and bandaging follows as with any open wound.

Deep partial thickness and full thickness wounds require surgical intervention. The wound is debrided to remove all nonviable and necrotic tissue. Over time, more tissue may lose its viability and require excision. Small wounds may be primarily closed at this time and large wounds may require grafting.

Frostbite

Lengthy exposure to the cold can cause hypothermic burns or frostbite. Areas most often affected are extremities and pinnae. Thin skin of the flank folds may also be injured. Iatrogenic damage may occur from misuse of a cryotherapy unit. Frostbite causes:

1 Tissue freezing: Ice crystals create intracellular and extracellular damage through disruption of the cell membrane and cell lysis

2 Hypoxia: cold causes vasoconstriction decreasing blood flow

3 Release of inflammatory mediators: activation of the inflammatory cascade causing clotting and intravascular thrombosis

Veterinary Burn Card

To calculate the burn percentage of the total body surface area (%TBSA):

1. Measure the burn with this card. How many cards are needed to cover the burn?
2. Weigh the patient. Convert the weight to surface area in m^2 using the conversion table on the back.
3. Apply numbers to the following:
    number of cards X $0.45/m^2$ = %TBSA burn

Example: 21kg dog, burn size 15.5 burn cards

15.5 X 0.45/0.76 = 9.2%TBSA

Weight to Surface Area

Dogs						Cats	
Kg	m^2	Kg	m^2	Kg	m^2	Kg	m^2
1	0.1	20	0.74	48	1.32	1.0	0.100
2	0.15	21	0.76	50	1.36	1.5	0.131
3	0.2	22	0.78	52	1.41	2.0	0.159
4	0.25	23	0.81	54	1.44	2.5	0.184
5	0.29	24	0.83	56	1.48	3.0	0.208
6	0.33	25	0.85	58	1.51	3.5	0.231
7	0.36	26	0.88	60	1.55	4.0	0.252
8	0.40	27	0.90	62	1.58	4.5	0.273
9	0.43	28	0.92	64	1.62	5.0	0.292
10	0.46	29	0.94	66	1.65	5.5	0.311
11	0.49	30	0.96	68	1.68	6.0	0.330
12	0.52	32	1.01	70	1.72	6.5	0.348
13	0.55	34	1.05	72	1.75	7.0	0.366
14	0.58	36	1.09	74	1.78	7.5	0.383
15	0.60	38	1.13	76	1.81	8.0	0.400
16	0.63	40	1.17	78	1.84	8.5	0.416
17	0.66	42	1.21	80	1.88	9.0	0.432
18	0.69	44	1.25			9.5	0.449
19	0.71	46	1.28			10	0.464

Figure 6.13 Veterinary Burn Card used to measure the area of the body that is burned. (Adapted from Bohling (2012).)

Frostbite treatment

Initial first aid includes rapid but gentle rewarming of the affected area. Lukewarm water (104–108 °F) immersion is the most effective treatment. This is not initiated if there is any chance of refreezing as a "freeze – thaw – freeze" cycle creates more damage. Along with thawing, fluid therapy is initiated to improve circulation and anti-inflammatory medications are provided. Final treatment of frostbite begins after the extent of injury is recognized. Debridement and open wound management is as described under thermal burns.

Chemical burns

Chemicals cause burns via a variety of actions. Acids (toilet bowl and drain cleaners) are oxidizers that disrupt the cellular protein structure. Alkaline or base chemicals (bleach and ammonia) are reducers causing a denaturing of proteins and other reactions that can lead to a thermal burn. Vesicants are blistering agents generally used in chemical terrorism. The chemotherapeutic drug doxorubicin shows tissue toxicity and blistering.

Chemical burn treatment

Neutralization of the agent is of primary importance. Until this happens, the burning continues. The chemical is neutralized via tissue components, another chemical, copious washing, and or dilution. Warning labels attached to household cleaning products, provide information for treatment of chemicals. Poison control hotlines are also excellent sources of information. Doxorubicin blistering treatment includes surgical removal, local treatment with hyaluronidase for dilution and infiltration of the site with dimethyl sulfoxide.

Following initial first aid, chemical burns are treated as with thermal burns dependent upon their degree and severity.

Electrical burns

Puppies and kittens suffer oral burns from chewing on cords. Other patients may receive electrical burns from improperly grounded electro-cautery units in surgery. Joule's law states that tissues with a higher electrical resistance (i.e., bone) will sustain greater damage than tissues with lower resistance (skin). Electrical wounds may appear superficial on the skin while underlying muscle, bone, and adjoining structures are severely injured as the electric energy met with resistance while traveling through the site. Surgical debridement of electrical wounds is required.

References

Bohling, M.W. (2012) Burns. In: Tobias, K.M. & Johnston, S.A. (eds), *Veterinary Surgery – Small Animal*. Volume II . Elsevier, St. Louis, MO, pp. 1291–1301.

Brown, C.B. (2012a) Wound infections and antimicrobial Use. In: Tobias, K.M. & Johnston, S.A. (eds), *Veterinary Surgery – Small Animal*. Volume 1. Elsevier, St. Louis, MO, pp. 628–646.

Brown, C.B. (2012b) Wound infections and antimicrobial Use. In: Tobias, K.M. & Johnston, S.A. (eds), *Veterinary Surgery – Small Animal*. Volume 1. Elsevier, St. Louis, MO, pp. 135–139.

Cornell, K. (2012) Open wounds. In: Tobias, K.M. & Johnston, S.A. (eds), *Veterinary Surgery – Small Animal*. Volume I. Elsevier, St. Louis, MO, pp. 125–129.

Demaria, M., Bryden, J.S., Hauptman, J.G. *et al.* (2011) Effects of negative pressure wound therapy on healing of open wounds in dogs. Veterinary Surgery, 40 (**2011**), 658–669.

Hosgood, G. (2012) Open wounds. In: Tobias, K.M. & Johnston, S.A. (eds), *Veterinary Surgery – Small Animal*. Volume II. Elsevier, St. Louis, MO, pp. 1210–1220.

Mangram, A.J., Horan, T.C., Pearson, M.L. *et al.* (1999). Guideline For Prevention Of Surgical Site Infection, Centers for Disease Control and Prevention, US Department of Health and Human Services 1999.The Hospital Infection Control Practices Advisory Committee.

McAnulty, J. (2014) Proceedings presented during Junior Surgery Lectures – University of Wisconsin School of Veterinary Medicine.

National Research Council Wound Classification System (2012) range of reported surgical infection rates in dogs and cats. In: Tobias, K.M. & Johnston, S.A. (eds), *Veterinary Surgery – Small Animal*. Volume 1. Elsevier, St. Louis, MO, pp. 135–139.

CHAPTER 7

Postoperative Care

All patients deserve quality care while hospitalized. Patients recovering from surgery have special needs to maintain their comfort. This includes both the immediate postoperative period of anesthesia recovery and any further hospitalization required until discharged. Postoperative pain control is essential to healing and patient well-being. Pain control is covered in Chapter 2 on Preoperative Planning.

Anesthesia recovery

Patients must be directly monitored while recovering from anesthesia. After stopping the flow of anesthetic gas, patients are maintained on an appropriate rate of oxygen flow until they are breathing well on their own. They are never left alone while an endotracheal tube is in place. Once a patient shows signs of consciousness, it is appropriate to deflate the endotracheal tube cuff and extubate the patient. Some patients may become very restless and begin thrashing during this time. It is important to assess the patient's pain level to determine if pain is causing the behavior. If pain is noted, appropriate pain medications are provided to maintain analgesia. If pain does not appear to be causing the patient distress, it is possible for the patient to be negatively reacting to anesthetic or analgesic medications. Many of these drugs can cause dysphoria. A tranquilizer may be indicated for these patients to calm them down while the drugs are dissipating from the body.

Even after the endotracheal tube is removed, patients recovering from surgery must be closely watched. (This is also a great time to trim toenails. Clients appreciate this extra benefit.) Patients' body temperature is monitored for changes. Hypothermia is very common, especially during long surgical procedures. The intraoperative and postoperative use of circulating hot water blankets, hot air warming units, blankets, towels, and so on lessens the incidence of hypothermia. Special care is taken when using microwaveable discs/packs or warm fluid bags. These products must be wrapped in a towel before applying to the patient to avoid contact burns. Patients are warmed to a body temperature of 99 °F before removing supplemental heating sources. Some patients, particularly cats, may develop hyperthermia after surgery. This appears to be an abnormal reaction to certain narcotic medications (Posner *et al.* 2007;.Niedfeldt and Robertson 2006) These patients are cooled by housing in a stainless steel cage with no bedding, applying cool, wet towels over the back or in the groin area, and by using fans. The patient is continuously monitored until a normal temperature is achieved.

While recovering from anesthesia, patients may not have good control of their bladder or bowels. Keeping the patient and cage clean are imperative to avoid contamination of the surgery site and to maintain patient comfort.

Once a patient is fully awake and able to stand (assuming it is expected to stand after surgery), it is safe to return the patient to its normal hospital cage. Dogs are walked, prior to returning to their cage or run, to urinate and defecate. Orthopedic and neurologic patients may need the assistance of a sling, towel, or blanket to aid their ambulation. Patients must not be allowed to slip and fall after any procedure.

Housing

Patients become stressed when not in their home environment and surrounded by their family. They are

Surgical Patient Care for Veterinary Technicians and Nurses, First Edition. Gerianne Holzman and Teri Raffel.
© 2015 John Wiley & Sons, Ltd. Published 2015 by John Wiley & Sons, Ltd.
Companion Website: wiley.com/go/holzman/surgical.

exposed to new smells, sounds, and handlers. Providing them with a comfortable and safe area, away from noise and hospital traffic, calms their fears and aids in healing.

Bedding

Many forms of bedding and housing are available to maximize patient care and comfort. Blankets and towels provide warmth and padding from cage and run floors. They must always be laundered and sanitized between patients. Monitor bedding frequently for patient soiling and change bedding as needed. Patients must never be allowed to reside in their urine, feces, or other body fluids. When soiled bedding is found, it is imperative to also check and clean the patient. Urine and feces left on the hair and skin may cause scalding and wound contamination. *Treat patients as one would want one's own pet taken care of.*

Pads

Foam rubber pads provide extra comfort for recumbent patients as well as those recovering from surgery. (Figure 7.1) To avoid cross-contamination between patients, the foam rubber is enclosed in an impermeable material. These pads can be custom made in sizes that partially or completely cover the floors of cages and runs. They are also made in a variety of thicknesses depending upon the depth of foam rubber interior. The pads are covered with waterproof material and should be cleaned and disinfected between patients. They are monitored for patient chewing or damage. If damaged, prompt repair is important to prevent patient

ingestion from chewing the internal foam rubber as well as contamination and wetting of this material.

Perforated mats

Rubber and plastic mats come in a variety of sizes and configurations. Commercially available mats are made in sizes specifically made for different brands of cages and runs or available by the roll – cut in clinic to custom sizes. They come ribbed or with circular holes to allow drainage (Figure 7.2). While they aid in keeping a patient out of urine, some urine may still be trapped between the mat and the patient. Close patient monitoring reduces this problem. These mats also provide traction for patients needing extra footing. However, they are generally hard plastic or rubber and provide minimal padding.

Other mats

Yoga and other commercially available mats are generally thin providing minimal padding. However, they are great for providing extra traction for patients in cages. They, also, are beneficial for performing patient exams – both for patient and technician/veterinarian comfort. Thin mats provide stability for standing exams. They provide padding for personnel standing, kneeling, or sitting while examining or restraining a patient.

Other bedding

A wide variety of beds is commercially available for added patient comfort. These include covered

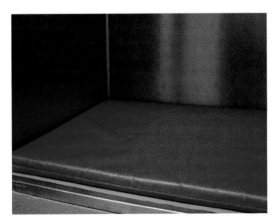

Figure 7.1 Cage pads provide comfortable conditions for patients. They must be impermeable and easy to disinfect.

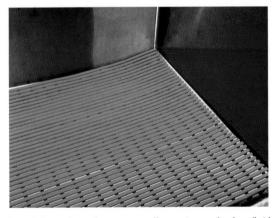

Figure 7.2 Perforated cage mats allow urine and other fluids to pass away from the patient; however they are not soft and provide minimal padding.

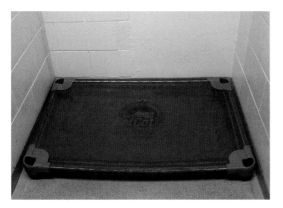

Figure 7.3 Hammock beds allow fluids to pass away from the patient, are soft and help to cool a patient with air circulating beneath the bed.

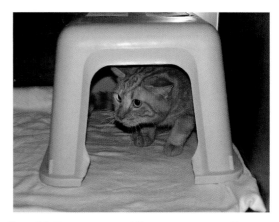

Figure 7.4 Boxes, crates, and litter pan covers provide a great secure "hiding place" for feline patients.

corrugated foam rubber to help prevent pressure sores. Four legged "hammock" type beds made of plastic mesh aid in keeping recumbent patients comfortable, allow urine flow, provide cooling, and air circulation (Figure 7.3).

Air and water mattresses are especially beneficial for preventing skin ulcerations. However, they are susceptible to leakage caused by patients' nails and teeth. They also do not allow urine to flow away from the patient. These mattresses provide the best patient comfort when covered with a blanket or towel. If any of these types of beds are not available, rotating a patient frequently helps to alleviate sores in recumbent patients.

Cage papers

Cages are lined with paper to provide patient traction and to absorb urine and spilled water. They also provide cold protection from the metal, plastic, or fiberglass cage floor. Commercially available cage paper can be ordered to custom fit cages. It does not cause staining as with newspaper and absorbs bodily fluids. While it is resourceful to recycle newspaper as cage lining, the ink can transfer to patients, especially when the paper gets wet. Newspaper, also, becomes smelly when moist.

Boxes/hiding spots

Plastic litter pans and covers, boxes, and crates provide stressed patients with comfort and help to keep small patients warm. Cats, especially, are anxious when hospitalized. Arranging a place for them to hide may help to calm them. Extra blankets or towels allow for

burrowing. The top of a covered litter pan placed on a blanket is a great place for a cat to hide (Figure 7.4). It can easily be lifted up to allow patient access. Simply covering the front of the cage with a towel can give a kitty a feeling of safety by lessening visual stimulation.

Blanket-lined boxes and large litter pans, either, upright or on their side give cats and small dogs a compact, warm-resting area. The sides of the box/pan must be low enough to allow the patient to move in and out. Caution is taken to monitor the patient for box chewing to avoid gastrointestinal obstruction.

Crates of assorted size and configuration provide a safe, warm, and closed environment for small dogs and cats. They also provide ease of transporting the patient around the hospital. If a patient arrives at the clinic with a crate, housing the patient in its own crate while in a cage is helpful. This is especially useful for calming stressed patients by providing them with the "smell of home." Placed in the patient's cage, the crate's door is left open for patient access. Crates are inspected and cleaned as needed to avoid post-op contamination and soiling.

Cage height

Housing cats in upper cages helps to relieve their stress. However, this is not practical with fractious patients – cats or dogs. These patients should always be housed in lower or mid-height cages to allow easier patient access and to protect personnel from injury. Patients in middle height cages can be coaxed onto a gurney at the same height level. Fractious and fearful patients are easiest to manage in low cages and runs. Patients will often walk out of an open cage or run door if they do not feel threatened. Minimal personnel in the area help the patient to feel less intimidated. When leaving an open lower cage or run door open, the surrounding kennel doors must be secure to avoid patient escape. When drastic removal measures are needed, e.g., rabies pole, the only safe area for accessing a patient is a lower cage or run.

Pheromones

Feline facial pheromones sprayed on blankets or as atomizers in rooms help to soothe cat patients. It calms and relaxes them during hospitalization and during venous catheterization (Carney *et al.* 2012). Canine pheromones as atomizers in kennels may calm anxious dogs.

Nutritional support

Patients are continually monitored for eating behavior both before and after surgery. Maintaining them on their home diet helps to encourage eating and reduces dietary upset from a change in the type of food. Trauma, surgery, pain, and the stress of hospitalization may lead to anorexia, as does the use of narcotics and anti-inflammatory medications. The body has a higher metabolic demand as it is recovering from surgery, infections, burns, and tumors (Fossum 2007). Long-term hospitalization accompanied with anorexia leads to malnutrition. The use of feeding tubes is advisable in these patients. Clients can be taught how to maintain the tube at home and provide parenteral nutrition.

Stress-related diarrhea might occur in surgical patients. Providing them with a bland but nutritional diet may aid in reducing diarrhea. Homemade diets of boiled hamburger or chicken and rice are bland but often enticing to the patient. Many commercially available diets provide excellent nutrition to fit a variety of metabolic conditions.

Urinary bladder care

Following surgery, especially involving the spinal cord, patients may develop the inability to urinate. Many techniques are available for emptying a bladder. While in the hospital, a patient may have an indwelling catheter or repeated catheterization episodes. Care is

taken to maintain sterile technique and minimize the risk of introducing bacterial cystitis. Catheterization of a male dog is much easier than a female dog and dogs are easier than cats. Using a catheter of the appropriate size for the patient provides the best results while limiting urethral trauma. Highly pliable red rubber and Foley catheters decrease the chance of bladder and urethral perforation when compared to stiff polypropylene catheters. Indwelling catheters are sutured in place. Attached to an administration set and empty intravenous fluid bag or urine collection bag creates a closed system for urine collection. Patients are monitored closely to keep from chewing the catheter and often need an Elizabethan collar.

Bladder expression is tailored to the individual patients. Cats and small dogs have easily palpable bladders that can be held in one hand. Grasping the bladder in one hand and providing gentle but firm compression may achieve the desired results. *Never attempt to express the bladder of a patient with a potential urethral stricture. Struggling to express the bladder in these patients may result in a bladder rupture.* For larger patients, a two-handed technique is required. The patient may be laying in lateral recumbency or standing with support. Using the flat surfaces of the hand, not the tips of the fingers, palpate the bladder. While isolating the urinary bladder, the hands are pushed together, while also pushing toward the patient's back. This traps the bladder between the hands and the back, thus allowing only one path for the urine – out the urethra.

Patients with bladder control are difficult if not impossible to express due to their sphincter control. Animals recovering from different types of intervertebral disc disease may have a neurogenic bladder – lacking bladder control. This includes under or over activity of the detrusor muscle and the urinary sphincter depending on the site of the protruding disc.

1 Lower motor neuron (LMN) signs originate from lesions in the sacral spinal cord. LMN bladders are distended and easily expressed. Over discharge of the sympathetic nerves to the urethral sphincter causes failure of urethral relaxation in LMN patients.

2 Upper motor neuron (UMN) signs come from lesions to the thoracolumbar spine as well as the brain and brain stem. UMN bladders are distended but difficult to express. An accurate diagnosis by the attending veterinarian provides appropriate medical management of these conditions to aid in bladder expression.

Patients with overly distended bladders may leak urine leading to misdiagnosis of their ability or inability to urinate. Unless a full voluntary stream of urine is observed, the presumption is the patient is experiencing overflow urination. Palpating the bladder's size, and/or imaging the bladder, confirms this assumption. Patients with overflow have a distended bladder. This must be addressed immediately to avoid permanent damage to the bladder musculature.

Bandages

External coaptation concepts (*Piermattei et al.* 2006)

External coaptation devices include external skeletal fixators (ESF), bandages, casts, splints, and slings. Most of these apparatus serve a specific purpose in orthopedic patient care. However, soft tissue patients require bandages for wound protection, active, and passive drainage control and for support. For example, a non-healing full thickness wound of the hock may heal better with a splint support that decreases bending and stretching of the wound while allowing wound healing. Figures 7.5 and 7.6 show an example of an Irish wolfhound with a nonhealing pressure sore treated with a custom-made orthotic splint. Multiple primary closure attempts were performed in this patient. However, due to the location of the wound, several incidences of dehiscence occurred.

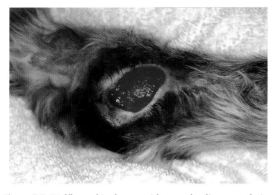

Figure 7.5 Wolfhound is shown with a nonhealing granulating wound on the lateral side of the foot. The patient laying on the wound and the motion within the foot decreased the ability to heal the wound. (Robert Hardie, University of Wisconsin Veterinary Care. Madison, WI. Reproduced with permission from Robert Hardie.)

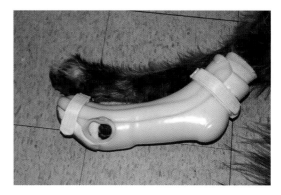

Figure 7.6 The same patient as seen in Figure 7.5 with an orthotic device to allow wound care, stop motion at the wound site and protect patient from lying on the wound. (Robert Hardie, University of Wisconsin Veterinary Care. Madison, WI. Reproduced with permission from Robert Hardie.)

The wound eventually closed by second intention after protection and support of the orthotic splint and topical therapy.

External coaptation serve the following functions:

1 Immobilizes a body part with external support: fractures, luxations, tendon ruptures, and wound protection all benefit from short-term or long-term protection. This may be temporary stabilization of a fracture prior to internal fixation or permanent support until healed such as a comminuted tibia fracture repaired with an external fixation device.

2 Provides control of fracture bending, some control of torsion but does not control compression or distraction. Fracture ends are still able to compress and distract within a cast or splint perhaps causing grinding and rounding of the fracture edges, ESF may provide control of all forces placed on a fracture.

To be effective in stabilizing a fracture, the entire bone must be supported. To do this requires the joint proximal and distal to the fracture to be immobilized. This is easily accomplished with injuries to the tibia/fibula by supporting the hock and the stifle and correspondingly fractures of the radius/ulna require immobilization of the carpus and elbow. Humerus and femur fractures require a spica splint for temporary stabilization. A spica bandage involves applying the bandage completely up the leg and incorporating the trunk. Splint material, extended from toes to body midline, is added to the bandage to keep the shoulder/hip from moving. If this type of bandage is impossible to apply, it is best to leave femur and humerus fractures with no protection. Coaptation that does not include the joint "above and below" the fracture may terminate at a fracture site thus creating a fulcrum and putting more pressure on the injury (Bohling 2012).

Types of support

Temporary support

Bandages, splints, and casts provide *temporary support*. Applied to a fracture prior to internal fixation, they control pain by limiting the movement of the fractured bones. Further soft tissue damage is decreased from any sharp fracture ends that may cut or puncture muscles, veins, arteries, and skin. Stabilization with a bandage or splint may keep a closed fracture from becoming open with the bones edges protruding through the skin. Provided as first aid; bandages, splints, and casts limit further trauma while allowing for safe transportation of the patient to a treatment facility.

Supplemental support

External coaptation delivers *supplemental support* when applied after internal fixation for fracture or tendon repair. ESF add stability and control rotational forces of intramedullary pin fracture repair. Acute tendon tear and laceration repair requires additional reinforcement to prevent bending and stretching as the tendon heals. Following many soft tissue and orthopedic procedures, postoperative bandages, applied for 24–48 hours, may control pain and swelling while keeping the incision clean and absorbing postoperative drainage. Recent studies show no reduction in swelling by bandaging patients after Tibial Plateau Leveling Osteotomy (TPLO) surgery (Unis *et al.* 2010).

Primary support

Casts, splints, and external skeletal fixation devices offer *primary support* of certain fractures and chronic tendon strains. A young animal with a nondisplaced fracture of the radius and an intact ulna may heal very well with a splint or cast. Greenstick or incomplete fractures also require less support than more serious injuries. However, petite dogs with a forelimb fracture often *do not* heal with only external coaptation (Welch *et al.* 1997). Patients with chronic strains of the calcaneal (Achilles) tendon or tendon repair benefit from long-term support via a bandage/splint combination or a custom made orthotic splint or brace (Figure 7.7). The orthotic can be made with a hinge to allow the ability to increase its range of motion over time.

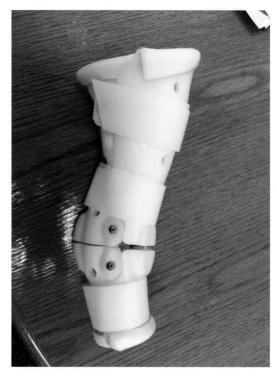

Figure 7.7 A custom-created orthotic with a hinge for treating a patient with a calcaneal tendon strain. The range of motion of the hinge is increased over time to allow more freedom of movement as the patient heals. (James T. Lewellen, University of Wisconsin Health Orthotics, Middleton, WI. Reproduced with permission from James T. Lewellen.)

Considerations

Not all orthopedic patients require external coaptation. Internal fixation of a fracture or ligament tear provides strong stabilization. They, most often, do not require any additional support other than a soft-padded bandage for 24 hours to control postoperative swelling. The veterinarian's decision to apply long-term external coaptation has several considerations.

1 Tolerance: Will a patient tolerate a bandage or an external fixator? Despite the use of an Elizabethan collar, dogs and cats may still aggressively try to pull a bandage apart or lick the pins of a fixator.

2 Wound care: The presence of open wounds often require daily or more frequent treatment. Applying a Robert Jones bandage that requires much staff time, materials, and potentially patient sedation may not be the best option for these patients. However, the use of an easily replaced bi-valved cast will provide

support of a fracture while allowing multiple quick bandage changes to attend a wound.

Very long-term wound care may benefit from a custom designed splint for support, ease of removal, and minimization of bandage sores.

3 Environment: The patient's home living conditions is a factor when determining the appropriateness of extended external coaptation. For example, dogs housed in outdoor pens and cats living on farms quickly soil bandages. Bandages that become wet and damaged provide no support and swiftly cause skin irritation. External skeletal fixation devices may become hooked on protruding home objects. These apparatus must also be kept clean from soil, water, and other contaminants. Other pets in the home may also be attracted to the patient's bandage, splint, and the like and must be monitored.

4 Client compliance: Veterinarians and veterinary technicians can provide the best care and support of the patient; however, it is imperative for the client to follow home care instructions. They must be educated in monitoring the external coaptation for problems. Clients also provide proper environmental conditions and monitor patients' tolerance. (See more information on home care in Chapter 8.) If a client cannot or will not deliver the patient's needs, external coaptation may not be appropriate.

Anatomy of a bandage

All bandages require the same "ingredients." As discussed with open wound management, these include the primary wound cover, a padding layer, a compressive layer, and a protective layer (Figure 7.8).

Additional components are added depending upon the patient's condition and the bandage's purpose. Splint or cast material is added for support and tape stirrups aid in decreasing bandage slippage on a limb. High-quality materials give high-quality results. Using inferior products or reusing materials may save money but cause frustration to the person applying the bandage as the material may tear and fray or not be able to be applied appropriately thus causing patient discomfort. Bandaging is a skill and an art that requires practice. *A poorly applied bandage may be worse than no bandage at all.*

Bandages applied to the abdomen, chest, and head are all soft-padded bandages. When used on the head, neck, and chest area, care is taken to avoid impeding

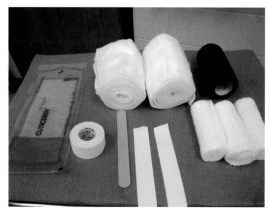

Figure 7.8 Anatomy of a bandage: (L–R) primary wound cover (oil emulsion gauze), tape stirrups (foreground), and tongue blade to keep stirrups separated, cast padding, elastic gauze (foreground), protective layer.

the ability to breathe and/or eat. Head and ear bandages are kept high enough to avoid eye irritation. If one or both ears may be left exposed, a figure of eight bandage is applied that aids in keeping the bandage in place. Likewise, chest bandages are often crossed over the front of the chest to keep the bandage from slipping back to the abdomen. Abdominal wraps are difficult to keep in place as they move around and slide backwards. A strip of adhesive bandage material or tape applied to the skin serves as an anchor. The rest of the bandage is created with one-half of the width of the anchor strip exposed. After the final layer of material is applied, another strip of adhesive tape is added to include the edge of the bandage and the anchor strip. This anchor tape is left in place for as long as the patient requires the bandage. This avoids excess trauma to the skin from repetitive removal of the adhesive. When no longer needed, the anchor strip is removed with the help of an adhesive remover.

Despite best efforts, chest and abdomen bandages are difficult to keep in place. A variety of commercial products are available to provide wound coverage and compression of these areas. They are made of tubular stretch gauze, neoprene, and other materials. Often they incorporate the legs or allow cutting of holes for legs. Product sizes vary and are custom fitted to individual patients. Some products include Velcro® straps to allow for more customization and others include no leg holes for use following amputation. Wraps are also available with pockets for portable monitoring devices.

Soft padded

These bandages provide varying degrees of support dependent upon the amount of padding material. More padding placed under robust compression provides increased stiffness and strong support. Modified Robert Jones (MRJ) or soft-padded bandages provide wound coverage and reduce swelling both preoperatively and postoperatively. They are lightweight with approximately 0.5–2 cm of padding thus giving only light support and nonrigid stability. However, due to the limited amount of padding, it is easy to apply excess compression thus causing a tourniquet effect on a limb or impeding breathing if applied over a thorax. There are many applications for this bandage for both short- and long-term use. It is the basis for all bandages. The patient lays in lateral recumbency, with the affected limb up, for orthopedic conditions and may be standing for other applications. The following section describes the application of a limb bandage, other wraps are similar but without the use of stirrups.

Application of a limb bandage

1 Apply tape stirrups to foot: (Figure 7.9) Application of stirrups to the medial and lateral side of the foot is more comfortable for the patient than application to the dorsal and palmer/plantar aspect. It avoids taping the pads together, adhesive material on the pads, and tape trauma to the tender skin over the toes. Location of stirrups may need adjustment to avoid taping over wounds.

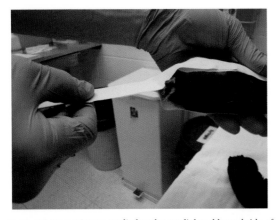

Figure 7.9 Tape stirrups applied to the medial and lateral side of the foot extend just to the carpus or tarsus. A tongue depressor placed between the two tape strips keeps them from sticking together.

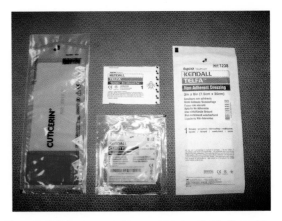

Figure 7.10 Primary wound cover examples: (L–R) oil emulsion gauze in two sizes and Telfa® pads in two sizes – both items are non-adherent.

Stirrups do not need to be long. Extending proximally to the carpus/tarsus and distally to about 10 cm beyond the toes is sufficient. Apply tape under – not over – a dewclaw to avoid compressing the nail into the foot causing a pressure sore. A tongue blade placed between the tape ends that extend beyond the foot keeps them from adhering to each other during bandage application. The tongue depressor is discarded after use.

2 Apply primary wound cover: (Figure 7.10) This may be adherent or nonadherent depending upon the patient's condition and needs. (See section on open wound management in Chapter 6 for more information.)

Care is taken while applying this layer to avoid wound contamination. The use of gloves and not handling the patient side of the primary wound cover decreases the spread of microbes to the lesion. If a wound is located proximally on a limb, delay application of the wound cover until the padding layer reaches its location to keep the wound cover in place.

3 Apply padding layer: (Figure 7.11) This layer provides wound protection and absorbs drainage. The thickness varies depending on the patient's needs. For a soft-padded bandage, moderate density is achieved with cast padding. This product is available in a wide variety of materials and widths. The patient's size determines the width of the bandage material. For example, do not use 6″ wide cast padding on a 2-kg patient and reversely while 2″ cast padding can be

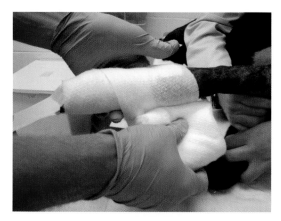

Figure 7.11 Begin by applying the padding layer of a soft-padded bandage. The roll stays next to the limb to control placement, the cast padding is unfurled off the "back" of the roll to maintain pressure.

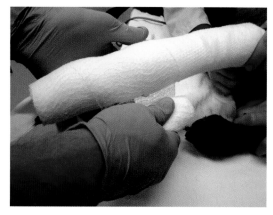

Figure 7.12 The compressive layer is placed over the padding layer to apply provide pressure to decrease edema and provide stability to the bandage.

used on a 60-kg patient; it will take much time and material to cover its leg.

Limb bandages begin at the toes to maintain pressure throughout the leg and to avoid a tourniquet effect. Starting distally also allows fluid to move away from the toes/limb and into the body. Always keep the roll of cast padding near the limb – unroll the material on the leg not in the air. Maintain pressure by unfurling off the "back" of the roll.

(In small animal practice, there is no preference to wrapping clockwise or counterclockwise. However, after determining a direction – continue in the same direction to avoid loosening underlying layers.) Begin by covering the foot twice with cast padding to secure the material to itself. Unless indicated by the patient's condition (i.e., toe injury), the two center toes of the foot remain exposed to monitor the foot for rotation, temperature change, swelling, redness, odor, and discharge. After securing the cast padding to the foot, continue wrapping the leg by overlapping the cast padding by about one-half of its width. Placing the material at an angle to the limb avoids creating a horizontal band and tourniquet effect. At the proximal end of the bandage, also wrap the limb twice to secure the cast padding at the top. Continue wrapping the leg moving proximally and distally until the desired amount of cast padding is applied. To maintain the angle of the material, a tuck or tear may be required. Even and constant pressure is used to apply the material while avoiding any bunching to

circumvent bandage sores. The cast padding is applied in even layers to maintain uniform pressure on the limb.

4 Apply compressive layer: (Figure 7.12) Compression adds some support to the limb by stiffening the padding layer. It also reduces wound swelling by moving fluid away from the limb into the rest of the body. The material of choice for this layer is stretch gauze. It comes in a variety of materials and widths. Veterinary technicians benefit from sampling different products for durability, stretch, and consistency to determine a personal preference. As with cast padding, the patient's size determines the width of the material to be applied.

Stretch gauze is applied over the cast padding beginning at the toes. A small edge of cast padding extends beyond the gauze at both the distal and proximal ends to keep the gauze from cutting into the skin. Cover the foot twice to adhere the gauze to the gauze. Continue proximally up the limb as with the cast padding while maintaining the gauze at an angle to the limb. Keep the roll of material directly next to the padding and unfurl along the limb, not in the air, to maintain even pressure. To increase/maintain compression, use the hand not holding the roll of gauze to compress the cast padding while bringing the gauze over the hand. For maximum compression over a large quantity of padding, the padding may be compacted from both directions.

As the stretch gauze is applied, lumps will appear in the bandage. Continue to apply layers of gauze overlapping one-half of the width of the material, moving distally to proximally, until the bandage is smooth and free of bulges. This may require several layers. Even pressure throughout the bandage is imperative to avoid pressure sores and a tourniquet effect – special attention is given to the toes to assure the bandage is as tight over the toes as through its entirety. The bandage should have a uniform firmness.

5 Attach tape stirrups to the gauze layer: The tongue depressor is removed from the ends of the tape stirrups that have been extending distal to the toes. The tape is twisted 180° to place the adhesive surface on the stretch gauze. If needed, the tape is gently pulled proximally to assure exposure of the two center toes.

6 Apply protective layer: The protective layer keeps the bandage clean and possibly a bit dry if exposed to a minimal amount of moisture. It is not meant to provide support or compression. Materials used for the protective layer include adhesive backed elastic tape, white adhesive tape, and self-adhering elastic tape. These products are available in a wide range of widths, colors, and materials. Personal preference has some bearing on choice although each product has its own advantages and disadvantages.

- adhesive backed elastic tape (sizes 1″, 2″, 3″, and 4″ width)
   ○ advantages: durable, adheres very well to underlying gauze and to skin
   ○ disadvantages: scissors required to cut, must cut to create smooth curves and edges, adhesive causes skin irritation, easy to over tighten, expensive
- white adhesive tape (sizes 0.5″, 1″, 2″, 3″ width)
   ○ advantages: durable, adheres well to underlying gauze less so to skin, tears without scissors, available in waterproof style, difficult to put on too tight, inexpensive
   ○ disadvantages: stiff and difficult to conform, strong adhesive makes it difficult to handle and to remove from roll
- self-adhering tape (sizes 2″, 3″, 4″ 5″ width)
   ○ advantages: easily conforms to body shape, variety of colors, does not adhere to skin, may tear without scissors, easy to decorate
   ○ disadvantages: not waterproof, easy to over tighten, moderate expense, prone to wear on bottom of foot

Apply the protective layer in the same manner as the cast padding and stretch gauze. Begin distally at the

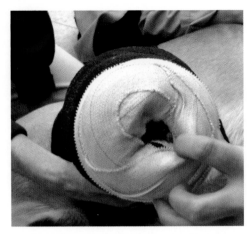

Figure 7.13 The protective layer of self-adherence or adhesive-backed bandaging tape keeps the bandage clean. Bandaging tape applied over the edge of the padding prevents the patient from pulling on the cast padding and may provide better friction for walking. (Jason Bleedorn, University of Wisconsin Veterinary Care, Madison, WI. Reproduced with permisison from Jason Bleedorn.)

toes, going around the toes twice to secure the bandage material. Leave a small amount of cast padding exposed at the distal and proximal ends of the bandage to avoid the protective layer cutting into the skin. Some patients tend to pull at the cast padding, covering the entire edge of the bandage may alleviate this problem (Figure 7.13). Additionally, bringing the edge of the protective layer over all bandage material and tucking in the edges assuring no direct contact with the skin may keep a patient from bothering the bandage. Elastic bandaging tapes can cut into the skin if applied incorrectly.

After covering the toes, continue proximally on the limb by overlapping the material by one-half of its width and proceeding at an angle to the leg. Cuts or tucks in the tape may be needed to go around curves. This material is *not* applied under tension as it provides protection only – not compression. One layer is usually sufficient. On rare occasions, adhesive elastic tape is applied at the proximal end of the bandage to keep it in place. This may occur if the injury is very proximal on the limb and a splint is not desired to keep the bandage from slipping down. However, most properly applied bandages do *not* need this extra adhesion and the adhesive tape causes skin irritation.

The most important parts of the bandage (primary wound cover, padding, and compression) are not what

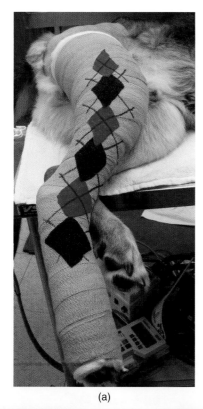

(a)

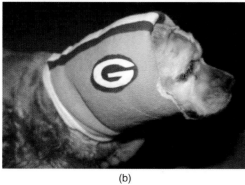

(b)

Figure 7.14 (a) The decoration on the bandage provides fun and entertainment for the client. (b) Showing home team spirit on a bandage.

the owners observe. However, the client may perceive the quality of the wrap by its external looks. Assuring the protective layer is smooth, wrinkle free, and clean provides the client with confidence. Adding decorative elements to the bandage creates an extra personal touch (Figures 7.14(a,b)).

Robert Jones (RJ)

The Robert Jones (RJ) bandage is bulky and cumbersome. Its size provides bending and some rotational stability to a fracture. The RJ also provides much compression to decrease swelling and apply pressure to a wound. It is used only for injuries distal to the elbows or stifles to provide stabilization of the joint above and below a fracture site. If applied to a femur or humerus injury, the proximal end of the bandage may rest at the fracture site, creating a very heavy fulcrum and causing greater injury to the patient. This bandage takes much time to apply and sedation of the patient may be required. The RJ is meant for short-term use.

The basic elements are the same as the padded or MRJ bandage except for the quantity of materials required. The other difference is to use roll cotton instead of cast padding as the padding layer. The stirrups and primary wound cover are applied as described under "padded/MRJ" bandage. As a full size roll of roll cotton is unrolled, it is torn in half (width) and rerolled creating two narrower rolls of cotton. This allows for easier handling and maneuvering around curves of the leg. The entire leg is wrapped, beginning distally at the toes with the two center toes exposed, while overlapping the cotton by one-half of its width. One or two layers of cotton may be needed as well as more rolls of cotton to create the required 4–8 cm of padding. The bandage is extremely bulky at this point.

Stretch gauze is applied in the same manner as for a MRJ – beginning at the toes. Due to the large quantity of cotton to be covered, using as wide a gauze as can be comfortably handled cuts down on the amount of time required to complete the compression. Alternate the gauze roll between the hands and use the opposite hand to compress the cotton. Many layers of gauze are needed to compact the cotton to one-half of its original size. Care is taken to provide even pressure throughout the bandage. When finished, the bandage should "thump like a watermelon." It is difficult, but not impossible, to apply too much pressure and compression to a Robert Jones bandage.

After compression, the stirrups are attached to the gauze and the protective layer is applied as with the MRJ bandage. Since this bandage takes an incredible amount of time and materials to complete, it is not meant for a wound requiring frequent attention. Again, it is only meant for temporary fracture stabilization.

Splints

Purposes

Splints have several uses in orthopedic surgery for temporary, supplemental, and primary support. Soft tissue patients may need splints to provide wound stabilization and following skin grafting to avoid tension on the wound/graft. The three main types of splints are as follows.

1 Limb splint: The most commonly applied splint

  (a) *Definitive* stabilization of fractures: young animals, minimally displaced, distal to elbow or stifle

  (b) *Temporary* stabilization of other fractures, luxations, and subluxations distal to elbow or stifle

  (c) *Supplemental* post-op support of above conditions

  (d) Must be well padded as previously described

  (e) Easy to overcompress due to moderate amount of padding

2 Spica splint: Less common, requires much practice to apply properly

  (a) Bandage extends from toes proximal to midline of torso

  (b) Includes scapula or hip

  (c) *Only* appropriate external coaptation for humeral or femoral fractures (stabilizes joint above and below)

  (d) *Temporary* or *supplemental* stabilization of fractures

  (e) *Definitive* fixation of greenstick fractures of humerus or femur in very young patients

  (f) Heavy sedation needed for application

  (g) Lengthy application time

  (h) Difficult to use in pelvic limb of male dogs to avoid incorporating the prepuce into the bandage and urine soiling

  (i) Cage confinement may be a better alternative if application is only for temporary support prior to internal fracture fixation of humerus or femur

3 Schroeder-Thomas splint: Not recommended (Figure 7.15)

  (a) Traction splint using aluminum rod and bandage material

  (b) *Definitive* treatment for minimally displaced mid-shaft tibia/fibula or radius/ulna fractures

  (c) Joints held in extension so causes joint stiffness requiring much rehabilitation following splint removal.

  (d) Much possibility of trauma from splint due to lack of padding

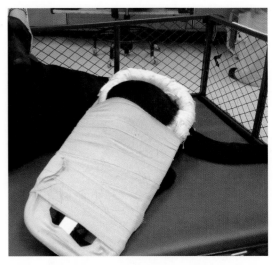

Figure 7.15 Schroeder-Thomas splints do *not* provide appropriate stability for fractures proximal to the stifle or elbow. They maintain the limb in an extended position. This type of splint *is not recommended*, as better splinting methods are available as described in the text.

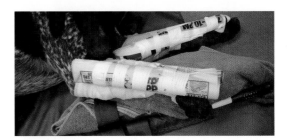

Figure 7.16 Newspaper splints for bilateral radius and ulna fracture provide *no stability* for these fractures.

  (e) *Never* used for femur or humerus fractures because the proximal end of the splint often rests at the fracture site creating a fulcrum

  (f) Not recommended – better splinting alternatives exist as previously described

Materials

Clinic-created splints are a soft padded bandage with the addition of a rigid material to provide immobilization. Rigid materials include fiberglass casting tape, thermoplastics, aluminum rods, as well as preformed plastic and metal splints. Each of the materials has its own advantages and disadvantages. Newspaper rolls *do not* provide enough support or length to support a fracture (Figure 7.16). The patient shown in Figure 7.16

suffered from bilateral radius and ulna fractures. The newspaper splints are not rigid and do not stabilize the joint proximal and distal to the fracture sites.

1 Fiberglass (2″, 3″, 4″, and 5″ width)

(a) Advantages: easily moldable and cuttable prior to curing; only water needed to cure quickly but may set up without water, easy to use

(b) Disadvantages: gloves needed to handle, leaves remnants on tables, power tools needed to cut after curing, may be expensive, cannot be reformed after cured

2 Thermoplastics (sheets and rolls, low and high temperature)

(a) Advantages: easily moldable and cuttable after heating, wide range of sizes and thicknesses available, light weight, no gloves needed, does not stick to surfaces, easy to use, can be reformed with reheating

(b) Disadvantages: hot water and source needed to soften, difficult to cut prior to heating, may be expensive

3 Aluminum Rods (1/8″, 3/16″, 1/4″ 5/16″, 3/8″ diameter)

(a) Advantages: smaller sizes easily bendable, inexpensive

(b) Disadvantages: not moldable, larger diameters require device to bend, large diameter required for rigid stability in large patient, challenging to keep in place

4 Preformed Plastic or Metal (variety of shapes and sizes)

(a) Advantages: rigid fixation if fits properly, no adjustments required, easy to use

(b) Disadvantages: not moldable or bendable to conform to patient, requires correct size for patient, difficult to immobilize joint proximal and distal to fracture, often misused, e.g., spoon splints used for radius/ulna fractures do not immobilize the fracture, expensive

Long-term – months or years of treatment – splints may be custom created from a variety of resources. They often include a neoprene type material, Velcro® straps for adjustment and may include a piece of thermoplastic for extra rigidity (Figure 7.17). Specific measurements, taken in-clinic, provide the manufacturer with the appropriate dimensions for splint creation. Each company has its own measuring policy that must be followed precisely to provide optimum fit and patient comfort.

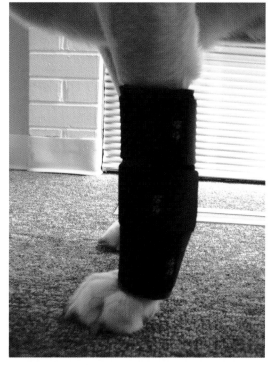

Figure 7.17 Commercially available carpal support, for long-term use, is comfortable, washable, and easily removed. (DoggLeggs Therapeutic and Rehabilitative Products, Reston, VA. Reproduced with permission from DogLeggs Therapeutic and Rehabilitative Products.)

Splint application

All clinic created splints begin with a soft-padded bandage as previously described. Prior to application of the protective layer, the splint is applied over the compressive layer. To provide maximum support, splint material must extend the full length of the bandage with a small (1/4″–1/2″) ridge of bandage material extending beyond the splint. This keeps sharp edges of the splint material from cutting into the skin. If using casting tape for splint material, after measuring the required length, the remainder of the roll can be unrolled on the patient or placed on a *covered* counter top – cage papers work well to cover the work area. (Fiberglass leaves semi-permanent remnants on uncovered tabletops.) Rounding the edges of fiberglass and thermoplastics aids in patient comfort. It is easiest to cut these materials prior to curing. Fiberglass, especially, is very sharp with very pointy end threads when hardened.

The splint is applied smoothly over the compressive layer, shaping moldable and bendable splint material into the desired position. Preformed splints must fit the patient perfectly. If this does not occur, the limb may be in the wrong position, not be properly supported, and the patient may develop bandage sores. Care is taken when applying a moldable splint to avoid indentations in the material. These may occur from inadvertently pushing on the splint material with the fingers or by creating a crease. Dents in the splint can cause a pressure sore on the patient's skin. After application of the splint material, it is held in place with an additional layer of stretch gauze or with the protective layer. Keeping one's thumbs upright when applying the final bandage layer(s) over the uncured splint material will avoid inadvertent indentations in the splint. Stirrups are moved into place over the stretch gauze after splint application but prior to adding the protective layer. If fiberglass or thermoplastics are used, the patient is kept immobilized until the product cures. This time varies with each individual material and manufacturer. Follow instructions on the package insert.

Splints applied to toe fractures provide a challenge. They must extend beyond the toes to provide stability. The patient walks on the splint not on its toes. In order to protect the footpads from cuts and abrasions from the distal edge of the splint material, the toes are often completely covered with bandage material. This eliminates the ability to assess the toes for swelling, odor, temperature change, and drainage. Stirrups may be added to provide some protection against slipping. They are applied as with a soft-padded bandage except kept separated with a tongue depressor on each distal end of the stirrup. "Spoon" splints, for toe and carpus fractures, may be manufactured with fiberglass or thermoplastics and are available premade. Care is taken for appropriate fitting of the splint with padding added to its distal end to protect the foot.

Spica splints

Create a special challenge with their application encircling the chest or abdomen. Their primary use is for patients that require stabilization of a humerus or femur fracture. Due to the length of time and manipulation needed to apply this bandage, the patient is generally under sedation. It is much better tolerated on the forelimb than rear limb. Therefore, this description is for a spica splint of the front leg. The bandage begins

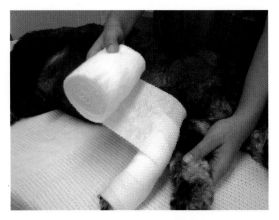

Figure 7.18 Begin a forelimb spica splint by wrapping counter-clockwise or from medial to lateral on the limb. A spica splint is the only method of temporarily stabilizing a fracture of the humerus or femur. It may also be used as supplemental support following internal fracture fixation of either of these bones.

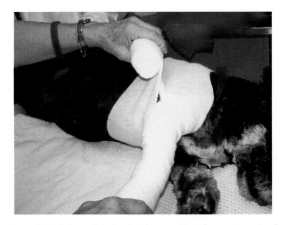

Figure 7.19 Spica splint step 1: After reaching the most proximal aspect of the limb, wrap the bandage material over the back and around the chest, bringing the bandage up behind the caudal side of the limb.

with stirrups and incorporates the same materials as any other limb bandage. The cast padding is applied in a medial-to-lateral (counter clockwise) direction going proximally up the leg (Figure 7.18).

As the axilla is reached, the roll goes over the back, around the chest then around the neck and back down the leg creating a half of a figure of eight or "spica" pattern (Figure 7.19 and 7.20). (The name Spica derives from Latin *spīca virginis* "Virgo's ear of grain" (usually

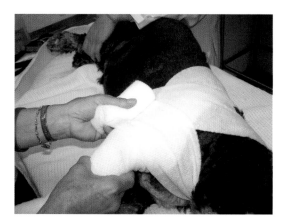

Figure 7.20 Spica splint step 2: Bring the bandage material over the back and around the neck creating a "V" or spica pattern. Continue to add cast padding in this pattern until the desired thickness is achieved. Secure the cast padding with stretch gauze placed in the same pattern.

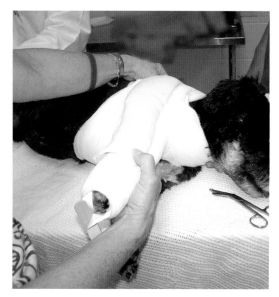

Figure 7.21 Spica splint step 3: Apply splint material to the lateral aspect of the limb; extending to the middle of the back.

wheat)[1] – the bandage material forms the same pattern as a wheat grain.) The cast padding applied over the back is spread out to provide padding to extend beyond the edges of the eventually applied splint material. (An assistant is needed to lift the patient as the chest encircling layers are applied. Cast padding is added until desired thickness is achieved. Stretch gauze is applied over the cast padding, again, moving in a medial to lateral pattern. As compression is applied, care is taken to not impede chest movements or compress the neck. However, in order to do its job, the wrap must be snug. One finger should fit between the first layer of the wrap and the chest. After the patient is awake and standing, tightness is rechecked, as this may be difficult to assess in a sedate, laterally recumbent patient.

After application of the compressive layer, the splint material is added. Fiberglass casting tape is the best material to use although splint rods may be employed if sufficiently bendable. The cast material extends from the distal end of the bandage to the midline of the back (Figure 7.21). One or more rolls of cast material may be needed to provide the desired rigidity. Speed is essential when combining two rolls of casting tape into one unit so the first roll does not begin to cure prior to the second roll's application. As with a regular splint, the edges are rounded to avoid points on the corners. Additional stretch gauze or the final protective layer is

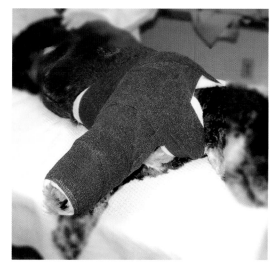

Figure 7.22 Spica splint step 4: Apply stretch gauze to maintain positioning of the splint. Cover with a protective layer in the same manner as the other bandage material.

added to keep the splint in place. Care is taken to avoid indentations in the splint and compression of the chest (Figure 7.22).

---

[1] http://en.wikipedia.org/wiki/Spica.

Spica splints take much time and materials to apply. They are not meant for daily changes unless necessary for the patient's condition. They take much practice to perfect the technique of application.

Casts

The purpose of a cast is to provide fracture stabilization or joint immobilization. They are meant for long-term use and therefore must be comfortable for the patient. Casts are initially applied while the patient is anesthetized or heavily sedated. They completely encircle the limb with a rigid material. It may seem counter intuitive but casts actually have less padding than a soft-padded bandage or a splint. While padding is needed to avoid skin irritation, it is the close conformity and proximity of the cast to limb that provides support. Casts may be used in patients requiring *supplemental* support following arthrodesis or ligament repair. In limited applications, casts may provide *definitive* stabilization for fractures meeting the following requirements.

- Minimally displaced
- Nonarticular
- Stable
- Transverse or incomplete greenstick
- Distal to elbow or stifle

The first layer of a cast is stockinette. This is sized to fit snugly to the leg and to extend a few centimeters beyond the cast in both directions. Cast application, then, follows as outlined under soft padded bandage except only one to two layers of cast padding is used. The compressive layer is minimal since there is little material to compress. Following label directions, fiberglass-casting tape is applied over the compressive layer. Gloves are worn to keep the fiberglass from adhering to the hands. The roll is unwound as with other materials with extreme care taken to avoid any imprints in the cast material. An assistant is needed to stabilize the limb during application. The assistant also wears gloves and only supports the limb with the flat part of the hands, not the fingers. After the initial layers of casting tape are applied to the foot, the assistant pulls up the distal end of the stockinette to create a "rolled-edge" to the cast. After reaching the proximal end of the cast, the stockinette is similarly pulled down to create the same softened edge. Casting tape then covers the stockinette up to the rolled-edge. Time is essential to apply all layers of the cast before any parts begin to cure to make the cast a cohesive unit. The cast must cure prior to the patient walking on it.

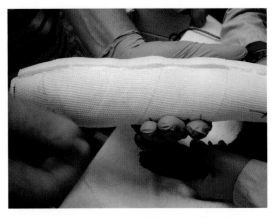

Figure 7.23 Cutting a cast in half (bi-valve) allows for wound care and easy replacement without the need to re-create the cast.

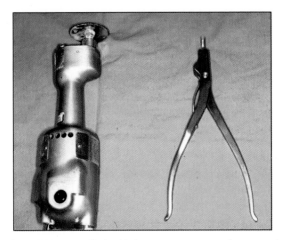

Figure 7.24 An oscillating blade cast saw cuts a cast for removal or bi-valving. The cast spreader opens up the two halves of the cast.

After application and curing, the cast can be cut on the lateral and medial side to create two pieces – like a clamshell (Figure 7.23). This is a bi-valve cast that can be removed, as needed, if skin wounds need attending. The two halves are kept together with an adhesive tape.

A cast saw and spreader is required to cut a cast either for bi-valving or for final removal (Figure 7.24). The oscillating blade of a cast saw limits the chance of cutting the underlying skin and is used in an "up and down" not sideways motion. When planning for a bi-valve cast, thin plastic applied over the stretch gauze,

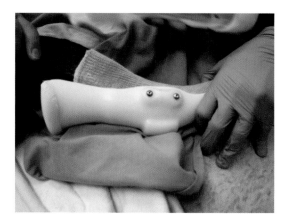

Figure 7.25 Patients requiring a long-term splint benefit from fitting with a custom-made orthotic device. This patient's calcaneal tendon laceration was repaired; however, the repair failed while waiting for the orthotic to be created.

prior to application of the cast, keeps the cast material from adhering to the compressive layer. Remove the plastic prior to reapplication of the cast.

For very long-term use, casts may be custom made by an orthotic specialist. Created from thermoplastics, they are well-padded and kept in place with straps and buckles (Figures 7.25 and 7.26). A strained but not severed calcaneus tendon is an example of the use of this cast. It takes many months to heal. The orthotic device is adjusted over time to allow the patient increased mobility and movement in the hock joint.

External coaptation complications and care

Bandages, splints, and casts require vigilant care to avoid wrap-induced trauma to the patient. Caregivers, in the hospital and at home, must check bandages daily. The skin adjacent to each edge of the bandage is especially susceptible to rubbing and prone to irritation. This varies from minimal redness to abrasions to full thickness wounds. Catching wounds early and correcting their cause prevents patient suffering and the potential for additional surgery. Bandages are checked daily for odor. This is especially important for limb wraps exposed to moisture and dirt. A smelly bandage may be just wet and need changing or may be a sign of infection. When possible, toes are left exposed to allow monitoring of swelling and temperature. Both of these may be indicative of a bandage being too tight and needing replacement. Clients are advised to compare

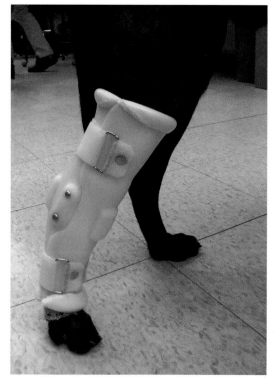

Figure 7.26 Patient seen in Figure 7.25 with the orthotic in place. Patient is able to stand normally and walks well.

the temperature of the toes, either hotter or colder, to the toes of the opposite limb. Too cold may mean decreased circulation to the feet and too hot may be another sign of infection. Any drainage at the edges of the wrap or soaking through (strike-through) the wrap is a cause for concern. Blood, purulent material, bandage sores, or normal wound drainage can all ooze into and through a bandage. Drainage at the foot of a limb wrap can also indicate wounds or necrosis of the feet from over tightness of the wrap or the patient chewing on the bandage. Casts, splints, and bandages must be kept clean and dry. If soiled, they must be changed to provide patient comfort and avoid contamination of any underlying surgical or traumatic wounds. When a bandage slips, it does not provide the patient with the desired stability. Bandages thus improperly located, lead to skin trauma and potentially harm to the patient's underlying condition. For example, if a cast slips, it may end directly at the fracture site creating a fulcrum for the fracture to bend.

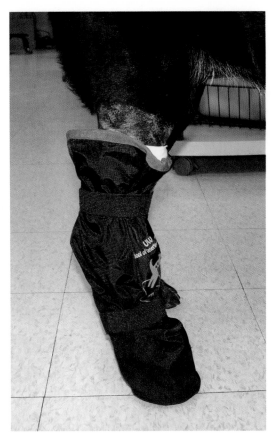

Figure 7.27 Many types of materials are useful for protecting bandages from the environment. Commercially available products are durable and kept in place with Velcro® straps. (Medipaw®. Reproduced with permission from Medivet Products.)

All wraps must be comfortable for the patient. If the dog or cat tries to chew or bite at a bandage, the source of irritation is investigated, which often includes removing a bandage to search for wounds. Patients with limb bandages that were walking well and then suddenly develop lameness may indicate a problem with the wrap. Clients are also advised to monitor their pet's attitude for changes suggestive of a problem.

When going outside, limb wraps must be protected from the elements. Plastic bags serve this purpose but are often thin so are checked at each use for holes and tears. They are only attached to the bandage with adhesive tape. While a rubber band will keep the bag in place, the rubber band may slip beyond the edge of the bandage and become a tourniquet on the limb. Used, dry intravenous fluid (IV) bags are great for covering smaller

bandages. The port end of the bag is cut off creating a thick plastic pocket. Slits are cut into the bag for lacing of roll gauze or umbilical tape. It is easily tied onto the foot. Commercially available bandage covers come in a variety of sizes, materials, and durability (Figure 7.27). They are longer and cover more of the bandage than plastic or IV bags. Attached straps keep them in place.

All bandage covers must be removed when the patient is indoors to avoid condensation and heat build-up within the wrap as well as to allow the bandage to "breath."

Some patients, despite the comfort of a bandage, will still chew the bandage or have fun pulling out the cast padding. Ingesting bandage material may cause gastrointestinal upset. Loss of integrity of the bandage, cast, or splint decreases its intended purpose. Elizabethan collars of a variety of materials, inflatable collars, and other assorted devices all keep patients from reaching their bandage. Cloth body covers, t-shirts, or scrub tops are useful to keep patients from thorax and abdominal wraps and wounds. Testing various techniques is often best to find the perfect solution for an individual patient.

The client checks the bandage, cast, or splint at least daily. Weekly clinic rechecks are often needed for bandage replacement and professional monitoring. The patient's condition determines bandage change intervals and the required length of time the wrap needs to stay in place. Casts may be downgraded, over time, to splints and soft padded wraps prior to allowing the patient full use of the limb.

Becoming proficient in the application of bandages, casts, and splints takes much time and practice. It is an art to be able to gauge the required pressure, compression, tension, and requirements of the wrap. Practicing on rubber models, staff owned pets, and patients is a valuable learning experience. However, veterinary technicians with bandaging skills become a treasured resource for veterinary surgeons.

External skeletal fixation (ESF) devices
Veterinarians apply ESF or fixation devices. Technicians assist the surgeons in their application and in postoperative care. ESF are employed for comminuted fracture repair, angular limb deformity correction, joint stabilization, tendon laceration immobilization and a variety of other injuries. The structure includes pins or wires inserted through the bone and held in place with an external device. These include bars, clamps, rings or

partial rings, and tubing filled with methylmethacrylate. Clamps and other structures do not contact the skin thus preventing irritation. The entrance of the pins and wires are cleaned at least daily with dilute chlorhexidine solution or saline to remove any crustiness. If oozing is present, the adjacent skin is cleaned to decrease scalding. Sterilized foam rubber sponges inserted between the bars and the skin provide postoperative compression to decrease swelling. Initially, a bandage is placed over the entire device to keep the sponges in place.

With time, this wrap can be decreased in size, as less compression is needed. Stockinette, stretch tube gauze, or a stocking with the foot removed is often the only protection needed for long-term use. This also allows the client easy access to the insertion sites for cleaning.

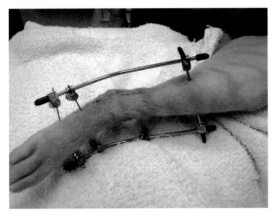

Figure 7.28 Surgical instrument "sharps" covers are perfect for covering sharp ends of external skeletal fixator pins.

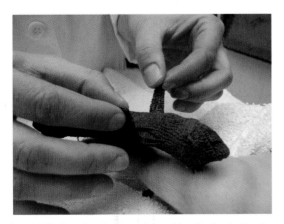

Figure 7.29 Covering the fixator bars with self-adhesive bandaging tape keep them from being caught on things and prevents patients from getting scratched.

All sharp ends of the pins are covered to avoid injury to the patient, client, or staff. Commercially available pin covers or "sharps" covers used for surgical instruments work well (Figure 7.28). Covering all sharp edges and protecting the bars helps to keep the bars from catching on objects and avoids scratches from the pointed ends of the pins (Figure 7.29).

Upon recheck exams, the ESF clamps and screws are tightened, as needed. Veterinary technicians may remove ESF devices. Radiographs provide important information regarding the fixator such as if pins are threaded, completely through both cortices of the bone, their location and if they have special removal requirements. External components of the devices may be cleaned, sterilized, and reused for another patient.

Slings

Slings maintain a limb in a specific angle and prevent weight bearing. An Ehmer sling on the hind limb provides abduction and inward rotation of the hip. Its most common use is following closed reduction of a coxofemoral luxation. Various techniques are used for application including adhesive tape with or without elastic gauze. The adhesive tape alone, however, is very irritating to the skin. Ehmer slings are often difficult to keep in place as they can slide off the butt. The commercially available DogLeggs Ehmer sling provides long-lasting comfort for the patient (Figure 7.30). Keeping a variety of sizes in the clinic allows for immediate postoperative use.

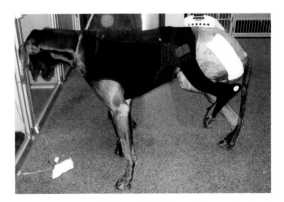

Figure 7.30 Commercially available Ehmer slings maintain the proper position of the rear limb following hip luxation surgery. (DoggLeggs Therapeutic and Rehabilitative Products, Reston, VA. Reproduced with permission from DogLeggs Therapeutic and Rehabilitative Products.)

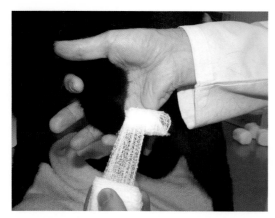

Figure 7.31 Velpeau sling step 1: Wrap stretch gauze several times around the front foot.

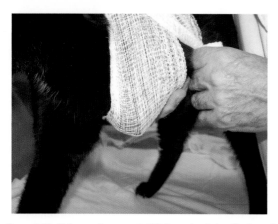

Figure 7.32 Velpeau sling step 2: While maintaining flexion of the carpus and elbow, create a figure of eight wrap to keep the limb close to the body.

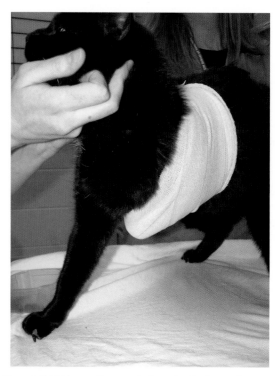

Figure 7.33 Velpeau sling step 3: Completed Velpeau sling on a domestic shorthair cat.

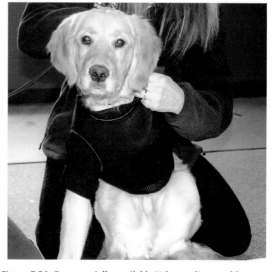

Figure 7.34 Commercially available Velpeau sling used for more long-term use and for patients able to get out of the traditional style of sling. (DoggLeggs Therapeutic and Rehabilitative Products, Reston, VA. Reproduced with permission from DogLeggs Therapeutic and Rehabilitative Products.)

Velpeau slings keep the forelimb in flexion and prevent weight bearing. It is primarily used after various shoulder surgeries where movement needs to be restricted – such as luxation, minimally displaced scapular fractures, and severe shoulder instability. The sling is created with stretch gauze.

1 Wrap the gauze around the toes. (Figure 7.31)
2 Flex the carpus and elbow while maintaining the shoulder in a neutral position.
3 Wrap the gauze around the chest behind the opposite forelimb while encompassing the carpus within the gauze. (Figure 7.32)
4 Apply multiple layers of gauze as needed to maintain the position of limb.
5 Apply the protective layer.(Figure 7.33)

Commercially available Velpeau slings are, also, available (Figure 7.34).

Patients tolerate slings well but they must be monitored weekly for skin irritation and wounds inflicted by the bandage. After 2 weeks, joint contracture may occur and further use of the sling may be contraindicated (Canapp *et al.* 2012). Physical rehabilitation of these patients helps to return them to normal function.

References

Bohling, M.W. (2012) Burns. In: Tobias, K.M. & Johnston, S.A. (eds), *Veterinary Surgery – Small Animal* Volume II. Elsevier, St. Louis, MO, pp. 1291–1301.

Canapp, S.O., Campana, D.M. & Fair, L.M. (2012) Orthopedic coaptation devices and small-animal prosthetics. In: Tobias, K.M. & Johnston, S.A. (eds), *Veterinary Surgery – Small Animal* Volume I. Elsevier, St. Louis, MO, pp. 628–637.

Carney, H.C., Little, S. *et al.* (2012) AAFP and ISFM feline-friendly nursing care guidelines. Journal of Feline Medicine and Surgery, 14, 337.

Fossum, T.W. (2007) *Small Animal Surgery*, 3rd edn. Mosby-Elsevier, St. Louis, MO, pp. 90–110.

Niedfeldt, R.L. & Robertson, S.A. (2006) Postanesthetic hyperthermia in Cats: a retrospective comparison between hydromorphone and buprenorphine. Veterinary Anaesthesia and Analgesia, 33, 381–389.

Piermattei, D.L., Flo, G. & DeCamp, C.E. (2006) *Handbook of Small Animal Orthopedics and Fracture Repair*, 4th edn. WB Saunders Co, Philadelphia, pp. 49–68.

Posner, L.P., Gleed, R.D. *et al* (2007) Post-anesthetic hyperthermia in Cats. Veterinary Anaesthesia and Analgesia, 34, 40–47.

Unis, M.D., Roush, J.K. *et al.* (2010) Effect of bandaging on post-operative swelling after tibial plateau leveling osteotomy. Veterinary and Comparative Orthopaedics and Traumatology, 23 (**4**), 240–244. doi:10.3415/VCOT-09-04-0046

Welch, J.A., Boudrieau, R.J. *et al.* (1997) The intraosseous blood supply of the canine radius: implications for healing of distal fractures in small dogs. Veterinary Surgery, 2657–2661.

CHAPTER 8

Aftercare and Home Care

Instructing and preparing clients for home care is essential for patient healing and return to well-being. This includes verbal and written discharge instructions as well as hands-on demonstrations of wound care, medication, and rehabilitation. Patient care, however, does not end when the animal walks out of the door. Following-up with clients within a few days of discharge provides an opportunity to monitor the patient's condition, answer clients' questions, assure compliance, and allay concerns.

Client instructions

Clients must receive home care instruction to provide their pet with the optimal healing experience. Communication is essential to patient care. Verbal instructions are important, but as with preparing for surgery, visual aids are helpful along with written instructions. Engaged clients retain and understand more information. While clients are anxious to be reunited with their pet, talking to them without this distraction is beneficial. Bringing a client to a quiet area such as an exam room eliminates other distractions and provides a private setting for a conversation. While providing oral instructions, it is beneficial to emphasize important points in the written instructions. Using a highlighting marker to stress certain aspects of the discharge underscores their importance for the client. When providing instructions for medications, asking the client to repeat the dosing schedule assures their understanding. It is important to provide information on when the next dose of medication is due after the patient is discharged.

Written instructions

Many studies, in human medicine, compare the appropriate reading grade level for discharge instruction comprehension and the actual reading level created (Bukata 2012). Studies indicate that the appropriate level of instructions be at the level of sixth grade reading (Somes 2003). While using medical terms is common knowledge for veterinary professionals, the general public may not understand them. Defining terms provides client education and understanding. For example, using the term "medial patella luxation or MPL" in a sentence is clear to the veterinarian and technician; however, a client may not recognize these words. Explaining this in layperson terms states this condition to be "the kneecap dislocates or moves to the inside of the knee." Use of acronyms, "MPL" in the above example, is also confusing and in need of explanation. Discharge instructions must be clear, concise, and free of errors. Creating a defined format for all clinic personnel provides consistency. When using a template, assure all pertinent information is correct for the individual patient. Include the following information:
- Patient and client names
- Client contact information
- Caregivers: veterinarian and technician
- Clinic/hospital/emergency contact information
- Diagnosis – medical and layperson terms
- Procedure-medical and layperson terms
- Medication(s)
  - name of drug (brand and generic)
  - dose (size in milligrams and quantity per dose)
  - route of administration (oral, transdermal, injection, topical, etc.)
  - frequency (how often to give)

Surgical Patient Care for Veterinary Technicians and Nurses, First Edition. Gerianne Holzman and Teri Raffel.
© 2015 John Wiley & Sons, Ltd. Published 2015 by John Wiley & Sons, Ltd.
Companion Website: wiley.com/go/holzman/surgical.

- number dispensed
- special precautions (give with food; do not mix with other medications, etc.)
- *example*: Rimadyl® (Carprofen) 25 mg, give one tablet by mouth – with food, twice daily
- Duration of medications – as needed, use all medications, etc.
- Feeding instructions – usual diet or special needs, when to start feeding
- Exercise – normal or restricted
- Tests and results – laboratory tests, imaging, etc
- General instructions for wound care, bandages, rehabilitation, etc.
- Follow-up – call, appointment, suture removal, bandage change, etc.

Using a larger font size (14 pt.) aids in readability. Break down the instructions into short paragraphs and bullet points for clarification. Providing extra space allows the client to make notes. Printing on a special color paper may help the client to find the discharge instructions when needed (Day 2012).

Hands-on demonstrations

Not all clients are proficient in or knowledgeable about medicating their pet. Providing a demonstration is important for client compliance. Asking the clients to also perform the task helps them to perfect their technique. Empty gel caps for oral medication and saline-filled syringes are great teaching aids. When bandaging is required at home, it is imperative to explain all steps and materials to the client as well as have them practice. Figure 8.1 shows a patient requiring slight compression on a neck incision. Using stretch stockinette as a "hood and shirt" allows the client to replace the gauze covering the wound.

Providing photos or videos helps clients who are visual learners. Anatomical models, electronic images, and hard copy books are additional aids to enhance client learning and understanding. Offer clients images of scoping procedures and radiographs. Explaining the images to clients enhances their experience. Reviewing charges with the client gives them a perception of all aspects of the surgery and its related costs. Through all stages of the discharge process, encourage and provide the client an opportunity to ask questions.

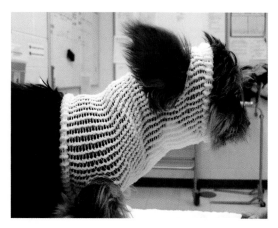

Figure 8.1 Patients may go home with a stockinette bandage, like this Yorkshire terrier following neck surgery. The bandage requires monitoring and changing by the client.

Feeding instructions

Patients may require special diets following their procedure. Short- or long-term needs are explained to the client. This information includes details of how to handle situations immediately after going home when food may need to be restricted to avoid vomiting due to anesthesia or pain medication–induced nausea. Patients are returned to their normal diet as soon as possible to avoid gastrointestinal upset. Some animals benefit from moistening dry kibble to be more palatable. Crushing the kibble prior to soaking in water hastens its water uptake. Patients reluctant to eat need coaxing with special foods such as commercially available canned pet food, baby food, boiled hamburger or chicken, water based tuna, and so on but not a high fat content food.

Long-term needs may include diet changes to comply with a specific medical condition, for example liver and kidney disease, degenerative joint disease as well as obesity. Pet obesity is on the rise in the United States. Recent studies indicate veterinarians classify 53% of dogs and 55% of cats as overweight (Association for Pet Obesity Prevention 2012). This study also shows that most pet owners are unaware of their pet's obesity. Providing clients information on weight-related conditions is imperative. These include kidney disease, breathing difficulties, hypertension, osteoarthritis, and type 2 diabetes. Showing and providing a body condition score and chart gives clients a visual aid in determining their pet's current and optimal fitness (Figures 8.2 and 8.3).

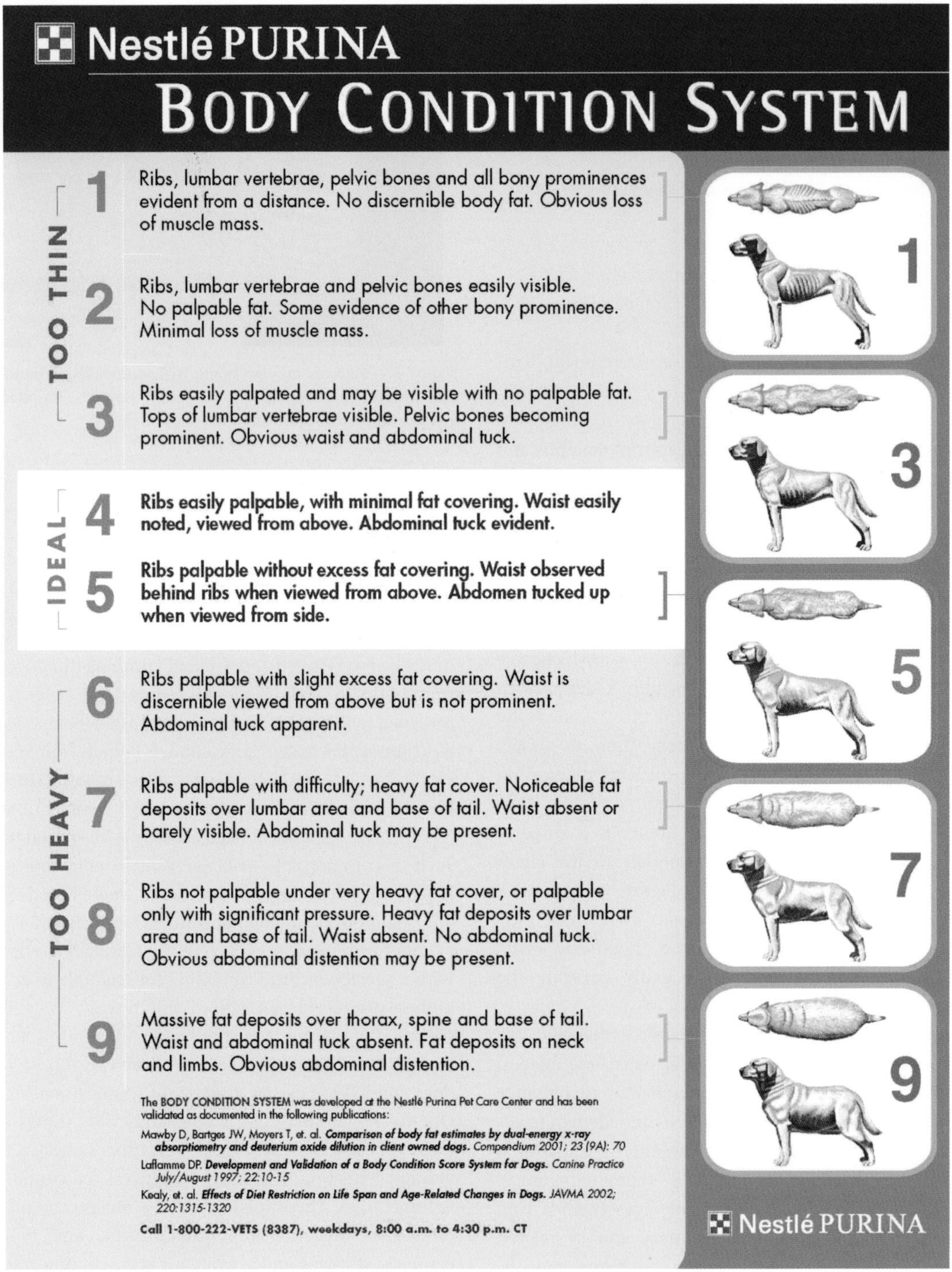

Figure 8.2 Canine body condition system scoring chart. (Courtesy of Nestle-Purina Petcare Company.)

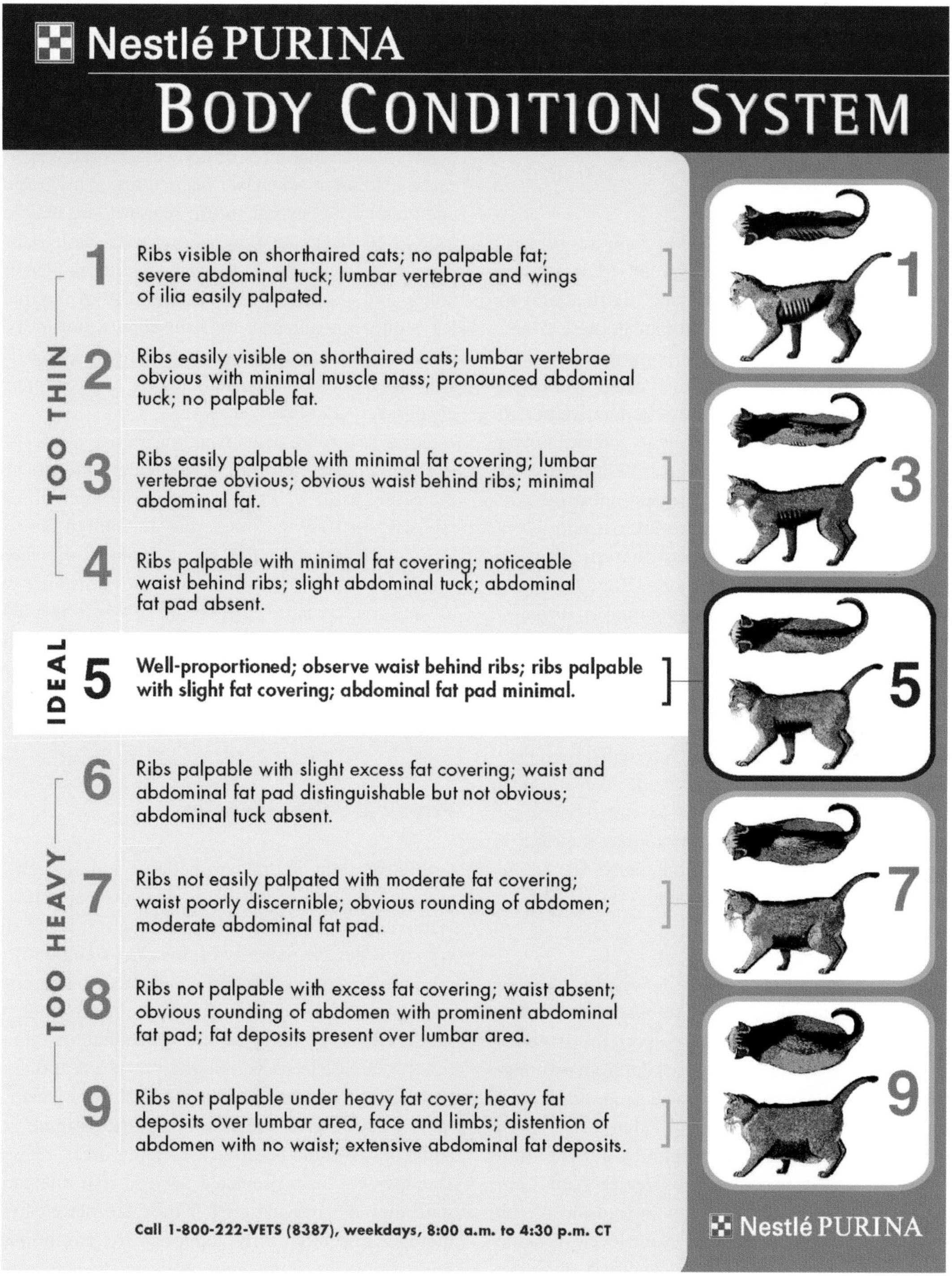

✦ Nestlé PURINA
BODY CONDITION SYSTEM

TOO THIN

1 Ribs visible on shorthaired cats; no palpable fat; severe abdominal tuck; lumbar vertebrae and wings of ilia easily palpated.

2 Ribs easily visible on shorthaired cats; lumbar vertebrae obvious with minimal muscle mass; pronounced abdominal tuck; no palpable fat.

3 Ribs easily palpable with minimal fat covering; lumbar vertebrae obvious; obvious waist behind ribs; minimal abdominal fat.

4 Ribs palpable with minimal fat covering; noticeable waist behind ribs; slight abdominal tuck; abdominal fat pad absent.

IDEAL

5 Well-proportioned; observe waist behind ribs; ribs palpable with slight fat covering; abdominal fat pad minimal.

TOO HEAVY

6 Ribs palpable with slight excess fat covering; waist and abdominal fat pad distinguishable but not obvious; abdominal tuck absent.

7 Ribs not easily palpated with moderate fat covering; waist poorly discernible; obvious rounding of abdomen; moderate abdominal fat pad.

8 Ribs not palpable with excess fat covering; waist absent; obvious rounding of abdomen with prominent abdominal fat pad; fat deposits present over lumbar area.

9 Ribs not palpable under heavy fat cover; heavy fat deposits over lumbar area, face and limbs; distention of abdomen with no waist; extensive abdominal fat deposits.

Call 1-800-222-VETS (8387), weekdays, 8:00 a.m. to 4:30 p.m. CT

✦ Nestlé PURINA

Figure 8.3 Feline body condition system scoring chart. (Courtesy of Nestle-Purina Petcare Company.)

Clients need instruction on measuring food intake, determining calorie content, and finding healthy treat alternatives such as raw vegetables. Advice is given on adverse foods not to be given as treats including products containing the artificial sweetener Xylitol, grapes and raisins, chocolate, avocados, garlic, onions, and macadamia nuts (Vetlearn 2011).

Elimination

The stress of hospitalization alone may cause gastrointestinal upset. Clients are warned to watch for vomiting, anorexia, constipation, and diarrhea and to contact the veterinarian or technician if these occur. This is especially true for patients prescribed narcotics and non-steroidal anti-inflammatory drugs (NSAIDs). Patients deprived from food in the perioperative period and receiving narcotics are less likely to produce bowel movements (Papich 2011) on a regular basis for a short period after discharge. This is generally not a medical concern. Providing clients with this information allays their concerns. However, patients that are unable to urinate require special attention. Often following spinal surgery, patients cannot voluntarily urinate. Carefully explaining the need to monitor urination and demonstrating bladder expression is essential in these patients. When clients are unable to express their pet's bladder, it may be advisable to continue hospitalization for expression or catheterization. Alternatively, repeat visits to the clinic may be required. Non-steroidal anti-inflammatory medications may cause vomiting and diarrhea. Clients are warned to contact the clinic if these occur, as it is imperative to stop the NSAID before the gastrointestinal condition worsens.

Exercise

Following any surgery, the patient is rested to provide an opportunity for the wound to heal. The extent of these restrictions is dependent upon the patient's individual condition. All patients are kept from running, jumping, and playing in the immediate postoperative period. This includes playing with other pets in the household. Exercise restriction continues, at least, until the incision is well healed and sutures or staples are removed. Clients are advised that the outside of the skin may quickly look healed but lower levels of tissue need additional time. Walking dogs on short (five foot or less) leashes with no off-leash exercise, keeping cats indoors and limiting activity inside the house all aid in

healing. Emphasizing the length of time and frequency of walks as well as the length of the leash improves client compliance. To avoid rambunctiousness, when unattended, the patient is restricted to a crate or small, unfurnished (e.g., bath or laundry) room during the client's absence.

Patients undergoing orthopedic procedures need more extensive exercise restrictions. This includes additional time beyond suture removal and may be as long as 10 weeks or more. Along with leash walking, support with a sling or towel keeps the patient from falling and aids in the use of stairs. Use of the injured leg is often encouraged; thus the sling is not meant to hold the patient off the ground. Patients going home with an Ehmer or Velpeau sling are the exception to encouragement of limb use.

Slowly returning patients to normal activity advances as their condition dictates. This includes incrementally increasing leash walks by 5–10 minute intervals every few days or weekly. Comparing an injured pet to an injured athlete gives the client a point of reference for increasing activity. For example, a runner with an anterior cruciate ligament (ACL) tear would not immediately run a marathon but would work up to that point. Similarly, a Labrador retriever recovering from a similar cranial cruciate ligament (CCL) injury does not immediately resume field trial work.

Physical rehabilitation

Orthopedic and neurologic patients require rehabilitation to return to normal or near-normal condition. While it starts in the hospital, oft times, it is the client who provides the majority of this care. Careful instruction is essential to provide the patient with appropriate rehab. Large referral practices may offer rehabilitation services by a certified canine rehabilitation therapist (CCRT). A CCRT is a veterinarian or physical therapist with special training. Veterinary technicians with the same training gain the title of certified canine rehabilitation assistant (CCRA). (In many areas, "Physical Therapy (PT)" is a protected term in that one cannot state they are providing PT if they are not a physical therapist and often only applies to treating humans.) In addition to immediate postoperative treatment, long-term therapy is beneficial for patients suffering from osteoarthritis and for conservative management

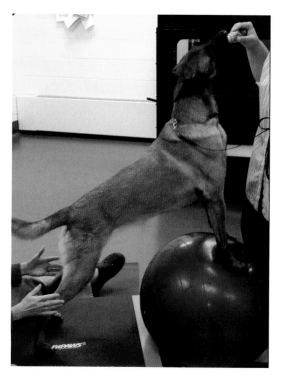

Figure 8.4 Patient receives strength and balance training while on a ball. (Courtney Arnoldy, University of Wisconsin Veterinary Care, Madison, WI. Reproduced with permission from Courtney Arnoldy.)

Table 8.1 Normal range of motion – flexion and extension.

Joint	Dog (degrees)	Cat (degrees)
Shoulder		
Flexion	60–70	60–70
Extension	65–75	90
Elbow		
Flexion	70–75	50–60
Extension	70–75	80–90
Carpus		
Flexion	155–160	130–140
Extension	20–30	30–40
Hip		
Flexion	70–80	50–60
Extension	80–90	100–110
Stifle		
Flexion	65–75	50–60
Extension	65–75	90
Tarsus		
Flexion	65–75	50–60
Extension	90–110	90–110

Adapted from Newton (1985). Reproduced with permission from Lippincott Williams & Wilkins.

of orthopedic and neurologic conditions. Providing strength and conditioning for working dogs helps healthy patients to maintain fitness (Figure 8.4). The goal of physical rehabilitation is to aid in recovery, improve function, and promote well-being.

An individual plan is developed for each patient to provide for its optimal rehabilitation needs. Timing of rehab is dependent upon the patient's condition. Following some joint surgeries (e.g., arthroscopy, osteochondritis dissicans, femoral head and neck ostectomy, extra-capsular stabilization of a cranial cruciate rupture), patients are strongly encouraged to immediately begin use of their limbs. Patients undergoing other surgeries (e.g., fracture repairs, osteotomies for cranial cruciate rupture, and intervertebral disc decompression) may benefit from more moderate therapy. Instituting the incorrect treatment at the wrong time may lead to poor outcomes (Arnoldy 2010). Pre-rehabilitation measurements of the affected joint's range of motion and the circumference of its accompanying muscles

provide a starting point for gauging effectiveness of treatment. The use of a goniometer and a tape measure are employed for these measurements. Knowledge of the normal range of motion of joints aids in determining a long-term goal for therapy (Table 8.1). Subsequently, after recovery, similar readings are taken for comparison. However, in the end, the goal is to have a comfortable, happy, and ambulatory patient. Physical rehabilitation is an excellent way for clients to be intimately involved with their pet's recovery.

Cryotherapy

Cryotherapy is one of the first stages of rehabilitation and is used in the acute stage of healing. Ice packing is done at specific intervals in the immediate postoperative period. It minimizes inflammation and provides pain relief. Cold applied to the skin causes vasoconstriction and decreases nerve conduction velocity. Muscles may cool by $1–4°C$ ($33–39°F$) and the skin by $12–13°C$ ($53–55°F$) (Knap *et al.* 2007). The effects of cryotherapy may last for 15–30 minutes. Bags of crushed ice, frozen peas, and commercially available freezer gel packs are great sources of cooling. A washcloth or paper towel is applied to the pack prior to application to the surgery site. Towels may be used but should not be too thick to impede the flow of cold to the skin. Incisions must be protected from cross-patient contamination in the hospital by cleaning the source of cold therapy, between patients, with a disinfecting solution. Cryotherapy is applied for 10–15 minutes up to every 4 hours depending on the client's schedule. This continues for the first 72 hours following surgery. Patients with cold sensitivity are monitored closely for distress.

Heat

Heat is used for long-term therapy beginning at day 3–4 of the postoperative period. It is not used when acute inflammation is present as it may increase hemorrhage and edema. Hyperthermia is not applied to active infections, tumors, or pregnant uteruses. Heat therapy creates vasodilation, muscle relaxation, and improves stretching ability. Hot packing provides superficial heating. (Deep heating may be achieved by a CCRT or CCRA with the use of therapeutic ultrasound.) Prior to application of a hot pack, the skin and incision are protected as with cryotherapy. Heat is applied with warmed towels or commercially available gel packs. This continues for 10–15 minutes, again, up to every 4 hours. The patient must be monitored closely for redness and skin irritation. Clients monitor the temperature of the pack by application to their own skin. If it is too hot for them, it is too hot for their pet. *Heating pads are never used for heat therapy as they become too hot and provide a focal point for potential burns.*

Massage

Massage soothes the patient and provides a bonding experience for the client. It improves the flow of the lymphatic system and in patients with distal edema aids in moving fluid from the extremities to the rest of the body. Massage also softens adhesions and relieves muscle contracture. Following hyperthermia treatment, massage prepares patients for exercises and stretching. Massage treatment always begins distally and works its way proximally. Beginning with soft strokes, the massage intensity increases to provide pressure to the muscles. The sessions proceed for 5–15 minutes as the patient tolerates.

Passive range of motion (PROM)

The passive range of motion exercises involve moving a joint through its full motion. It increases joint flexibility while providing extension to the surrounding muscles, tendons, and ligaments. Passive Range of Motion improves nutritional support of the synovium and increases blood flow. PROM is beneficial to maintain mobility and avoid joint contracture. However, to improve strength and reduce muscle atrophy, active range of motion is indicated. This includes the patient walking on its own with assistance, underwater treadmills, swimming, and other exercises outlined below. To perform PROM, the limb is grasped distal to the joint of interest. The limb is supported proximal to the joint with the other hand. With the leg maintained in an even plane, the joint is slowly flexed and extended (Figures 8.5 and 8.6).

Initially, it may not be possible to reach a full range of motion – the patient's comfort dictates the extent of movement. As each motion (flexion or extension) is reached, it is held for 15–30 seconds. Twenty repetitions performed three to four times daily are sufficient. Each individual joint of the affected limb is taken through a PROM. "Bicycling" movements by grasping the foot

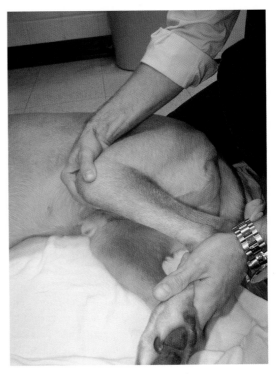

Figure 8.5 Passive range of motion: stifle flexion.

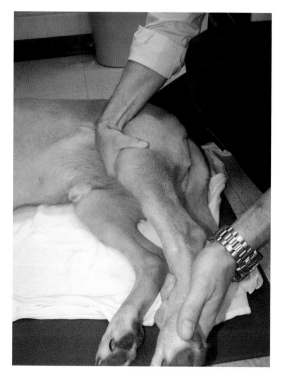

Figure 8.6 Passive range of motion: stifle extension.

and imitating a walking movement *does not* provide full range of motion to all of the joints.

Therapeutic exercises

Therapeutic exercises may be performed by a CCRT or CCRA and can be incorporated into home care. Exercise improves a patient's attitude, range of motion, muscle strength, and limb use. As with all rehabilitation methods, therapeutic exercise is individualized for the patient. As the patient improves, exercise is increased in repetitions, duration, and intensity. Simply standing with assistance improves patient balance, muscle tone, and patient attitude. The patient is helped to stand on an even, stable, nonslippery surface. Sufficient time is allowed between standing exercises to allow the patient to rest. As the patient's condition improves, standing time is increased, while support is decreased. Therapeutic round and peanut-shaped balls assist in-clinic standing and balancing exercises.

Sit–to-stand and down-to-stand exercises improve muscle strength of the quadriceps, semimembranosus, semitendinosus as well as the biceps and triceps. Range of motion and joint mobility is improved. If a patient is

unable to stand or rise on its own, the patient is assisted with sling support. When performing this exercise, the patient is encouraged to sit/stand symmetrically without tilting to either side. As with all training, the use of treats rewards the behavior. Begin this exercise slowly (1–5 repetitions) twice daily until the animal is able to sit/stand squarely. As the patient tolerates, more repetitions are added.

Veterinary hospitals with rehabilitation facilities may offer clients in-house rehabilitation with the use of an underwater treadmill. While manufactures differ slightly, underwater treadmills use a holding tank and filtration system that warms and chlorinates the water for recirculation during the patient's session. (The water is changed between patients.) A leak-proof, clear-sided chamber encloses the treadmill. Depending on the particular product, adjustments are available for speed and incline. The chamber is filled with water and the level of the water depends on the kind of patient. The water is deep enough to provide buoyancy but still keep the patient's feet on the treadmill – generally to the height of the sternum (Figure 8.7).

This reduction in gravity provides for a lower impact exercise. The reduced stress on joints allows for ease of movement, longer strides, and extended range of motion. Walking against the flow of water aids in muscle strengthening while the warmth of the water relaxes muscles and eases pain. Over time, the level of the water may be lowered to provide more impact.

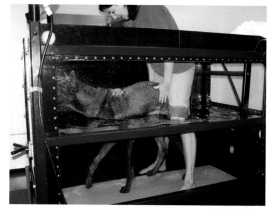

Figure 8.7 Underwater treadmill provides an active range of motion to all four limbs, while the water lessens the impact of the exercise. (Courtney Arnoldy, University of Wisconsin Veterinary Care, Madison, WI. Reproduced with permission from Courtney Arnoldy.)

Underwater therapy does not begin until all incisions are healed. Patients are always attended when in a treadmill; small or nonambulatory animals are assisted with a technician in the water with the patient. Flotation devices provide extra safety for all patients. The exercise begins slowly in very short sessions of 1–2 minutes gradually increasing by 5-minute intervals as the patient tolerates. The patient is monitored very closely for signs of fatigue and the exercise stopped immediately when this is noticed. Clients with land treadmills in their homes, with time and patience, may be able to teach their pet to use these devices between sessions in the underwater treadmill.

Swimming is a great exercise for rehabilitation, active range of motion, strengthening, and coordination. This low-impact activity improves muscle mass and stamina. Swimming occurs in an underwater treadmill, pool, lake, or other body of water. Most four-legged dogs swim primarily with their front legs. However, patients missing one forelimb swim well with their back legs providing extra strengthening exercises for their remaining legs. Dogs not used to the water, must slowly be acclimated and some patients will never accept swimming. Flotation devices provide safety and allow the patient to rest. The animal is accompanied in the water or within very close proximity. During rehab, dogs are encouraged to walk into the water and not jump from a dock or pier to minimize the impact on their joints. As with the underwater treadmill, patients are monitored closely for fatigue.

Another exercise, requiring more impact, includes controlled walks at a slow pace. When forced to move at a leisurely pace, pets are more likely to use all of their limbs. When trotting or running quickly, animals have more momentum to allow walking on three legs and carrying the injured leg. (Watching an amputee's walk demonstrates this phenomenon well. Three or even two-legged veterinary patients move better at a faster speed and are more easily fatigued at a slower pace.) Walking provides an active range of motion exercise to increase joint mobility as well as muscle strengthening. Additionally, walking over and around obstacles provides more thoughtful movement as the patient navigates the impediment. Stair climbing and walking on an incline or decline strengthen muscles and forces flexion of the joints. No impact activities are instituted until the patient is sufficiently healed from surgery. For less ambulatory patients, sling support is

beneficial. Clients are advised to gradually introduce the exercises and slowly increase their duration. Varying rehabilitation techniques provide more stimulation for the patient, less boredom for the client and different joints put through range of motion while different muscles are strengthened.

Follow-up

Clients are often stressed and nervous when caring for their recuperating pet. They may not want "to bother" the veterinarian with a call. They may not understand or remember some of the instruction provided at discharge. Patient follow-up is important to monitor progress, answer client questions, and assure compliance with discharge instructions (Figure 8.8).

A phone call or email to the client within 24–72 hours of surgery (SironaHealth 2013) conveys concern for the patient's welfare. Little problems caught early can avoid major complications. This provides an opportunity to confirm dosing schedules, rehabilitation plans, and discuss wound care. Clients are quizzed on the appearance of an incision and its surrounding skin – is it red, warm, swollen, or is there any drainage – clear, bloody, purulent? (Figure 8.9)

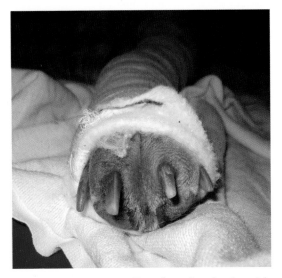

Figure 8.8 Postoperative swelling of toes from bandage tightness. Following bandage application, clients monitor toes daily for problems. (Susan Schaefer, University of Wisconsin Veterinary Care, Madison, WI. Reproduced with permission from Susan Schaefer.)

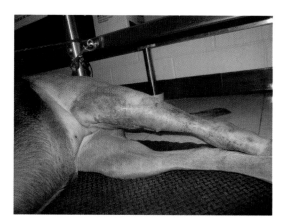

Figure 8.9 Observing the skin, every day, for redness, bruising, drainage, and irritation prevent severe problems. (Jason Bleedorn, University of Wisconsin Veterinary Care, Madison, WI. Reproduced with permisison from Jason Bleedorn.)

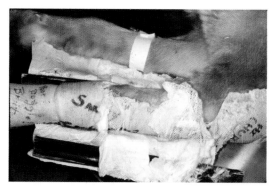

Figure 8.10 Without protection, patients chew bandages and casts. A chewed wrap may indicate an underlying problem and needs to be investigated. (Susan Schaefer, University of Wisconsin Veterinary Care, Madison, WI. Reproduced with permission from Susan Schaefer.)

What is the condition of any bandages that were placed? Is the animal bothering the bandage? Clients may need additional instructions for wound and bandage care. If there is a problem, a return visit to the clinic/hospital is in order (Figure 8.10).

Monitoring a patient's eating and elimination is especially important when prescribed many medications. Antibiotics, non-steroidal anti-inflammatories and narcotics may all cause nausea, anorexia, and/or abnormal urination or defecation. Diarrhea may be present from some treatments and advising clients to monitor for blood in the stool and to call if evident can prevent serious complications. Providing dietary suggestions, such as a bland diet of boiled hamburger or chicken and rice in the event of vomiting and diarrhea helps clients to provide nourishment for their pet. If a fentanyl patch or adhesive bandage has been placed, clients may need advice on their removal. (Send patient home with odor-free adhesive remover packets.)

Follow-up communication provides an opportunity for scheduling suture/staple removal along with recheck exams and client updates. It also gives the client an opportunity to discuss any new symptoms that may have arisen after the patient went home. Clients are always encouraged to call with other questions and provided with emergency contact information. Experienced veterinary technicians may answer most of a client's questions; however, they must never hesitate to seek the advice of the attending surgeon. Keeping all members of the surgical team informed and updated provides the best patient care.

References

Arnoldy, C. (2010) Rehabilitation for dogs with cranial cruciate ligament rupture. In: Muir, P. (ed), *Advances in The Cranial Cruciate Ligament*. John Wiley and Sons.Inc, Ames, IA, pp. 249–253.

Association for Pet Obesity Prevention (2012) petobesityprevention.com, Calabash, NC [accessed on 8 November 2014].

Bukata, R. (2012) With Discharge Instructions, Less is More. *Emergency Physicians Monthly* 01/2012

Day, D. (2012) 5 ways to help patients recall their post-visit discharge instructions. The Care Transitions Journal Sirona Health, South Portland, ME, see web: http://www.caretransitions.com/health_call_center_blog/bid/57106/5-Ways-to-Help-Patients-Recall-Their-Post-Visit-Discharge-Instructions [accessed on June 20 2012].

Knap, K., Johnson, A.L. & Schulz, K. (2007) Fundamentals of physical rehabilitation. In: Fossum, T.W. (ed), *Small Animal Surgery Textbook*, 3rd edn. Mosby Elsevier, St. Louis, MO, pp. 111–129.

Papich, M.G. (2011) *Saunders Handbook of Veterinary Drugs*, 3rd edn. Saunders Elsevier, St. Louis, MO.

SironaHealth,(2013) *7 Steps to Successful Post Discharge Follow Up Care – Using Inbound and Outbound Calling Programs* e-book, SironaHealth, South Portland, ME

Somes, J. (2003) Reading levels of ED patients compared to level of discharge instructions. In: *Emergency Nurses Association*. Virginia Henderson International Nursing Library, Indianapolis, IN.

Vetlearn (2011) Human Foods That Are Dangerous for Dogs and Cats Care Guide Vetlearn.com, Vetstreet Inc., Yardley, PA [accessed on 8 November 2014].

Glossary

A

Abrading: removal of the superficial later of the skin

Abrasion: skin wound less than full skin thickness

Acetabulum: "socket" part of the hip joint

Adhesions: fibrous bands of scar tissue that form between internal organs and tissues, joining them together abnormally

Aerosolized: converted from liquid or solid state to a gaseous state

Alopecia: lack of hair

Ambulation: ability to walk

Analgesic: medication or treatment that reduces pain without inducing unconsciousness

Anesthetic: medication administered to reduce the perception of pain; it may (or may not) produce unconsciousness

Anomalous: deviation from normal

Antibiotic: medication to kill or inhibit the growth of bacteria

Anti-inflammatory: reducing inflammation

Anti-microbial: agent that kills or suppresses growth of microorganisms

Appose: bringing edges of a wound together

Arrhythmia: an abnormal heart rhythm

Arthrocentesis: joint tap, obtaining synovial fluid via syringe with needle inserted into the joint

Arthrogram: radiographic demonstration of the joints employing contrast media

Arthroscopy: internal visualization of a joint through a camera and employing instruments through ports to perform intra-articular surgery or for diagnosis

Aseptically: perform without introducing microorganisms into the area or field

Atrophy: wasting away or decreasing in size of an organ or body part such as muscle from lack of use

Aural: of the ear

Austenite: a solid solution of ferric carbide or carbon in iron

Autogenous: originating from the host, self-generating

Avascular: without blood flow or blood supply

Avulsion: tearing away

B

Biceps tenosynovitis: inflammation of the biceps brachii tendon and its synovial sheath

Box lock: the joint or point of union of two sides of a ring handled instrument

Bradycardia: slow heart rate

C

Calculi: plural of calculus; abnormal concretions (stones) formed of minerals in the kidney, urinary bladder or gallbladder; calcified plaque on the teeth

Cancellous: bone having a lattice like or spongy structure

Cardiovascular: of the heart and blood vessels

Cavitation: action of an ultrasound to produce small bubbles that then burst when they contact an item, to clean the item

Celiotomy: surgical incision into the abdominal cavity

Cerclage: to encircle a bone with wire to aid in the repair of a fracture

Cesarean section (C-Section): incision into the uterus (hysterotomy) to remove fetuses, may be performed with an ovariohysterectomy

Circumferential: encircling, peripheral

Coaptation: fitting together of two parts

Cortex: the outer layer of a long bone

Cortical: pertaining to the outer layer of a bone

Cryotherapy: cold treatment to reduce inflammation and pain e.g. ice packing

Cystic: relating to the urinary bladder, gall bladder or a cyst

Cystocentesis: obtaining a urine sample using a syringe with a needle through the abdominal wall into the bladder

Cystogram: radiographic demonstration of the bladder employing contrast media

Cytotoxic: causing a toxic effect on cells

Surgical Patient Care for Veterinary Technicians and Nurses, First Edition. Gerianne Holzman and Teri Raffel.
© 2015 John Wiley & Sons, Ltd. Published 2015 by John Wiley & Sons, Ltd.
Companion Website: wiley.com/go/holzman/surgical.

D

Debridement: surgical removal of dead, devitalized, or contaminated tissue and/or foreign material

Deciduous: primary teeth or first set of teeth

Decompression: to release or remove pressure

Decubital ulcer: skin wound from compression

Degloving: loss of skin and underlying tissue

Dehiscence: rupture or break open (surgical wound)

Developmental: occurring during growth

Diaphysis: shaft of a long bone

Disinfectant: product that kills many, but not all, microorganism on an inanimate object

Dissection: to cut apart or separate

Distal: away from the center or point of attachment

Distended: swollen, expanded

Dominant: strongest or most commonly used

Dosimeter: instrument used to measure and indicate the amount of radiation absorbed over a certain period of time

E

Echocardiogram: image produced from ultrasonic waves examining the structures and function of the heart

Ectropion: eyelid turning out and away from the eye

Edema: swelling of organs, skin or other body parts due to fluid accumulation

Efficacy: how efficient or well something performs

Effusion: fluid escaping from blood or lymphatic vessels into tissue or spaces

Emaciated: extremely thin, usually related to disease or lack of food

Endothelin: proteins that constrict blood vessels and raise blood pressure

Enterogram: radiographic demonstration of the intestines employing contrast media

Entropion: eyelid turning inward and toward the eye

Erythema: redness

Esophogram: radiographic demonstration of the esophagus employing contrast media

Everting: edges of the wound turning outward

Exteriorization: to remove or bring out of a body cavity

Extravasation: accumulation of fluid outside of the joint

Extruded: protruded out from the original position

F

Fenestrated: solid sheet of material that has a window of material purposefully removed

Fissure: crack, tear or groove in a body part

Fragmented medial coronoid process: portion of medial coronoid process of ulna separates from parent bone

G

Gastric dilatation volvulus (GDV or bloat): stomach is twisted causing enlargement (may have simple dilatation without volvulus (twisting)

Gastro-intestinal (GI): relating to the stomach and intestines

Granulation: small, fleshy protuberances on the surface of a healing wound

H

Hematocrit: percentage by volume of red blood cells in a sample of blood after centrifugation

Hematoma: a lump or swelling filled with blood that is not flowing

Hemilaminectomy: decompression of the spinal cord via removal of a portion of a vertebral body to relieve pressure, provides access for removal of extruded intervertebral disc material

Hemoglobin: iron-containing substance in red blood cells that transports oxygen from the lungs to the rest of the body

Hemostasis: control of blood loss

Hip dysplasia: genetic disorder where the hip is malformed and the head of the femur does not sit properly in the acetabulum

Hyperextension: extending beyond the normal range of motion of a joint

Hyperflexion: flexing beyond the normal range of motion of a joint

Hypertension: elevated blood pressure

Hyperthermia: higher than normal body temperature

Hyperthyroid: over active thyroid gland

Hypoextension: extending less than the normal range of motion of a joint

Hypoflexion: flexing less than the normal range of motion of a joint

Hypotension: low blood pressure

Hypothermia: lower than normal body temperature

Hypothyroid: under active thyroid gland

I

Ileus: mechanical or functional bowel obstruction

Infestation: large number of external parasites causing damage

Inflammation: protective tissue response to injury

Insufflation: infusing gas into a body cavity to aid in visualization i.e. during laparoscopy

Insufflator: machine used to perform insufflation

Integrity: whole or undivided

Integument: outer covering of the body: skin, hair, etc

Intraoperative: time during surgery

Inverting: edges of the wound turning inward

L

Laceration: skin wound with sharp edges

Laminar Air Flow: system of circulating filtered air in parallel-flowing planes

Laparoscopy: examination of the abdominal cavity using an endoscope

Larynx: opening at the proximal trachea to control breathing and prevent food from entering the trachea

Lavage: act of washing

Ligation: use of suture to tie around a vessel or tissue mass to achieve hemostasis or closure

Locomotion: ability to move

Longevity: length of time something survives

M

Martensitic: formed in stainless steel by rapid quenching, consisting of a supersaturated solid solution of carbon in iron

Memory: ability of suture to return to its packaged form

Menace (reflex): poking finger toward eye to test vision, normal response is closing of the eye

Modulation: synapse of the neurons in the nucleus caudalis in the medulla of the brain

Monofilament: single strand of suture

Multifilament: multiple strands of suture braided together to form a single strand

Musculoskeletal: muscles and bones

N

Neoplasia: tumor, new tissue

Neuromuscular: condition affecting the nerves and the muscles

Nociception: an unpleasant sensation which may be associated with actual or potential tissue damage and which may have physical and emotional components; pain

Nystagmus: rapid, involuntary eye movements

O

Obtunded: mentally dull

Occlude: to prevent the passage of

Onychectomy: declaw, removal of the third phalanx of each digit

Orchiectomy: (Neuter/castration)

remove testicles to sterilize a male dog and prevent breeding

Orthotic: orthopedic appliance used to support a body part

Ossification: the formation of bone from fibrous tissue

Ostectomy: removing all or part of a bone

Osteoarthritis: degenerative joint disease, joint inflammation characterized by cartilage degeneration

Osteochondritis dissicans: incomplete endochondral ossification causes cartilage to remain; fissure in this cartilage creates a flap that may loosen causing a "joint mouse"

Osteotomy: cutting a bone

Ovariohysterectomy: (OHE, neuter, spay) remove ovaries and uterus to sterilize a female dog and prevent breeding

P

Palmar: underside of the front foot

Palpation: feeling parts of the body to determine normal or abnormal conditions

Parameters: measurable factors

Pathogen: disease-causing microorganism

Penetrating: poke through or into

Perineal urethostomy: – (PU)

penile amputation to alleviate chronic urethral obstruction not relievable by other means

Perineum: area of the body including the rectum and urogenital openings

Perioperative: period of time surrounding surgery including preoperative, intraoperative and postoperative

Pharynx: funnel shaped structure in the back of the oral cavity including the larynx, esophagus, tonsils, etc.

Pheromones: chemical secreted by an animal that affects behavior of the members of the same species

Pitting: creation of small dents or "pits" on a surface e.g. pitting edema

Plantar: underside of the rear foot

Plaque: biofilm on the teeth containing bacteria and glycoproteins

Platelet: disc shaped portion of blood that aids in clotting

Pliability: ease of suture workability

Polydipsia: increased thirst

Polyuria: increased urination

Portosystemic shunt (PSS): blood vessels bypass the liver and drain from the stomach, intestines, spleen and pancreas directly into the circulatory system thus partially eliminating the liver's filtering properties, may be intrahepatic or extrahepatic

Postoperative: time after surgery

Povidone: iodine infused into a product

Preoperative: time preceding surgery

Proprioception: awareness of one's movement based on sensations

Proximal: nearer the center of the body or attachment

Puncture: penetrating injury

Pyoderma: skin infection

R

Ratchet: toothed tabs that interdigitate and lock as on a ring handled instrument.

Rehabilitation (rehab.): treatment of physical conditions to restore normal function

Renal: of the kidneys

Residual effect: duration of efficacy after application

S

Seroma: local accumulation of serum within a tissue or organ

Serrated: cutting edge of a scissors that has small teeth for grasping then cutting tissue

Sphincter: a circular muscle constricting an orifice

Splenectomy: surgical removal of the spleen

Stabilization: secure to eliminate movement

Stenotic nares: nostrils with very narrow openings

Sterilization: act of removing or killing microorganisms, unable to reproduce

Supplemental: in addition to the regular amount

Synovial fluid: joint fluid

T

Tachycardia: fast heart rate

Tensile strength: amount of tension that can be withstood before the breaking

Thoracotomy: surgical incision into the chest wall between two ribs or through the sternum

Thrombin: protein in blood that aids in clotting by converting fibrinogen to fibrin

Tranquilizer: sedative

Transduction: conversion of the unpleasant sensation into electrical impulses by a free afferent nerve ending

Transmission: transports electrical impulses along nerve fibers to the nucleus caudalis of the brain

Transverse: horizontal plane of a surface; crossing from side to side

Tympanic membrane: eardrum

U

Ultrasound: sound waves greater than 20,000Hz/second

Ununited anconeal process: anconeal process does not attach to proximal ulna

Urinalysis: laboratory analysis of urine to aid in the diagnosis of a medical condition

Urogenital: relating to the urinary and genital organs and their functions

V

Valgus: outward turning of a bone

Varus: inward turning of a bone

Viability: ability of an item or organism to live or survive

Visualization: ability to see a structure

X

Xyphoid: caudal end of the sternum

Index

Note: Page numbers in *italics* refer to Figures; those in **bold** to Tables

---

Surgical Patient Care for Veterinary Technicians and Nurses, First Edition. Gerianne Holzman and Teri Raffel.
© 2015 John Wiley & Sons, Ltd. Published 2015 by John Wiley & Sons, Ltd.
Companion Website: wiley.com/go/holzman/surgical.